# PERSPECTIVES ON THE CLASSIFICATION OF SPECIFIC DEVELOPMENTAL DISORDERS

## NEUROPSYCHOLOGY AND COGNITION

VOLUME 13



The purpose of the Neuropsychology and Cognition series is to bring out volumes that promote understanding in topics relating brain and behavior. It is intended for use by both clinicians and research scientists in the fields of neuropsychology, cognitive psychology, psycholinguistics, speech and hearing, as well as education. Examples of topics to be covered in the series would relate to memory, language acquisition and breakdown, reading, attention, developing and aging brain. By addressing the theoretical, empirical, and applied aspects of brain-behavior relationships, this series will try to present the information in the fields of neuropsychology and cognition in a coherent manner.

*The titles published in this series are listed at the end of this volume.*

# PERSPECTIVES ON THE CLASSIFICATION OF SPECIFIC DEVELOPMENTAL DISORDERS

Edited by

JAN RISPENS

*Utrecht University, the Netherlands*

TOM A. VAN YPEREN

*NIZW, Utrecht, the Netherlands*

and

WILLIAM YULE

*University of London, U.K.*

KLUWER ACADEMIC PUBLISHERS

DORDRECHT / BOSTON / LONDON

A C.I.P. Catalogue record for this book is available from the Library of Congress.

ISBN 0-7923-4871-0

Published by Kluwer Academic Publishers,
P.O. Box 17, 3300 AA Dordrecht, The Netherlands.

Sold and distributed in the U.S.A. and Canada
by Kluwer Academic Publishers,
101 Philip Drive, Norwell, MA 02061, U.S.A.

In all other countries, sold and distributed
by Kluwer Academic Publishers,
P.O. Box 322, 3300 AH Dordrecht, The Netherlands.

*Printed on acid-free paper*



Printed in the Netherlands.

LIST OF CONTRIBUTORS

H. AMOROSA, Heckscher Klinik München-Solln, Wolfratshauser Str. 350, Haus 5, D-8000 München 71, Germany.

A. L. BARNETT, School of Education, University of Wales at Cardiff, 21 Senghennydd Road, Cardiff CF2 4YG, United Kingdom.

D. V. M. BISHOP, MRC Applied Psychology Unit, 15, Chaucer Road, Cambridge, CB2 2EF, United Kingdom.

G. P. VAN GALEN, Nijmegen Institute for Cognition and Information NICI, Nijmegen University, P.O. Box 9104, 6500 HE Nijmegen, The Netherlands.

S. E. HENDERSON, Department of Psychology and Special Needs, Institute of Education, University of London, 25 Woburn Square, London, WC1H OAA, United Kingdom.

K. HENNIGHAUSEN, Department of Child and Adolescent Psychiatry, Philipps-University Marburg, Hans-Sachs-Str. 6, D-35033 Marburg, Germany.

A. F. KALVERBOER, Developmental and Experimental Clinical Psychology, University of Groningen, Grote Kruisstraat 2/1, 9712 TS Groningen, The Netherlands.

B. MAUGHAN, Institute of Psychiatry, Dept. of Child and Adolescent Psychiatry, De Crespigny Park, London SE5 8AF, United Kingdom.

H. REMSCHMIDT, Department of Child and Adolescent Psychiatry, Philipps-University Marburg, Hans-Sachs-Str. 6, D-35033 Marburg, Germany.

J. RISPENS, Dept. of Educational Sciences, Utrecht University, P.O. Box 80140, 3508 TC Utrecht, The Netherlands.

M. RUTTER, Institute of Psychiatry, Dept. of Child and Adolescent Psychiatry, De Crespigny Park, London SE5 8AF, United Kingdom.

L. S. SIEGEL, Ontario Institute for Studies in Education, University of Toronto, 252 Bloor St. West, Toronto, Ontario, Canada M5S 1V6.

M. M. SCHOEMAKER, Developmental and Experimental Clinical Psychology, University of Groningen, Grote Kruisstraat 2/1, 9712 TS Groningen, The Netherlands.

G. SCHULTE-KÖRNE, Department of Child and Adolescent Psychiatry, Philipps-University Marburg, Hans-Sachs-Str. 6, D-35033 Marburg, Germany.

B. C. M. SMITS-ENGELSMAN, Nijmegen Institute for Cognition and Information NICI, Nijmegen University, P.O. Box 9104, 6500 HE Nijmegen, The Netherlands.

K. E. STANOVICH, Ontario Institute for Studies in Education, University of Toronto, 252 Bloor St. West, Toronto, Ontario, Canada M5S 1V6.

T. A. VAN YPEREN, Netherlands Institute of Care and Welfare, P.O. Box 19152, 3501 DD Utrecht, The Netherlands.

W. YULE, Institute of Psychiatry, Dept. of Child and Adolescent Psychiatry, De Crespigny Park, London SE5 8AF, United Kingdom.

TABLE OF CONTENTS

MICHAEL RUTTER

# FOREWORD

It has been recognized for a long time that severe and persistent difficulties in spoken language, reading, spelling, and motor coordination not infrequently occur in children of normal general intelligence, without any obvious neurological disorder, who come from an unremarkable family background, and who have had apparently adequate schooling and other educational experiences. At first, the terminology applied to these marked, but seemingly isolated, problems reflected concepts derived from adult neurology - word blindness, developmental dysphasia, developmental dyspraxia, dyslexia and the like. During the 1960s however, researchers and clinicians of all disciplines (medical and nonmedical alike) became increasingly uneasy with diagnostic terms that implied a neurological syndrome in the absence of convincing evidence that the difficulties always rose as a result of some kind of structural brain pathology (see e.g., Rutter, 1969). This unease was strengthened by epidemiological studies showing marked variations between geographical areas in reading difficulties (Berger, Yule, & Rutter, 1975) and similar variations between schools (Rutter, Maughan, Mortimore, Ouston, & Smith, 1979). The implication seemed to be that psychosocial risk factors and quality of schooling might play a part in aetiology. A preference developed for more descriptive terms that seemed to involve fewer assumptions about pathology. Descriptions such as specific reading retardation, developmental language disorders and the 'clumsy child' syndrome were used increasingly. Initially, they seemed theoretically neutral, simply serving as a useful starting point from which to investigate the nature, causes, course, and outcome of the difficulties they described.

In the event, they aroused as much controversy as the medical terms they replaced. In part, this reflected a sea change in attitudes to classification. Prior to the 1960s, few people paid much attention to classification of mental disorders and diagnostic issues were mostly ignored or bypassed by clinicians and researchers alike - especially in the U.S.A. The situation today could scarcely be more different. The scientific journals are full of papers on diagnostic and classificatory issues; the classificatory schemes developed by the World Health Organization (1992), ICD-9 and the ICD-10, and the American Psychiatric Association (1994), DSM-III, DSM-III-R, and now DSM-IV, occupy a prominent role in most training schemes; and the A.P.A. diagnostic manuals have proved to be the biggest money-spinners that the organization has ever had. Much of this represents real and important progress. It has greatly facilitated communication between professionals, it has sharpened diagnostic concepts and it has improved research. But the very process of specifying diagnostic criteria and of seeking to operationalize them, has also served to highlight the paucity of the evidence on which they are based, the arbitrariness of many of the cut-off points, and the lack of empirical validation of some of the diagnostic distinctions. This has, not surprisingly, led to extensive questioning, not only of the specifics, but also of the basis of psychiatric classification itself (see Rutter & Shaffer, 1980). Nowhere is this more evident than in the field of developmental disorders of specific psychological functions.

But, quite apart from these broader concerns over approaches to classification, there has been vigorous dispute over the very few assumptions involved in what was meant to be a straightforward pragmatic set of descriptors of a few key subdivisions that might prove useful in research. None has aroused such a passion as the notion that it might be helpful to differentiate between reading difficulties that were part of a more general cognitive impairment and those that were not. In part, the objections have seemed to stem from a general aversion to any use of IQ measures or concepts; in part from a concern over problems of measurement; in part from a reluctance to separate extreme categories from their associated normally distributed dimensions; and in part from the lack of good empirical evidence to resolve these issues. Yet, it is clear that some sort of descriptive terms must be available and it is necessary to decide how to move ahead in research and clinical practice with respect to this group of disorders.

That is just what this set of empirically based, but theoretically informed essays seeks to achieve. It is extremely timely to have overviews of the issues surrounding concepts of specific developmental disorders and this volume serves a most useful purpose in its provision of critical, but constructive, accounts of the history of the ideas, the empirical research findings, and the practical implications that follow from classification decisions. Reading retardation, speech/language disorders, and motor coordination impairment are used as case examples to indicate the conceptual, measurement, and validation issues, and to discuss possible ways ahead. Quite deliberately, the authors were selected to represent a range of views and it is evident that a consensus has not yet been achieved. The Scottish 'not proven' verdict is needed with respect to almost all the views expressed. Nevertheless, it is also apparent that there has been considerable progress in narrowing the areas of dispute and in agreeing the kinds of research findings that might resolve the remaining areas of dispute. Therein lies the most important contribution of this provocative, but informative, volume.

Because all of the chapters focus on one or other of the three chosen examples of developmental disorders, there is perhaps a danger of readers assuming that the problems are peculiar to this field, but they are not. Even a brief glance at the literature on other disorders makes *that* clear. The battles over whether of not the statistical curve of reading discrepancy scores shows a 'hump' at the extreme bottom end was preceded nearly half a century ago by the disputes over a comparable issue with respect to hypertension. Statisticians have now come to agreement that the shape of distributional curves provides a most uncertain guide to whether or not there are one, two of three groups within it. The need, as always, is for external validation of the proposed diagnostic distinctions. Although, of course there are some special considerations with respect to specific developmental disorders, most of the issues are much more pervasive, with obvious parallels in many other fields of medicine and of psychology. Accordingly, in this foreword, it may be useful to set the scene for what follows in the book itself by outlining some of the key considerations.

The most basic point is one put succinctly by the philosopher Sir Karl Popper (1972) when he argued that definitions should be read from right to left. In other words, the starting point has to be the phenomenon to be accounted for, and not the diagnostic term. Popper's predecessor 'Humpty Dumpty' made the point forcefully in his claim that you could make words mean whatever you wanted them to mean (Through the Looking Glass, Lewis Carroll, 1872).

So what is the phenomenon? Clearly, it is the occurrence of severe and specific impairments in particular psychological functions that ordinarily follow a developmental course, impairments that arise as relatively isolated deficits against a background of otherwise unremarkable general cognitive functioning. That is, more or less, what the specific reading retardation and specific developmental disorders of language are meant to cover.

Given that there is immense individual variation in the timing of all developmental milestones (consider, for example, the differences among children in the age at which teeth erupt or puberty is reached), it should be no surprise that there is equal variation in the acquisition of spoken language and of reading skills. The question is whether extremes in such variation have any clinical meaning. Follow-up findings make it abundantly clear that they do. Thus, although many children with a marked delay in speech acquisition catch up by the time they start school and show no apparent later sequelae (Bishop & Edmundson, 1987), many do not and indeed show important social impairments that are still evident in adult life (Rutter & Mawhood, 1991). The former may reasonably be considered normal, albeit marked, variations; whereas the latter clearly represents a disorder of some kind. Similarly, follow-up studies continued into adult life have indicated that few children with severe reading difficulties in middle childhood later catch up in reading (Maughan, Hagell, Rutter, & Yule, 1994). Most, instead, continue to exhibit quite marked reading and spelling difficulties many years after most of their peers have achieved mastery of these skills. Again, the presence of continuing impairment justifies the concept of disorder.

The same longitudinal data, however, have brought out a further key point: namely, that the manifestations change with age to an important extent. Thus, with very few exceptions, even the children with the most severe forms of developmental language disorder will be talking in full sentences in adult life. On the other hand, many will show more subtle language problems, often there are reading difficulties, and frequently social relationships are impaired. Similarly, people may improve considerably in their reading but nevertheless be left with major problems in spelling. Any adequate set of diagnostic criteria will have to take these variations in account.

Non-medics are sometimes inclined to view this 'fuzziness' as a reflection of the supposed woolliness of psychology, or the inadequacy of the tools for psychological measurement, or as a indication that developmental disorders cannot be 'proper' diseases. All are misguided assumptions. Even single gene Mendelian medical disorders show amazing variability. Thus, tuberose sclerosis may be manifest by gross handicap accompanied by mental retardation, epilepsy, and calcified masses of the brain or only by subtle skin lesions that require an expert to detect them. Even monozygotic twins both of whom have autism may differ in IQ by over 50 points as well as in numerous details of symptomatology (Le Couteur et al., 1996). The validity of a diagnostic concept had nothing to do with homogeneity in symptom pattern or in clinical course, despite frequent claims that these are required: extensive medical findings indicate otherwise. Of course, equally, validity does require some external evidence that there is an essential unity (in pathophysiology or cause) despite variation. For the most part, such evidence is lacking in the case of developmental disorders, although as several chapters in this volume note, there are some possible leads to follow (see also Tallal, Miller, & Fitch, 1995). None, however, mention the potential of molecular genetics which may well provide the breakthrough that is much needed (see Plomin & Rutter, submitted; Rutter & Plomin, submitted).

Psychologists (and psychiatrists) who have used psychometric definitions of developmental disorders (e.g. a skill at least 2 standard deviations below expectation for chronological age, or for chronological age and intelligence) have done so to provide comparability across studies and to ensure that meaningful levels of disorder were being studied. Unfortunately, this has often been misunderstood as meaning that lesser degrees of severity are either not meaningful or are qualitatively different in some respect. The validity in both the pattern and severity of manifestations of even clear-cut diseases indicates that no such supposition is warranted. Psychometric definitions have their utility but they are essentially arbitrary and it is extremely implausible that they will coincide with the true boundaries of the disorder as indicated by either pathophysiology or cause.

Many would accept that arbitrariness of psychometric cut-offs but would object to the assumption of 'disorder' on the grounds that they are no more than the extremes of a normal distribution. In that connection, it is important to appreciate that many medical diseases are either in themselves an extreme (as e.g., with hypertension), or are based on dimensional risk factors (as e.g., with coronary artery disease and cholesterol levels, or epilepsy and convulsive threshold). In these cases, the extremes are regarded as diseases or disorders because being at the extreme sets in motion abnormal pathophysiologic mechanisms (as with malignant hypertension) or is associated with impairment that warrants treatment (as with epilepsy). Nevertheless, it is still meaningful to ask if the difference between the extreme and the middle of the range is qualitative or quantitative. The fact that the trait of characteristic involves similar components at all points on the range is not helpful one way or the other. That would be so with intelligence, for example but, despite that, the causes and consequences of severe mental retardation are quite different from those associated with variations in the middle of the IQ range (Cantwell & Rutter, 1994; Simonoff, Bolton, & Rutter, 1996). Accordingly, the finding that the cognitive components of reading seem similar in all groups does not aid classification.

As almost all chapters in this volume note, associations with IQ dominate all considerations of specific developmental disorders of psychological functions. The issues are real enough and it has to be accepted that they have not yet been resolved. However, the true issues are not quite the same as they are sometimes portrayed. Thus, the concern cannot be any supposed expectations that IQ as measured provides a true, unbiased estimate of general intelligence. It does not, but exactly the same applies to tests of reading or language. Similarly, the concern cannot be the discredited notion that IQ sets a ceiling on achievement. Indeed there is as much interest in special isolated 'idiot savant' skills above the overall level of intelligence as in the special deficits below that overall level. Also, despite reading retardation (i.e. a disorder defined in terms of a discrepancy between reading and the expectation based on chronological age and IQ) truly differs from general reading backwardness (i.e., a disorder using an expectation based only on chronological age). To begin with, there is huge overlap between the two so that any contrast would have to involve this third, overlap, group. But much more crucially, almost all protagonists do take IQ into account one way or another. Some do so by excluding those with an IQ below some set level (e.g., 70 or 80 or 85) and some by focusing on discrepancies defined in terms of regression equation predictions. It might be meaningful to ask which approach works best but both presuppose a difference from general mental retardation.

The more basic question is whether that presupposition is valid. Certainly it is with respect to severe mental retardation (because the causes are so different), but does specific reading retardation differ meaningfully from mild mental retardation? Do both these extremes differ from variations within the normal range (Rutter, Simonoff, & Plomin, 1996)? And do the different varieties of special skill deficits (reading, spelling, mathematics, motor coordination, language) differ from one another? It is usually supposed that they do, if only because the cognitive patterns differ somewhat, but it would be premature to conclude that the matter is settled. The question has been opened up by the growing body of evidence that the special skills defined by the list of developmental language disorders are not as quite as 'pure' as used to be supposed. Thus, developmental language disorders are associated with a range of important cognitive deficits that extend outside language as traditionally defined (Bishop, 1992). Also, genetic evidence suggests that, to an important extent, the same genetic liability underlies a range of specific cognitive skills (Plomin, DeFries, McClearn & Rutter, 1997). That is scarcely surprising, however, in view of the substantial intercorrelations between supposedly separate skills and between each of these and general intelligence. The more crucial question is whether, in addition to these general factors, there is something different about the causes (genetic or environmental) of severe developmental deficits. The answer to that question has still to be obtained.

Finally, as discussed in several of the chapters, it needs to be borne in mind that classification is needed for several quite different purposes and these may require rather separate approaches. Thus, it is often advantageous in research to define groups in ways that match the hypotheses to be tested, frequently it will be helpful to focus on extreme 'typical' categories (to avoid false positives), and it is of little concern that the approach may leave many patterns unclassifiable. By contrast, classifications for clinical purposes need to be based on what is known to work in practice, and the aim must be to classify as high a proportion of patterns possible. Practical considerations also may take priority over scientific ones. For example, even if the distinction between specific reading retardation and general reading backwardness proved to be scientifically valid, if the teaching needs were similar for the two groups, practitioners might not wish to make the distinction. Conversely, if mathematical and reading difficulties turned out to have the same genetic or environmental causal factors, it would still be useful to separate them diagnostically because they require a different focus in teaching.

With this aperitif of conceptual considerations to whet the appetite, readers need to move on now to the more substantial meal provided by the thoughtful and well-informed discussions that are provided in the chapters that follow. Hopefully, it will be appreciated that they may serve as a basis for a problem-solving set of both research strategies and practical steps that will ensure real resolution of the dilemmas outlined here.

December, 1996

Michael Rutter,
University of London, United Kingdom

## REFERENCES

American Psychiatric Association (1994). *Diagnostic and statistical manual of mental disorders* (4th ed.). Washington, DC: American Psychiatric Association.

Berger, M., Yule, W., & Rutter, M. (1975). Attainment and adjustment in two geographical areas: II The prevalence of specific reading retardation. *British Journal of Psychiatry, 126*, 510-519.

Bishop, D. & Edmundson, A. (1987). Language-impaired 4-year olds: Distinguishing transient from persistent impairment. *Journal of Speech and Hearing Disorders, 52*, 156-173.

Bishop, D. (1992). The underlying nature of specific language impairment. *Journal of Child Psychology and Psychiatry, 33*, 3-66.

Cantwell, D. P. & Rutter, M. (1994). Classification: Conceptual issues and substantive findings. In M. Rutter, E. Taylor, & L. Hersov (Eds.), *Child and adolescent psychiatry: Modern approaches* (3rd ed., pp. 3-21). Oxford: Blackwell Scientific.

Le Couteur, A., Bailey, A., Goode, S. Pickles, A., Robertson, S., Gottesman, I., & Rutter, M. (1996). A broader phenotype of autism: The clinical spectrum in twins. *Journal of Child Psychology and Psychiatry, 37*, 785-801.

Maughan, B., Hagell, A., Rutter, M., & Yule, W. (1994). Poor readers in secondary schools. *Reading and Writing: An Interdisciplinary Journal, 6*, 125-150.

Plomin, R., DeFries, J., McClearn, G. E., & Rutter, M. (1997). *Behavioural Genetics* (3rd ed.). New York: W. H. Freeman.

Plomin, R. & Rutter, M. (submitted). *Child development and molecular genetics: What do we do with genes once they are found?*

Popper, K. R. (1972). *Objective knowledge: An evolutionary approach.* Oxford: Oxford University Press.

Rutter, M. (1969). The concept of dyslexia. In. P. Wolff & R. MacKeith (Eds.), *Planning for better learning* (pp. 129-139). London: S.I.M.P./ William Heinemann Medical Books.

Rutter, M., Maughan, B., Mortimore, P., Ouston, J., & Smith, A. (1979). *Fifteen thousand hours: Secondary schools and their effects on children.* London/ Cambridge, MA: Open Books, Harvard University Press.

Rutter, M. & Mawhood, L. (1991). The long-term psychosocial sequelae of specific developmental disorders of speech and language. In M. Rutter & P. Casaer (Eds.), *Biological risk factors for psychosocial disorders* (pp. 233-250). Cambridge: Cambridge University Press.

Rutter, M. & Plomin, R. (submitted). *Opportunities for psychiatry from genetic findings.*

Rutter, M. & Shaffer, D. (1980). DSM-III: A step forward or back in terms of the classification of child psychiatric disorders? *Journal of the American Academy of Child Psychiatry, 19*, 371-394.

Rutter, M., Simonoff, E., & Plomin, R. (1996). Genetic influences on mild mental retardation: Concepts, findings and research implications. *Journal of Biosocial Science, 28*, 509-526.

Simonoff, E., Bolton, P., & Rutter, M. (1996). Mental retardation: Genetic findings, clinical implications and research agenda. *Journal of Child Psychology and Psychiatry, 37*, 259-280.

Tallal, P., Miller, S., & Fitch, R. H. (1995). Neurobiological basis of speech: A

case for the pre-eminence of temporal processing. *The Irish Journal of Psychology, 16*, 194-219.
World Health Organization (1992). *The IDC-10 classification of mental and behavioural disorders: Clinical descriptions and diagnostic guidelines.* Geneva: World Health Organization.

# SECTION 1

# INTRODUCTION

JAN RISPENS, TOM A. VAN YPEREN & WILLIAM YULE

# PERSPECTIVES ON THE CLASSIFICATION OF SPECIFIC DEVELOPMENTAL DISORDERS: AN INTRODUCTION

## INTRODUCTION

This volume deals with the classification of specific developmental disorders. The concept of specific developmental disorder (SDD) refers to developmental delays that cannot be explained in terms of intellectual retardation, physical handicap, or adverse environmental conditions. For example, the diagnosis 'specific developmental expressive language disorder' implies that children (unexpectedly) lag behind in the development of their expressive language abilities despite normal intelligence, and in the absence of physical or sensory handicaps (Bishop, 1992). The assumption is that SDD differs in certain ways, such as prognosis or course of the disorder, from other types of developmental delays. Specific developmental disorders are described in terms of a discrepancy between the observed level of development compared to the developmental level that may be expected, given the child's capacities. In other words, children with SDD lag behind in their development without any apparent reason.

Specific developmental disorders may be present in the developmental domains of language development, motor coordination, and the acquisition of scholastic skills. Also, a combination of developmental delays may be present. The prevalence of the various categories of SDD is relatively high. Figures vary from three percent (SDD of language) to six percent (SDD of motor coordination), in the age range from 5 to 11 years (Rutter, 1989).

Categories of SDD have become part of classification systems such as the ICD-10 Classification of Mental and Behavioural Disorders (ICD-10, World Health Organization [WHO], 1992) and the Diagnostic and Statistical Manual of Mental Disorders, fourth edition (DSM-IV, American Psychiatric Association [APA], 1994). These official classifications contain descriptions of numerous mental disorders. Each description includes a number of diagnostic criteria. A classification system serves as a diagnostic tool that offers clinicians a standardized language for describing a clinical picture.



*J. Rispens et al. (eds.),*
*Perspectives on the Classification of Specific Developmental Disorders*, 3–13.

Although the categories of SDD are well known to clinicians and researchers and are widely applied in clinical practice, they are subject to much debate. For example, the adequacy of the description of the various categories of SDD in terms of a discrepancy between observed and expected developmental level is questioned (Fletcher, Francis, Rourke, Shaywitz, & Shaywitz, 1992). Also, the operationalization of the diagnostic criteria causes much trouble (Siegel, 1992). The results of recent studies have led some researchers to doubt the very existence of categories of specific developmental disorders (Shaywitz, Fletcher, Holahan, & Shaywitz, 1992). They argue that in some studies no difference has been found between SDD and other types of developmental delays. These critical remarks suggest that a closer look at the concept of SDD and its role in classifications systems is needed.

It is the aim of this volume to take up this challenge and to discuss the concept of SDD from the perspective of classification. The following chapters deal with questions such as the reliability and external validity of the categories of SDD, the adequacy of diagnostic criteria and descriptions of the various categories in existing classification systems, and the problem of heterogeneity within a single category and the division into subtypes. Although critical about the current status of the concept, the authors have endeavoured to contribute toward further development of classification by suggesting possible improvements.

In this first chapter we briefly introduce the two concepts that play a crucial role in the following chapters, namely the idea of classification and the notion of SDD.

## ISSUES IN THE CLASSIFICATION OF SPECIFIC DEVELOPMENTAL DISORDERS

Clinical practice has undergone important changes during the last decades, partly due to a certain standardization of diagnostic procedures. The introduction of classification systems such as DSM and ICD has contributed significantly to this process. Classification refers to the process of ordering phenomena into groups or types (Achenbach, 1985). Classification systems describe disorders in a standardized language (Rutter & Gould, 1985) and order these descriptions into a coherent and hierarchical system. They offer a standard for the communication about disorders, which is important for clinicians since it may help them to describe a clinical picture, while for researchers the standardized descriptions of the categories of disorders are especially useful for sample selection. Classification systems play an increasingly important role in clinical practice.

DSM and ICD are the two major official classification schemes that are most often used in clinical practice and research. It should be noted that attempts to construct generally accepted systems for the classification of mental disorders are relatively new. The first edition of the ICD, developed by the World Health Organization, appeared in 1899. This edition was primarily a classification of somatic diseases, meant to promote the communication between countries with respect to the prevalence of health problems and causes of death. There were only 11 categories for psychiatric disorders. The first edition of the DSM appeared in 1952. This system was developed by the American Psychiatric Association, for the classification of mental disorders. DSM-I contained 127 categories, organized under eight headings. From then on new versions of both systems have appeared regularly. The latest version of the ICD, ICD-10, appeared in 1992, while DSM-IV appeared in 1994. In every new version there is not only an increase of the number of categories of disorders, but also a further refinement of the diagnostic criteria of each disorder.

Classification systems contain numerous categories of disorders. Categories that refer to related disorders are grouped together under the umbrella of a uniting concept. Also, some categories are divided into subcategories. For example, ICD-10 has under the heading 'Disorders of psychological development' seven categories of developmental disorders. They share a number of common features, such as onset of the disorder during infancy or childhood, and the notion that the impairment is strongly related to biological maturation of the central nervous system. Four of these categories refer to specific developmental disorders, namely 'SDD of speech and language' (with six subcategories), 'SDD of scholastic skills' (also with six subcategories), 'SDD of motor function', and finally the category of 'Mixed specific developmental disorders'. These categories of SDD all share the same pattern of diagnostic criteria, based on the notion of a discrepancy between the expected and the observed level of development. The three remaining categories of disorders of psychological development in ICD-10 are: 'pervasive developmental disorders' (that includes eight subcategories, for example childhood autism), the category 'other disorders of psychological development' (that includes developmental agnosia), and finally the category 'unspecified disorder of psychological development', that is meant for those cases of developmental delays that do not fit into the other categories.

An important difference between DSM and ICD is that the former is multi-axial. Axes represent different domains of information about the clinical picture. DSM-IV has five Axes, namely: Axis I: Clinical disorders; Axis II: Personality Disorders and Mental Retardation; Axis III: General Medical Conditions; Axis IV: Psychosocial and Environmental Problems; Axis V: Global Assessment of Functioning.

The two systems also share a number of important features. In both schemes the basis for classification is not theory, but clinical expertise (Cantwell, 1996). New versions are based on the consensus of large groups of clinical experts. Furthermore, both systems apply a categorical approach. Disorders are described in such a way that the clinician must decide whether or not the patient meets the criteria for the disorder. One of the advantages of a categorical system is that most clinical decisions are categorical, such as a yes or no decision with respect to the selection of a treatment of a certain type. Hence, categorical classification is easily related to clinical decision making (Cantwell & Rutter, 1994). However, categorical systems also have disadvantages. For example, the notion of a forced choice gives no room for uncertainties and doubt. In a dimensional system a patient is described as a set of scores on a variety of aspects that constitute a multi-dimensional space. An advantage of this approach is that it allows a description of a diversity of symptoms in one patient, while another disadvantage of a categorical system is that comorbidity, implying that more that one category is applicable, is more difficult to handle. Also, the reliability of dimensional systems is generally higher (Cantwell, 1996).

Various evaluative criteria are used to describe the quality of a classification system (Cantwell, 1996; Cantwell & Rutter, 1994). First, the scheme should not be based on a controversial theory. Instead, it should be theoretically unenterprising, which means that it must be based on concepts that are generally accepted. We already mentioned that ICD and DSM are based on clinical consensus. These systems try to avoid controversial theoretical notions. However, this does not imply that theoretical concepts and findings from empirical research are not integrated into the definitions of the categories. Second, a scheme must have a logically consistent structure. It should be clear which choices were made in constructing the system and why these choices were preferred. Third, reliability, validity and clinical utility are important criteria.

## THE CONCEPT OF SPECIFIC DEVELOPMENTAL DISORDERS

Clinicians have long been aware of the existence of various subgroups within the group of children with developmental delays. For example, from early on school psychologists have suggested that not learning to read despite normal intelligence and in the absence of other explanations of poor performance, should be distinguished from poor reading that may be ascribed to limited intellectual capacities or adverse home conditions. The first clinical descriptions of this specific type of developmental disorders appeared at the beginning of this century. Terms such as 'dyslexia' (specific developmental reading retardation), 'dysphasia' (specific developmental language disorder), and 'the clumsy child syndrome' (specific motor coordination disorder) were coined to denote this class of children who unexpectedly manifest a developmental delay. The term SDD has evolved as a concept that serves as an umbrella covering the various categories of specific developmental disorders. The notion of SDD is widely used in clinical practice.

The concept of SDD not only reflects clinical expertise and intuition. Since the Twenties, a rapidly growing number of empirical studies exploring the concept of SDD has appeared. Most of these studies were devoted to the category of specific reading disorder. Initially, the categories of SDD were studied primarily from a medical perspective. An important aim of this research was to describe each of these disorders in terms of a specific aetiology, such as neurological factors or heritability. Furthermore, not much attention was paid to the developmental perspective. A developmental perspective implies that a proper understanding of a developmental delay must be based on insight into the qualitative changes in behaviours over time that are inherent to the notion of development (Cicchetti & Cohen, 1995). Early research on SDD frequently mentions an analogy or even a relationship between a certain type of SDD and adult cerebral disorders. For example, Kinsbourne and Warrington (1966) in their (clinical) study of a group of children with reading difficulties suggested that the problems of some of these children were analogous to those of adults with a cerebral cortical disorder, namely the Gerstmann syndrome, characterized by difficulties in right-left discrimination, writing and naming the fingers. In the same vein, various researchers assumed an analogy between specific language disorders and aphasia.

An interesting conclusion from most of these studies was that in each of the categories of SDD there is a considerable heterogeneity with respect to aetiology and symptomatology. As a consequence, attempts to define each of the categories in terms of one or more causal factors were not very successful. Categories of SDD were defined negatively, by stating what was not the cause of the disorder. For example, in 1970 the World Federation of Neurology defined specific developmental dyslexia as: "A disorder manifested by difficulties in learning to read despite conventional instruction, adequate intelligence and sociocultural opportunity. It is dependent upon fundamental cognitive disabilities which are frequently of constitutional origin" (Critchley, 1970, p. 11). This kind of definition has been criticized for lack of specificity and clarity. Definitional issues have remained a matter of debate (Bishop, 1992; Stanovich, 1994).

Surprisingly, in the initial research not much attention was paid to the external validity of the concept of SDD. The question how SDD differs from other types of developmental disorders was virtually neglected until the beginning of the Seventies, when the results of the Isle of Wight study appeared. In this groundbreaking epidemiological study, Rutter and his co-workers (Rutter & Yule, 1970; Rutter & Yule, 1973) demonstrated that children with a specific reading disorder differ from children with another type of reading delay, labelled 'general backwardness in reading', with respect to correlates such as sex ratio, presence of neurological signs, and prognosis. Another important aspect of this study was the application of a descriptive definition of the specific reading disorder, without reference to causal factors. SDD of reading was defined as a discrepancy between observed and expected reading performance of more than two standard errors of prediction, while general backwardness in reading referred to a significant deviation from the average reading score of the age group. The Isle of Wight study provided a formula for computing discrepancies that takes statistical artifacts into account.

Nearly a century of research and clinical application have made it increasingly clear that the categories of SDD do not represent a single condition, with a known neurological basis (Bishop, 1992; Rutter, 1989; Stanovich, 1994). SDD represents a fuzzy concept, implying that there is a nucleus of 'pure' cases surrounded by a much larger band of subjects who manifest the typical characteristics of SDD in various degrees. Furthermore, each category of SDD may contain various subtypes, differing in symptoms, course and underlying cognitive deficiencies that may be related to different brain pathologies. Some researchers even suggest that various categories of SDD, such as specific developmental language disorder and specific developmental reading disorder, may be manifestations of the same underlying cognitive deficit (Tallal, Sainburg, & Jernigan, 1991).

This state of affairs, not uncommon in scientific and applied disciplines, causes a number of practical problems that are not easily solved. For example, how is a disorder to be defined if there is no one single cause to which it can be described? Are stringent diagnostic criteria required, in order to exclude subjects who do not belong to the nucleus group? Is there a qualitative difference, for example in terms of underlying cognitive capacities or deficiencies, between this core group and other children who manifest a developmental delay? Given the available data, these questions cannot be answered with certainty as yet.

A practical solution, that solves part of these problems is to define SDD in terms of a discrepancy between observed and expected level of performance without further reference to underlying pathology. For example, in ICD-10 an expressive language disorder is described as: "A specific developmental disorder in which the child's ability to use expressive language is markedly below the appropriate level for his or her mental age, but in which language comprehension is within normal limits" (WHO, 1992, p. 237). These descriptive and psychometric definitions of the various categories of SDD have generally been accepted, and they contribute to the comparability of clinical and research samples. Nevertheless, some definitional issues remain a matter of concern.

First, the definition produces some difficult technical problems, especially with respect to the operationalization of the notion of a discrepancy. What exactly is meant by 'markedly below'? Application of stringent diagnostic criteria (for example: 'markedly below' implies at least 2 sd's below the average score of the age group) may have far reaching practical consequences regarding eligibility for treatment. There is ample evidence that the number of children classified as SDD varies as a function of diagnostic criteria (Rispens, Van Yperen, & Van Duijn, 1991). The application of too stringent criteria may result in the exclusion of some children from remedial treatment.

Another much discussed issue pertains to the question whether an estimate of expected performance (which is required to determine the discrepancy with observed performance) should be based on mental age, as suggested in the WHO definition. Both in research and in practice a discrepancy is generally defined as 'performance below the expected level, given the child's IQ'. However, one may argue that IQ is an inadequate measure of potential performance.

One reason is that IQ may have been affected negatively by the developmental delay (Siegel, 1992).

Although psychometric definitions of the categories of SDD clearly have a certain merit, they do not solve the fundamental problems that arise from the fuzzy character of the concept of SDD. Even the application of a narrow interpretation of the notion of a discrepancy may result in the inclusion of children who do not belong to the core group (Rutter, this volume). The reason is that defining SDD in terms of a discrepancy will result in an overlap between SDD and other types of developmental delays. In the Isle of Wight study a considerable number of children diagnosed as specific reading disordered also obtained the classification 'general backwardness in reading' (Rutter & Yule, 1973). This finding has been replicated in several other studies (Fletcher et al., 1994; Stanovich & Siegel, 1994). On the basis of these results, some researchers conclude that there are no qualitative differences between the two groups (Shaywitz et al., 1992). They argue that the concept of SDD simply represents the lower end of the continuum of scores on tests in domains such as reading, language or motor development, and that there is no such thing as dyslexia. Opinions such as these fuel the ongoing debate about the concept of SDD and its categories.

However, another interpretation of these findings is also defendable. One could argue that the descriptive definitions that are in use lack sufficient sensitivity to discriminate between the core group and its surrounding broad band of children who manifest the problems of the core group to some extent, but who probably do not share the same underlying deficits. An improved definition of SDD in terms of underlying processes, typical symptoms, differing prognosis, and specific treatment that the condition requires, is needed in order to properly identify children with SDD. In other words, an improved definition should be explicit about what is specific about specific developmental disorders (Rispens & Van Yperen, 1997).

Classification systems are the result of the ongoing process of the integration of research findings and clinical expertise into more sophisticated and refined schemes. For that reason new versions will continue to appear. The ongoing debate about the status of the concept of SDD must be reflected in the development of new classification systems. A possible outcome of this discussion may be the inclusion of improved definitions of the categories of SDD, based on recent research findings, and further differentiation and specification of the diagnostic criteria.

## GLOBAL THEMES

The aim of this volume is to contribute to the debate about improved classification of SDD in future versions of classification systems. It is important to note that this issue is discussed from the perspective of existing classification systems. The starting point is the concept of SDD as it is currently represented in these systems. Although a critical attitude prevails in each section, it is not the intention of this volume to argue that existing classification systems should be changed completely or to propose a classification of SDD that cannot fit into the format of the schemes that are in use.

The volume is divided into three sections, according to the subdivision of SDD into three categories, namely disorders of scholastic skills, language disorders, and developmental motor disorders. The section on disorders of scholastic skills deals exclusively with specific reading disorders. The basic outline of each section is as follows.

First, in each of the chapters general questions that arise in the discussion about the categories of SDD are presented. To some extent those problems are inherent in the format and structure of the existing classification schemes. We already noted that a categorical system implies a forced choice: the patient either does or does not meet the diagnostic criteria. Consequently, the specificity and adequacy of diagnostic criteria give rise to much concern. Since classification systems are not based on explicit and grounded theories about disorders, criteria cannot be derived from a theoretical framework underlying the description of the disorder. Furthermore, issues such as comorbidity and heterogeneity pose problems that are not easily solved in a categorical system. For that reason much attention is devoted to this issue in the various chapters of this book.

Second, in existing classification systems the concept of SDD is a higher-order concept, that serves as an umbrella covering the various categories of SDD. However, it is conceivable that future developments will not be the same for all categories. For example, it may be that based on the results of research and clinical practice the traditional psychometric and descriptive definition of one the categories will be replaced by a description in terms of underlying processes, while other categories remain unchanged. Hence, one may wonder whether it will be possible to retain the concept of SDD as a unifying concept.

Third, in each section various questions are presented that are relevant to each particular category of SDD. These questions pertain to definition, external validity, subtyping, and the cause of the disorder. These are the stepping stones that may contribute to an improved description of the categories of SDD.

## REFERENCES


Achenbach, T. M. (1985). *Assessment and taxonomy of child and adolescent psychopathology*. Newbury Park: Sage.

American Psychiatric Association (1994). *Diagnostic and statistical manual of mental disorders* (4th ed.). Washington, DC: American Psychiatric Association.

Bishop, D. V. M. (1992). The underlying nature of specific language impairment. *Journal of Child Psychology and Psychiatry, 33,* 3-66.

Cantwell, D. P. (1996). Classification of child and adolescent psychopathology. *Journal of Child Psychology and Psychiatry, 37,* 3-13.

Cantwell, D. P. & Rutter, M. (1994). Classification: Conceptual issues and substantive findings. In M. Rutter, E. Taylor, & L. Hersov (Eds.), *Child and adolescent psychiatry: Modern approaches* (pp. 3-22). Oxford: Blackwell.

Cicchetti, D. & Cohen, D. J. (1995). Perspectives on developmental psychopathology. In D. Cicchetti & D. J. Cohen (Eds.), *Developmental psychopathology: Vol. I* (pp. 3-23). New York: Wiley.

Critchley, M. (1970). *Developmental dyslexia.* London: Heinemann.

Fletcher, J. M., Francis, D. J., Rourke, B. P., Shaywitz, S. E., & Shaywitz, B. (1992). Validity of discrepancy-based definitions of reading disabilities. *Journal of Learning Disabilities, 25,* 546-548.

Fletcher, J. M., Shaywitz, S. E., Shankweiler, D. P., Katz, L., Liberman, I. Y., Stuebing, K. K., Francis, D. J., Fowler, A. E., & Shaywitz, B. A. (1994). Cognitive profiles of reading disability: Comparisons of discrepancy and low achievement definitions. *Journal of Educational Psychology, 86,* 6-23.

Kinsbourne, M. & Warrington E. K. (1966). The developmental Gerstmann syndrome. In J. Money (Ed.), *The disabled reader* (pp. 325-349). Baltimore: John Hopkins Press.

Rispens, J. & Van Yperen, T. A. (1997). How specific are 'specific developmental disorders'? The relevance of the concept of specific developmental disorders for the classification of childhood developmental disorders. *Journal of Child Psychology and Psychiatry, 38,* 351-365.

Rispens, J., Van Yperen, T. A. & Van Duijn, G. A. (1990). The irrelevance of IQ to the definition of learning disabilities: Some empirical evidence. *Journal of Learning Disabilities, 24,* 434-438.

Rutter, M. (1989). Isle of Wight revisited: Twenty-five years of child psychiatric epidemiology. *Journal of the American Academy of Child and Adolescent Psychiatry, 28,* 633-653.

Rutter, M. & Gould, M. A. (1985). Classification. In M. Rutter & L. Hersov (Eds.), *Child and adolescent psychiatry: Modern approaches* (2nd ed.) (pp. 304 -325). London: Blackwell.

Rutter, M. & Yule, W. (1970). Neurological aspects of intellectual retardation and specific reading retardation. In M. Rutter, J. Tizard, & K. Whitmoore (Eds.) *Education, health and behaviour* (pp. 54-74). London: Longman.

Rutter, M. & Yule, W. (1973). Specific reading retardation. In L. Mann (Ed.), *The first review of special education* (pp. 1-51). Philadelphia: JSE Press.

Shaywitz, B. A., Fletcher, J. M., Holahan, J. M., & Shaywitz, S. E. (1992). Discrepancy compared to low achievement definitions of reading disability: Results from the Connecticut longitudinal study. *Journal of Learning Disabilities, 25,* 639-648.

Siegel, L. S. (1992). An evaluation of the discrepancy definition of dyslexia. *Journal of Learning Disabilities, 25,* 618-629.

Stanovich, K. E. (1994). Does dyslexia exist? *Journal of Child Psychology and Psychiatry, 35,* 579-597.

Stanovich, K. E. & Siegel, L. S. (1994). Phenotypic performance profile of children with reading disabilities: A regression-based test of the phonological-core variable-difference model. *Journal of Educational Psychology, 86,* 24-53.

Tallal, P., Sainburg, R. L., & Jernigan, T. (1991). The neuropathology of developmental dysphasia: Behavioural, morphological and physiological evidence for a pervasive temporal processing disorder. *Reading and Writing, 3,* 363-377.

World Health Organization (1992). *The ICD-10 classification of mental and behavioural disorders: Clinical descriptions and diagnostic guidelines.* Geneva: World Health Organization.

JAN RISPENS AND TOM A. VAN YPEREN

# THE ROLE OF SDD IN CLASSIFICATION SYSTEMS: HISTORICAL OVERVIEW AND CURRENT STATUS

## INTRODUCTION

Categories of specific developmental disorders (SDD) are part of current classification systems such as ICD and DSM. The term SDD refers to impairments in three domains of development, namely language and speech (communication), scholastic skills, and motor coordination, that cannot be explained in terms of intellectual retardation, physical handicap, or adverse environmental conditions. The categories all share the same pattern of diagnostic criteria:

A: The disturbance interferes significantly with academic achievement or activities of daily living that require language, speech, scholastic or motor ability.

B: Performance in the developmental domain is substantially below what could be expected, given the person's chronological age, measured intelligence, and (in case of learning disorders) age-appropriate education. In other words, there is a discrepancy between the observed and the expected performance.

C: In the case of language difficulties, the disorder does not meet criteria for a pervasive developmental disorder. In the case of motor coordination problems, criteria for a pervasive developmental disorder are also not met, and the problems are not due to a general medical condition.

D: In the case of learning difficulties: if a sensory deficit is present, the difficulties in learning are in excess of those usually associated with a sensory deficit.
In the case of language disorders: if mental retardation, a speech-motor or sensory deficit, or environmentally deprivation is present, the language difficulties are in excess of those usually associated with these problems.
In the case of motor disorders: if mental retardation is present, the motor difficulties are in excess of those usually associated with mental retardation. Furthermore, the disturbance is not



*J. Rispens et al. (eds.),*
*Perspectives on the Classification of Specific Developmental Disorders,* 15–37.

due to a general medical condition and does not meet the criteria for a pervasive developmental disorder.

In these classification schemes the concept of SDD plays a role as a higher-order concept. It serves as a unifying umbrella, covering various categories of specific developmental disorders, contributing to the standardization of the definition of the various categories of SDD, since they are all based on the notions of discrepancy and exclusion that are inherent to the concept of SDD. As a consequence, a higher-order concept may positively affect the reliability of the classification of the disorders that are subsumed under this umbrella (Gould, Shaffer, Rutter, & Sturge, 1988).

The prevalence of these disorders is relatively high. For example, in DSM-IV (APA, 1994) the prevalence of reading disorder is estimated at 4 percent; estimates of the prevalence of expressive language disorder range from 3 to 5 percent, while the prevalence of the clumsy child syndrome (Developmental Coordination Disorder) is estimated to be 6 percent (in the age range from 5 to 11 years). Therefore, specific developmental disorders are well known in clinical practice.

It is interesting to note that the role of the concept of SDD has increased in the various versions of ICD and DSM. For example, DSM-I (APA, 1952) included a limited number of categories of developmental disorders, and only one those referred to SDD, namely the category of 'Learning disturbance'. In each new version the number of categories of SDD increased, and the notion of SDD as a higher-order concept was introduced. In this chapter we describe the role of the concept in successive versions the of classification systems. From this description it will become clear that its role has changed considerably. We also will pay attention to research regarding the reliability and validity of the categories of SDD in the various versions of the systems, in order to get an impression of its clinical relevance. In the second section we briefly discuss the possible future of the concept of SDD, given the many theoretical and practical problems that need to be solved.

## HISTORICAL OVERVIEW

### *Introduction*

The history of the concept of SDD and the role it has played in the development of classification systems can be divided into three phases. In the first phase, disorders such as dyslexia and dysphasia were treated as unrelated entities, and it was assumed that they were part of broadly defined categories of developmental deviations each including a heterogeneous variety of disorders. As a consequence, the unifying concept of SDD was not applied in the early versions of classification systems such as DSM or ICD. In the second phase, the domain of the disorder was narrowed to a specific and more or less homogeneous set of learning, language, speech and motor disorders, and the unifying concept of SDD was introduced. The disorders were organized in the classification systems under one heading, called 'specific developmental disorders'. The third phase was one of the further breakdown of this set of disorders into more refined categories. At the same time, less emphasis is put on the conceptual unity of the disorders.

### *First Phase: Separate Entities and Broad Concepts*

Early classification schemes such as ICD-7 and DSM-I included a limited number of categories of specific developmental disorders. They were part of broad sections, encompassing a heterogeneous variety of disorders. We briefly discuss (a) the ICD-7 and DSM-I; (b) DSM-II and the GAP-scheme; (c) the scheme for the classification of child and adolescent disorders proposed by Rutter and his colleagues in 1969.

#### *a. The Start: ICD-7 and DSM-I*

The concept of SDD originates from clinical notions about disorders such as word blindness, word deafness and clumsiness. The first descriptions of developmental reading disorders, as opposed to acquired disorders, appeared at the end of the 19th century. In an overview of the early literature, Critchley (1970) shows that from the beginning it was stressed that developmental reading disorders implies an inability to learn to read despite normal intelligence. Hinshelwood (1917) used the term 'congenital word-blindness' to refer to cases of pure reading disabilities, as opposed to 'congenital dyslexia', which implies mildly backward reading in relatively dull children, and 'congenital alexia', referring to inability to read due to mental retardation. In the literature the term congenital word-blindness has been replaced by the concept of dyslexia or specific developmental reading disorder, while other types of poor reading are often referred to as the 'garden variety' of poor reading (Gough & Tunmer, 1986).

'Dysphasia' or 'word deafness' is another term that originates from clinical practice (McCall, 1911). It was used to express the belief of clinicians that language disorders in children with no apparent sensory disorders and a normal family background should be distinguished from other types of language delays such as acquired loss of language.

In these early notions of deviations in motor development, language and academic skills, no attention was paid to possible interrelations between these disorders. In other words, they were considered as separate conditions. Hence, the classification schemes that were developed during the fifties usually included these developmental deviations in broad sections, together with disorders

TABLE 1

DSM-I (1952) and ICD-7 (1957)

| DSM-I | ICD-7 |
|---|---|
| Special Symptom Reaction | Other and unspecified character, behaviour and intelligence disorders |
| Learning disturbance | Specific learning defects |
| Speech disturbance | Stammering and stuttering |
| Enuresis | Other speech impediments |
| Somnambulism | Acute situational maladjustment |
| Other | Other and unspecified |

of a quite different nature. Table 1 demonstrates that in DSM-I (APA, 1952) the main category 'Special Symptom Reaction' contained four disorders. Two of those, namely Learning disturbances and Speech disturbances are forerunners of later categories of SDD, but in DSM-I no mention is made of an interrelation between the two. The concept of SDD is not used.

ICD-7 (WHO, 1957) offered a very broad category for developmental disorders, titled 'Other and unspecified character, behaviour, and intelligence disorders'. Three categories for learning and speech disturbances were included, but again with no mention of possible interrelations. In both schemes, no further reference was made regarding the specific nature of these disorders.

### *b. DSM-II and the GAP-scheme*

The second edition of DSM-II (APA, 1968), like the first, provided categories for learning and speech disturbance (stuttering) in a special symptoms section. The number of categories for specific developmental disorders remained unchanged, and again no mention was made of the higher order concept of SDD. However, as Table 2 shows, the number of disorders in the domain of 'Special Symptoms' increased, since tics, disorders of sleep and feeding, encopresis and cephalalgia were included also.

TABLE 2

GAP (1966) and DSM-II (1968)

| GAP | DSM-II |
|---|---|
| Developmental Deviations | Special Symptoms |
| In Maturational Patterns | Speech disturbance (stuttering) |
| | Specific learning disturbance |
| In specific dimensions | Tic |
| Motor | Disorders of sleep |
| Sensory | Feeding disturbance |
| Speech | Enuresis |
| Cognitive | Encopresis |
| Social | Cephalalgia |
| Psychosocial | |
| Affective | |
| Integrative | |
| Other developmental deviation | |

Two years before the appearance of DSM-II, another definition of the concept of SDD had been developed. The Group for the Advancement of Psychiatry (GAP, 1966) proposed a classification scheme which described developmental deviations more or less as a conceptual unity. The disorders were defined as deviations in personality development that occur at a time, in a sequence, or degree not expected for a given age level or stage of development. Biological factors were seen as important contributors to these disorders. Three main categories were mentioned: (a) deviations in maturational patterns, which included the broader retardations in maturational steps; (b) deviations in specific dimensions of development; and (c) other. The concept of the 'developmental deviations in specific dimensions' may be considered as a direct forerunner of the concept of SDD, used as a higher order concept that covers disorders in various developmental domains. The domain of this category was much broader than it is today. It was used to cover a wide range of disorders, including various aspects of development, such as motor development (e.g. hyperactivity, coordination, handedness), sensory development (e.g. overreactiveness to stimuli), speech (articulation, rhythm, phonation, comprehension), cognitive aspects of development (reading, writing, arithmetic), social development (e.g. separation capacity, control of aggression), psychosexual development (e.g. appearance of sexual curiosity), affective dimensions of development (e.g. emotional lability given developmental level) and integrative functions (e.g. impulse control, frustration tolerance).

### *c. The Work of Rutter et al. (1969)*

The generic concept of 'Specific developmental disorders' was used for the first time in the scheme proposed by an international committee on the classification of child and adolescent disorders of the World Health Organization (Rutter et al., 1969). The committee described specific developmental disorders as "related to biological maturation", "generally much commoner in boys", and "not secondary to any other psychiatric syndrome" (Rutter et al., 1969, p. 48). Although this description can be interpreted as another step towards explaining the specific character of SDD, the term still covered a heterogeneous group of disorders, including the hyperkinetic syndrome, enuresis, encopresis, tics, and stuttering (see also Table 3).

TABLE 3

Part of the scheme proposed by Rutter et al., (1969)

| |
|---|
| Specific Developmental disorders |
| The hyperkinetic disorder |
| Speech and language disorder |
| Specific learning disorder |
| Abnormal clumsiness |
| Enuresis |
| Encopresis |
| Tics |
| Stuttering |

## *Second Phase: Narrowing the Concept*

The second phase in the development of the concept of SDD and its role in classification consisted of a narrowing of the concept. In this phase the notion of SDD was used to denote disorders in a relatively limited domain of developmental issues. A number of schemes were introduced, in which SDD was presented as a unifying concept. We will discuss four schemes that were developed during this period.

### *a. The Isle of Wight Studies and the Proposal by Rutter, Shaffer, and Shepherd*

An important impetus for the further development of the concept of SDD came from the epidemiological studies conducted by Rutter and his colleagues in the sixties, known as 'the Isle of Wight Studies'. Rutter and Yule (1973, 1975) divided reading difficulties into two categories. The term 'reading backwardness' was used for children whose reading was behind the average achievement for that age. The term 'specific reading retardation' denoted a specific disability in reading. The term 'specific' implied that the reading difficulties were not explicable in terms of the child's general intelligence. A comparison of groups of retarded readers with groups of backward readers yielded empirical evidence to support the validity of the distinction.

The influence of these new ideas can be recognized in a new proposal for the classification of specific developmental disorders, presented by Rutter, Shaffer, and Shepherd in 1975. They suggested adding to the description of SDD that "... the disorders with developmental delay have a conceptual unity and also there is substantial empirical evidence linking them as a group and separating them from other conditions", that "a delay in one skill is often associated with lesser delays in other skills", and that "there is a characteristic and similar age trend in all disorders (improvement with increasing age)" (Rutter et al., 1975, p. 58). Here, the notion of SDD is applied for the first time as a higher order concept, uniting various disorders. They suggested that enuresis, encopresis, stuttering, tics, and hyperkinesis should be excluded from the category of specific developmental disorders. In other words, the concept of SDD is applied here to a limited number of developmental disorders. The result is shown in Table 4.

TABLE 4

The categories in Rutter et al. (1975), MAS and ICD-9 (1978)

| |
|---|
| Specific delays in development |
| Specific reading retardation |
| Specific arithmetical retardation |
| Other specific learning difficulties |
| Developmental speech or language disorder |
| Specific motor retardation |
| Mixed developmental disorder |
| Other |

### *b. ICD-9 and MAS*

The proposal by Rutter, Shaffer, and Shepherd was adopted by the World Health Organization and was included in the next version of the ICD, namely the ICD-9. In the MAS, the multi-axial version of their scheme (Rutter, Shaffer, & Sturge, 1979), the categories for specific delays in development were placed on a separate axis. The glossary (Rutter et al., 1979, p. 4) stated that "codings on this axis are descriptive and not aetiological", and that a coding should be made without regarding its nature or causation. Furthermore, the glossary specified that " ... a child who shows the syndrome of infantile autism associated with serious language impairment should have the former coded on the first axis (i.e. Clinical psychiatric syndrome - JR/TvY) and the latter coded on this axis. However, to be coded there must be a *specific* delay in some aspect of development, so that a mentally retarded child with a general delay should receive a coding of '0' (no specific delay)" (Rutter et al., 1979, p. 4). Included were developmental areas that were assumed to be related to biological maturation. However, non-biological influences were assumed to be present also. Excluded were disorders explicable in terms of a general intellectual retardation, a neurological disorder, or - in the case of disorders of scholastic skills - exclusively due to poor schooling.

### *c. DSM-III*

DSM-III (APA, 1980) followed more or less the same course as ICD-9, but also showed some differences. In the glossary, developmental disorders were defined as one of the five classes of disorders in a large section called 'Disorders usually first evident in infancy, childhood, or adolescence'. These classes were (APA, 1980, pp. 35-36): I. Intellectual disorder (mental retardation); II. Behavioural disorder (attention deficit disorder, conduct disorder); III. Emotional disorder (anxiety disorders of childhood and adolescence, other disorders); IV. Physical disorder (eating disorders, stereotyped movement disorders, other disorders with physical manifestations - including enuresis and encopresis); and V. Developmental disorder (pervasive developmental and specific developmental disorders). Thus, although the scheme used the concept of SDD, it suggested that on a higher level of abstraction specific developmental disorders are related to the pervasive developmental disorders, since both belong to a higher-order category of developmental disorders. However, this relation was not expressed in the way the various categories were located in the system. The section for developmental disorders was divided over two Axes. Pervasive developmental disorders were placed on Axis I (Clinical syndromes), while the specific developmental disorders were placed on Axis II, together with the personality disorders. Table 5 lists the categories for specific developmental disorder that were included on Axis II. The glossary did not offer any further explanation of the nature of the higher order unity of the developmental disorders or the reasons for spreading the categories over two Axes.

TABLE 5

| DSM-III (1980) |
|---|
| Specific Developmental Disorders |
| Developmental Reading Disorder |
| Developmental Arithmetic Disorder |
| Developmental Language Disorder |
| Developmental Articulation Disorder |

A second difference with the ICD-9 was that the DSM-III approach was more restrictive in defining the domain of specific developmental disorders and more detailed in its description of diagnostic criteria. The glossary opened with the statement: "This subclass is for disorders of specific areas of development not due to another disorder" (APA, 1980, p.92). The section included reading, arithmetic, language and articulation disorders. No separate category was defined for motor disorders. Diagnostic criteria for the disorders in reading and arithmetic stated that performance on standardized, individually administered tests of reading skill or arithmetic achievement should be significantly below the expected level, given the individual's schooling, chronological age, and mental age (as determined by an individually administered IQ test). In addition, the child's performance on tasks requiring reading or arithmetic skills had to be significantly below his or her intellectual capacity, according to the concept of specific reading retardation or underachievement developed in the sixties and seventies.

Language disorders were divided into an expressive and a receptive type. Here, the diagnostic criteria stated that there should be a failure to develop language skills, that is not due to mental retardation, a pervasive developmental disorder, a hearing impairment, or trauma.

The categories of specific developmental disorders in DSM-III did not represent a broad consensus on the classification of impairments in scholastic skills, language/speech development, and motor coordination. On the contrary, during the preparation of DSM-III, serious problems regarding the operationalization and the validity of the concept of SDD were discussed in the literature. Especially the question of how to measure and interpret underachievement - based on the notion that a *specific* disorder may be defined as a developmental delay that cannot be explained in terms of the child's IQ - led to an enormous controversy (Rutter, 1978; Reynolds, 1981). Various authors argued that the concept of specific developmental disorders introduces measurement problems that cannot be solved (Epps, Ysseldyke, & Algozzine, 1983; Stevenson & Richman, 1976; Van Dellen, 1986; Willson & Reynolds, 1984). Moreover, several investigations (Rodgers, 1983; Silva, McGee, & Williams, 1985; Van der Wissel & Zegers, 1985) failed to replicate the findings of the epidemiological studies from which the concept originated. As a consequence, doubt arose about the validity of the concept of SDD. The sense and nonsense of the concept of SDD as a nomological entity became a heavily debated issue, with specific reading retardation at the focus of the discussion. These discussions continue to date (Shaw, Cullen, McGuire, & Brinckerhoff, 1995).

### *d. DSM-III-R and ICD-10*

The debate about the scientific status of the concept of SDD did not affect the revision of DSM-III (APA, 1987). On the contrary, in

DSM-III-R the concept was elaborated and refined. Specific developmental disorders were (again) placed within a higher order section for Developmental disorders. Table 6 gives an overview of the categories included. The glossary now explained that this section comprised impairments that usually first become evident in infancy, childhood, or adolescence, in which "(...) the predominant disturbance is in the acquisition of cognitive, language, motor, or social skills." The course was described as being "chronic", while "in many mild cases, adaption or full recovery may occur." (APA, 1987, p.28). Included in this section of Developmental disorders were specific developmental disorders, as well as mental retardation and pervasive developmental disorders. All these disorders were placed on Axis II of the scheme (together with personality disorders). The subclass of specific developmental disorders now included the developmental motor coordination disorder. The criteria for each category were adapted and followed the same pattern as in the categories for learning disorders. As a result, the notion that performance should be significantly below what could be expected, given the child's age and intellectual capacity, became part of the criteria of language and motor disorders also.

TABLE 6

DSM-III-R and ICD-10

| DSM-III-R (1987) | ICD-10 (1992) |
|---|---|
| Developmental Disorders | Disorders of psychological development |
| Mental retardation | SDD of speech and language |
| Pervasive Developmental Disorders | Specific speech articulation disorder |
| Specific Developmental Disorders | Expressive language disorder |
| Academic Skills Disorders | Receptive language disorder |
| Dev. Arithmetic Disorder | Acquired aphasia with epilepsy |
| Dev. Expressive Writing Disorder | Other developmental disorders of speech/language |
| Dev. Reading Disorder | Dev. disorders of speech/language, unspecified |
| Language and Speech Disorders | SDD of scholastic skills |
| Dev. Articulation Disorder | Specific reading disorder |
| Dev. Expressive Language Disorder | Specific spelling disorder |
| Dev. Receptive Language Disorder | Specific disorder of arithmetical skills |
| Motor Skills Disorder | Mixed disorder of scholastic skills |
| Dev. Coordination Disorder | Other developmental disorders of scholastic skills |
| Specific Developmental Disorder NOS | Dev. disorders of scholastic skills, unspecified |
| Other Developmental Disorders | SDD of motor function |
| Developmental Disorder NOS | Mixed specific developmental disorder |
| | Pervasive developmental disorders |
| | Other disorders of psychological development |
| | Unspecified disorder of psychological development |

The WHO, in their revision of the ICD, followed approximately the same course as the APA. In the newly published ICD-10 (WHO, 1992), the section Specific developmental disorders is likewise considered as a subclass of a higher-order concept. Together with the categories for Pervasive developmental disorders, this section comprises the cluster of the 'Psychological disorders' (see Table 6). The main ingredients for this higher order concept are: "(a) an onset that is invariably during infancy or childhood; (b) an impairment or delay in the development of functions that are strongly related to biological maturation of the central nervous system; and (c) a steady course that does not involve the remission and relapses that tend to be characteristic of many mental disorders." (WHO, 1992, p. 233). Furthermore, it is stated that the impairments tend to lessen with increasing age, there is a marked tendency for the disorders to be more common in males, and there is often a familial loading for similar or related disorders. The aetiology in most cases is held for unknown, but "there is presumptive evidence that genetic factors play an important role in the aetiology of many (but not all) cases." (WHO, 1992, p. 233).

Within this broad cluster of disorders, the classification criteria for specific developmental disorders are based on considerations regarding the severity of the disorder (more than two standard-deviations below average), course (a history of severe impairment), pattern (deviance and/or delay), and associated features (e.g. emotional or behavioural disorders). Meeting all of these four aspects, however, is not necessary for classification (e.g. Rutter, 1989a; 1989b). In the case of SDD, performance in a developmental domain should be clearly below the expected level, given the child's mental age. Also, poor performance should not be the consequence of mental retardation, and not directly attributable to a physical handicap or a specific diagnosable neurological condition (e.g. visual or auditory handicaps, abnormalities of the speech apparatus, cerebral palsy). Disorders in language development and scholastic skills should not be due to a pervasive developmental disorder, environmental deprivation, or inadequate schooling (e.g. Rutter, 1989a; WHO, 1992).

In DSM-III-R and ICD-10 the concept of SDD has become very complex. The categories have been placed in a conceptual hierarchy that at a higher level connects these disorders explicitly with pervasive developmental disorders and, in the case of the DSM-III-R, with mental retardation as well. This is in contrast with the schemes that were developed during the first phase, when different types of disorders were simply placed together without much clarification.

The framework in DSM-III-R and ICD-10 is sometimes weakened by inconsistencies. For example, acquired aphasia is included in the ICD-10 category of specific developmental language disorders (Schmidt, 1987). Nevertheless, categories are defined in an explicit theoretical framework, linking one type of disorder to another.

Another feature of this second phase in the development of the concept of SDD is that the diagnostic criteria have become very complicated. The attempt to formulate these criteria in a uniform pattern has led to a generalization of rules that were originally used to define specific reading disorder. It is far from clear to what extent these complicated criteria are applied in clinical practice.

### *Third Phase: Leaving the Idea of a Conceptual Unity*

The most recent scheme, DSM-IV (APA, 1994) reduces the complexity of the concept of SDD to a certain extent. The APA has abandoned the notion that specific developmental disorders are part of a higher order conceptual unity. Instead, the SDD categories have become part of the section 'Disorders Usually First Diagnosed in Infancy, Childhood, or Adolescence', under three separate headings: Learning disorders, Motor skills disorder and Communication Disorders. These three headings have not been combined, as in earlier versions, into a higher-order class 'specific developmental disorder', and no mention is made of relations between these disorders and mental retardation or pervasive developmental disorders. Interrelations between these three types of disorders may be derived from statements concerning differential diagnoses. Table 7 offers an overview of the new classification. The reasons for dropping the notion of SDD as a unifying concept are not explained in the glossary. Interestingly, the category of stuttering, usually not included in the section of developmental disorders, has become part of the section communication disorders, together with language and speech disorders, that are typically examples of developmental disorders. This may be another sign that DSM-IV has abandoned the idea that the general concept of SDD is a useful umbrella covering various development disturbances.

However, not much has changed in the diagnostic criteria of each of the learning, language and motor disorders. In other words, although the unifying concept is gone, the uniform structure of the

TABLE 7

| DSM-IV |
| --- |
| Learning disorders |
| Reading disorder |
| Mathematics disorder |
| Disorder of written expression |
| Learning disorder NOS |
| Motor skills disorder |
| Developmental coordination disorder |
| Communication disorders |
| Expressive language disorder |
| Mixed receptive-expressive disorder |
| Phonological disorder |
| Stuttering |
| Communication disorder NOS |

definition has been retained in almost all of the categories in this part of the scheme. Disorders are still defined in terms of a discrepancy between observed and expected level of performance. For example, in DSM-III-R (APA, 1987, p. 47) the first diagnostic criterion for Developmental Expressive Language Disorder is: "The score obtained from a standardized measure of expressive language is substantially below that obtained from a standardized measure of nonverbal intellectual capacity (as determined by an individually administered IQ test)". This criterion demonstrates that the notion of a discrepancy is the key feature in the classification of a specific developmental disorder. Furthermore, it illustrates the inadequacy of the operationalization of this concept into a clear diagnostic procedure, since the criterion does not state what is meant by 'substantially below'.

In DSM-IV (APA, 1994, p. 58) the concept of SDD is no longer used. The former category of 'Developmental Expressive Language Disorder' has been renamed 'Expressive Language Disorder'. However, the first diagnostic criterion has not changed dramatically: "The scores obtained from standardized individually administered measures of expressive language development are substantially below those of both nonverbal intellectual capacity and receptive language development. (....)". The concept of a discrepancy is still the core of the diagnostic criterion, and its operationalization has not been improved.

In other words, abandoning the concept of SDD has not resulted in a substantial change of diagnostic criteria. Therefore, also DSM-IV has not accounted for the criticism regarding the concept of SDD.

## THE PSYCHOMETRIC QUALITIES OF THE CATEGORIES OF SDD

Thus far, we discussed the content of the successive versions of classification schemes. Another way of looking at the history of the concept of SDD and its role in classification is to consider the psychometric properties of the categories of SDD in various versions of classification schemes. Traditionally, reliability and validity are important criteria for evaluating the quality of a classification system (Rutter & Gould, 1985). However, studies of the psychometric qualities of the categories of SDD have focused exclusively on interrater reliability. Very few validity studies have been conducted, mostly in the field of specific reading disorders. Another problem is that in many studies definitions of SDD have been used that were not in line with those of the official classification schemes. We will briefly review the studies on interrater reliability of the systems we described earlier.

The first study on the interrater reliability of the SDD categories is by Freeman (1971), who evaluated agreement between clinicians using the GAP scheme. The qualifications used to indicate the level of reliability were in terms of 'majority agreement' and 'minority agreement'. For the overall category 'Developmental deviation' a minority agreement was found. In a similar vein, Beitchman, Dielman, Landis, Benson, and Kemp (1978) assessed the reliability of the GAP-scheme. Again, the interrater reliability of the 'Developmental deviation' section was low: they found an intraclass correlation of .11.

The reliability of the MAS scheme has been studied by Klijn (1983). Results were expressed in terms of the overall agreement in the classification of the categories on Axis II of this scheme (Specific developmental disorders). Klijn found 80 percent agreement. Remschmidt, Schmidt, and Göbel (1983) and Remschmidt (1988) studied the reliability of the MAS in two conditions, namely with and without the use of the glossary. In their study expert child psychiatrists diagnosed 28 written case summaries. Again, results were expressed in terms of overall agreement. An average of 81% was found in the condition without the glossary, and 75% when the glossary was used. In a Dutch study on the classification of specific developmental disorders, Van Yperen (1990) reanalysed the Remschmidt et al. data, and computed kappa's for each Axis II category separately. Table 8 shows that the kappa's varied. In the condition without the glossary, moderate to substantial reliability was found. In the condition with the glossary reliability was merely fair. In another study, Skovgaard, Isager and Jorgensen (1988) found an overall interrater agreement of 70 percent.

Several studies report data about the reliability of the DSM-III categories for specific developmental disorders, but data on the particular categories are scarce. Russell, Cantwell, Mattison and Will (1979) found an overall reliability of 80% for the Axis II categories of SDD. A re-analysis, excluding cases classified as 'no disorder', resulted in an overall interrater agreement of 78%.

TABLE 8

Reliability categories Axis II of the MAS:
A re-analysis of the Remschmidt et al. data[a]

| Category | without glossary | | | with glossary | | |
|---|---|---|---|---|---|---|
| | n | p | k | n | p | k |
| No specific delay | 25 | .65 | .64 | 27 | .66 | .49 |
| Specific reading retardation | 8 | .15 | .66 | 10 | .12 | .41 |
| Specific arithmetical retardation | 0 | . | . | 0 | . | . |
| Other specific learning difficulties | 7 | .03 | .00 | 4 | .02 | .02 |
| Dev. speech/language disorder | 4 | .02 | .05 | 6 | .06 | .26 |
| Specific motor retardation | 2 | .01 | .06 | 1 | .01 | .09 |
| Mixed developmental disorder | 9 | .15 | .57 | 10 | .13 | .32 |

**Legend**

[a] Computations based on raw data presented by Remschmidt et al., 1983, p. 66;
n = Number of cases with category coded by at least one rater;
p = Overall proportion of ratings in a category (total N of ratings = 294);
k = Kappa after Fleiss & Cuzick (1979)

Studies of the reliability of the section of SDD of two DSM-III drafts (APA, 1980) yielded an overall kappa of .77 for the first, and of .51 for the second draft. Mezzich, Mezzich and Coffman (1985), using the 1978 pre-final draft, found a kappa of .27 for the category of specific reading disorder. Rey, Plapp and Stewart (1989) found a kappa of .76 for the Axis II section of specific developmental disorders.

Few reliability studies have been conducted regarding the SDD section of ICD-10. Koot (1993) reports a kappa of .37 for the overall category of SDD. Regier, Kaelber, Roper, Rae, and Sartorius (1994) showed that reliability was fair for the ICD section that includes SDD and pervasive developmental disorders (F8). They do not report separate data for the overall category of SDD and its subcategories. To our knowledge, no data are available about the reliability of the three DSM-IV categories of developmental disorders.

In all, our brief review shows that, although the history of the classification of SDD goes back for more than two decades, psychometric data on the categories of SDD are very scarce. There are only a few validity studies that used conceptualisations and definitions of SDD that correspond with the official classification schemes (Rispens, this volume). Although research on the interrater reliability is more common, we rarely find results that pertain to specific categories. Nearly all studies concentrate on the overall concept of SDD. It remains unclear whether this overall picture gives a fair impression of the reliability of the subcategories of SDD. Moreover, over the years the content of the section of SDD has varied considerably. Data about the most recent schemes are even more scarce, and the interrater reliability of the current sections of SDD cannot be derived from the older data. Hence, we must conclude that despite a history of more than twenty years, the psychometric qualities of the categories of SDD included in various classification schemes are still virtually unknown.

## CONCLUSION

In this section we discussed the history and the role of the concept of SDD in classification. The concept of SDD was first used as a generic term that denoted delays in a broad variety of areas of development. Later, disorders such as hyperactivity, enuresis, and tics were excluded from the category in a process of further refinement of the content of the concept of SDD. SDD was used as a higher-order concept, uniting impairments in the domains of language, scholastic skills and motor coordination. 'Specific' implied that the disorder could not be explained by the child's IQ, a physical handicap or other disorders. On a higher conceptual level, the impairment was assumed to be related to other types of disorders, such as mental retardation or pervasive developmental disorder, because they all shared the notion of development.

Successive versions of classification systems such as ICD and DSM have incorporated various categories and subcategories of SDD. The number of subcategories has increased considerably, especially in the domains of scholastic skills and language development. An interesting new development in DSM-IV is that the unifying concept of SDD is no longer mentioned. However, various categories of developmental disorders, subsumed under the heading SDD in earlier versions, are still included in the system and diagnostic criteria have not been changed substantially.

Our historical review does not suggest that there was a gradual clarification, both theoretically and empirically, of the notion of SDD over the years. Rather, it seems as if the idea of specificity has been elaborated unsystematically. Hence, successive versions of DSM and ICD do not represent more sophisticated interpretations of the notion of SDD.

Another conclusion is that the subsequent versions of the ICD and DSM do not reflect the fact that the SDD concept is beset with controversies. In each version the concept and each of the categories were elaborated and refined, despite the well-known problems with the operationalization of the diagnostic criteria and the lack of data about the validity of the concept. Reliability studies report satisfactory interrater agreement at the overall level, but data are still scarce and incomplete. In the few studies that report data on subcategories, reliability is only modest. A serious drawback is that investigations that evaluate specific subcategories are extremely rare. Therefore, we conclude that to date we have gained only very limited insight in the value of the categories of specific developmental disorders.

## HOW ARE WE TO PROCEED WITH THE CONCEPT OF SPECIFIC DEVELOPMENTAL DISORDERS?

### *The State of the Art is Unsatisfactory*

The relevance of the concept of the specific developmental disorder as part of a classification system depends on its reliability, validity and clinical utility (Skinner, 1986; Rutter & Gould, 1985). However, the improvement of diagnostic categories should be part of a broader movement, that aims at critical analysis of both the classification model and each of its categories. Skinner (1986) provided a theoretical framework for such an evaluation. He suggests that the development of a classification system implies an ongoing process of theory formation, followed by internal and external validation. Both the classification model, and each of the categories, should be based on theories that are subjected to a process of empirical validation.

From this perspective several critical remarks must be made. First, based on our historical overview, we conclude that the various operationalizations of the concept of SDD in successive versions of classification systems fail an empirical test. Data about reliability are scarce and not very convincing. Moreover, most reliability data pertain to earlier versions of DSM and ICD. No data pertaining to the recent versions of both systems are available. The situation regarding external validation, which refers to studies about various aspects of validity, is even worse. Systematic studies, aiming at an evaluation of construct validity or the predictive validity of the categories of specific developmental disorders in ICD and DSM, have not been undertaken. Validity studies were virtually always conducted outside the context of the official schemes, mostly using different concepts and definitions. The outcomes of these investigations are of marginal relevance to the further development of classification schemes. Finally, the clinical utility of the section of SDD has not been investigated. In all, it is difficult to evaluate the degree to which the categories of SDD in DSM and ICD meet the criteria of adequate classification.

Second, there are several empirical problems that affect the clinical relevance of the concept of SDD negatively. Heterogeneity and coexistence are examples of those problems. There is sufficient evidence of a considerable heterogeneity within the various categories of SDD (Bishop, 1992; Henderson & Barnett, this volume). The same holds for coexistence of specific developmental disorders. For example, in cases of specific reading disorder a specific arithmetic disorder is also often present (Geary, 1994). Many children with a specific learning disorder also suffer from language problems (Catts, 1993). One possible answer to this problem might be the development of a subclassification within each of the categories. Although various subtypes have been proposed, no consensus has been reached and a generally accepted subclassification in the domains of disorders of scholastic skills and language disorders is not available.

In the previous section we already noted that both the WHO and the APA seem to ignore data that point to the controversial nature of the categories of specific developmental disorder. Despite this apparent lack of data, classifications are refined, new categories are added, or categories move to other classes, without empirical justification. However, it will be clear that in the end this is not a satisfactory answer to the many critical remarks that have been made during the last decade.

### *The Need for a Rigorous Conceptual and Empirical Test*

How are we to proceed with the concept of specific developmental disorder? One solution, implicitly proposed in DSM-IV, might be to simply abandon the overall concept and focus on a (limited) number of categories such as dyslexia or dysphasia. However, all categories are controversial to a certain extent. Hence, this procedure does not solve the problems that are inherent to the categories of SDD. Therefore, we propose an alternative approach that implies a rigorous conceptual and empirical test of the concept of SDD.

Firstly, the idea that somehow developmental delays of intellectually bright children from a normal environment differ from developmental arrests of dull children with a deprived background has an intuitive appeal. For that reason, the notion of the specific developmental disorder has become popular in clinical practice. A careful conceptual analysis of the concept is needed in order to clarify the core of this notion. What do we mean by the concept of SDD?

Secondly, the validity of the concept of specific developmental disorders must be put to a rigorous empirical test. The notion of a diagnostic residue, which implies that the observed level of development lags behind the expected level, given the child's abilities and aptitude, should be approached critically. We already mentioned a number of studies which yielded data that are not concordant with the Isle of Wight findings. In several of the following chapters the validity of this notion of discrepancy, which is at the heart of the concept of specific developmental disorders, is questioned in the light of recent empirical investigations.

Based on a detailed conceptual an empirical study, it might be possible to purify the various categories of developmental disorders. The next chapters are devoted to this idea.

## REFERENCES

Algozzine, B. & Ysseldyke, J. E. (1987). In defense of different numbers. *Remedial and Special Education, 8*, 53-56.

American Psychiatric Association. (1952). *Diagnostic and statistical manual of mental disorders*. Washington DC: American Psychiatric Association.

American Psychiatric Association. (1968). *Diagnostic and statistical manual of mental disorders* (2nd ed., Rev.). Washington DC: American Psychiatric Association.

American Psychiatric Association. (1980). *Diagnostic and statistical manual of mental disorders* (3rd ed.). Washington DC: American Psychiatric Association.

American Psychiatric Association. (1987). *Diagnostic and statistical manual of mental disorders* (3rd ed., Rev.). Washington DC: American Psychiatric Association.

American Psychiatric Association. (1994). *Diagnostic and statistical manual of mental disorders* (4th ed.). Washington DC: American Psychiatric Association.

Beitchman, J. H., Dielman, T. E., Landis, J. R., Benson, R. M., & Kemp, P. L. (1978). Reliability of the Group for Advancement of Psychiatry diagnostic categories in child psychiatry. *Archives of General Psychiatry, 35*, 1461-1466.

Beitchman, J. H., Inglis, A., & Schachter, D. (1992). Child psychiatry and early intervention: III. The developmental disorders. *Canadian Journal of Psychiatry, 37*, 240-244.

Bishop, D. V. M. (1992). The underlying nature of specific language impairment. *Journal of Child Psychology and Psychiatry, 33*, 3-66.

Catts, H. W. (1993). The relationship between speech-language impairments and reading disabilities. *Journal of Speech and Hearing Research, 36*, 948-958.

Critchley, M. (1970). *Developmental dyslexia*. London: Heinemann.

Epps, S., Ysseldyke, J. E., & Algozzine, B. (1983). Impact of different definitions of learning disabilities on the number of students identified. *Journal of Psycho--educational Assessment, 1*, 341-352.

Fletcher, J. M. (1992). The validity of distinguishing children with language and learning disabilities according to discrepancies with IQ: Introduction to the special series. *Journal of Learning Disabilities, 25*, 546-548.

Freeman, M. (1971). A reliability study of psychiatric diagnosis in childhood and adolescence. *Journal of Child Psychology and Psychiatry, 12*, 43-54.

Geary, D. C. (1994). *Children's mathematical development: Research and practical applications*. Washington DC: APA.

Gould, M. S., Shaffer, D., Rutter, M., & Sturge, C. (1988). UK/WHO Study of ICD-9. In M. Rutter, A. H. Tuma, & I. S. Lann (Eds.), *Assessment and diagnosis in child psychopathology* (pp. 37-66). London: David Fulton.

Gough, P. B. & Tunmer, W. E. (1986). Decoding, reading and reading disability. *Remedial and Special Education, 7*, 6-10.

Group for the Advancement of Psychiatry. (1966). *Psychopathological disorders in childhood: Theoretical considerations and a proposed classification* (Report No. 62). New York: Group for the Advancement of Psychiatry.

Hinshelwood, J. (1917). *Congenital word-blindness*. London: Lewis.

Klijn, W. J. L. (1983). *Het multi-axiale classificatie-systeem voor kinder- en jeugdpsychiatrische stoornissen*. Unpublished manuscript. Oegstgeest: Kinder-psychiatrisch Centrum Curium.

Koot, J. M. (1993). *Problem behaviour in Dutch preschoolers*. Doctoral dissertation, Erasmus Universiteit Rotterdam, Rotterdam.

McCall, E. (1911). Two cases of congenital aphasia in children. *British Medical Journal, 110*, 1407.

Mezzich, A. C., Mezzich, J. E., & Coffman, G. A. (1985). Reliability of DSM-III vs. DSM-II in child psychopathology. *Journal of the American Academy of Child Psychiatry, 24*, 273-280.

Morris, R. D. (1988). Classification of learning disabilities: Old problems and new approaches. *Journal of Consulting and Clinical Psychology, 56*, 789-794.

Regier, D. A., Kaelber, C. T., Roper, M. T., Rae, D. S., & Sartorius, N. (1994). The ICD-10 clinical field trial for mental and behavioural disorders: Results in Canada and the United States. *American Journal of Psychiatry, 151*, 1340-1350.

Remschmidt, H. (1988). German study of ICD-9. In M. Rutter, A. H. Tuma, & J. S. Lann (Eds.), *Assessment and diagnosis in child psychopathology* (pp. 66-83). London: David Fulton.

Remschmidt, H., Schmidt, M., & Göbel, D. (1983). Erprobungs- und Reliabilitätstudium zum multiaxialen Klassifikationsschema für psychiatrische Erkrankungen im Kindes- und Jugendalter. In H. Remschmidt & M. Schmidt (Hsgr.), *Multiaxiale Diagnostik in der Kinder- und Jugendpsychiatrie: Ergebnisse empirischer Untersuchungen* (pp. 43-75). Bern: Huber Verlag.

Rey, J. M., Plapp, J. M., & Stewart, G. W. (1989). Reliability of psychiatric diagnosis in referred adolescents. *Journal of Child Psychology and Psychiatry, 30*, 879-888.

Reynolds, C. R. (1981). The fallacy of "two years below grade level for age" as a diagnostic criterion for reading disorders. *Journal of School Psychology, 19*, 350-358.

Rispens, J., Van Yperen, T. A. & Van Duijn, G. A. (1991). The irrelevance of IQ to the definition of learning disabilities: Some empirical evidence. *Journal of Learning Disabilities, 24,* 434-438.

Rodgers, B. (1983). The identification and prevalence of specific reading retardation. *The British Journal of Educational Psychology, 53*, 369-373.

Russell, A. T., Cantwell, D. P., Mattison, R., & Will, L. (1979). A comparison of DSM-II and DSM-III in the diagnosis of childhood psychiatric disorders. *Archives of General Psychiatry, 36*, 1223-1226.

Rutter, M. (1978). Prevalence and types of dyslexia. In A. L. Benton & D. Pearl (Eds.), *Dyslexia: An appraisal of current knowledge* (pp. 3-28). New York: Oxford University Press.

Rutter, M. (1989a). Child psychiatric disorders in ICD-10. *Journal of Child Psychology and Psychiatry, 30*, 499-513.

Rutter, M. (1989b). Isle of Wight revisited: Twenty-five years of child psychiatric epidemiology. *Journal of the American Academy of Child and Adolescent Psychiatry, 28*, 633-653.

Rutter, M. & Gould, M. A. (1985). Classification. In M. Rutter & L. Hersov (Eds.), *Child and adolescent psychiatry: Modern approaches* (2nd ed.) (pp. 304-325). London: Blackwell.

Rutter, M., Lebovici, S., Eisenberg, L., Sneznevsky, A. V., Sadoun, R., Brooke, E., & Lin, T. (1969). A tri-axial classification of mental disorders in childhood. *Journal of Child Psychology and Psychiatry, 10*, 41-61.

Rutter, M., Shaffer, D., & Shepherd, M. (1975). *A multi-axial classification of child psychiatric disorders: An evaluation of a proposal.* Geneva: World Health Organization.

Rutter, M., Shaffer, D., & Sturge, C. (1979). *A guide to a multi-axial classification scheme for psychiatric disorders in childhood and adolescence* (3rd ed.). London: Department of Child and Adolescent Psychiatry, Institute of Psychiatry.

Rutter, M. & Yule, W. (1973). Specific reading retardation. In L. Mann & D. A. Sabatino (Eds.), *The first review of special education* (pp. 1-51). Philadelphia: JSE Press.

Rutter, M. & Yule, W. (1975). The concept of specific reading retardation. *Journal of Child Psychology and Psychiatry, 16*, 115-125.

Schmidt, M. H. (1987). Klassifikation kinder- und jugendpsychiatrischer Störungsbilder in der ICD-10: Zum Stand der Diskussion. *Zeitschrift für Kinder- und Jugendpsychiatrie, 15*, 208-223.

Shaw, S. F., Cullen, J. P., McGuire, J. M., & Brinckerhoff, L. C. (1995). Operationalizing a definition of learning disabilities. *Journal of Learning Disabilities, 28,* 586-597.

Siegel, L. S. (1989). IQ is irrelevant to the definition of learning disabilities. *Journal of Learning Disabilities, 22*, 469-478, 486.

Siegel, L. S. (1992). An evaluation of the discrepancy definition of dyslexia. *Journal of Learning Disabilities, 25*, 618-629.

Silva, P. A., McGee, R., & Williams, S. M. (1985). Some characteristics of 9-year-old boys with general reading backwardness or specific reading retardation. *Journal of Child Psychology and Psychiatry, 26*, 407-421.

Silva, P. A., Williams, S., & McGee, R. (1987). A longitudinal study of children with developmental language delay at age three: Later intelligence, reading and behaviour problems. *Developmental Medicine and Child Neurology, 29*, 630-640.

Skinner, H. A. (1986). Construct validation approach to psychiatric classification. In T. Millon & G. L. Klerman (Eds.), *Contemporary directions in psychopathology: Toward the DSM-IV* (pp. 307-330). New York: The Guilford Press.

Skovgard, A. M., Isager, T., & Jorgensen, O. S. (1988). The reliability of child psychiatric diagnosis: A comparison among Danish child psychiatrists of traditional diagnoses and a multi-axial diagnostic system. *Acta Psychiatrica Scandinavica, 77*, 469-476.

Stanovich, K. E. (1994). Does dyslexia exist? *Journal of Child Psychology and Psychiatry, 35*, 579-597.

Stanovich, K. E. & Siegel, L. S. (1994). Phenotypic performance profile of children with reading disabilities: A regression-based test of the phonological-core variable-difference model. *Journal of Educational Psychology, 86*, 24-53.

Stevenson, J. & Richman, N. (1976). The prevalence of language delay in a population of three-year-old children and its association with general retardation. *Developmental Medicine and Child Neurology, 18*, 431-441.

Van Dellen, T. (1986). *Response processing and movement organization in clumsy children: An experimental approach.* Ph.D. thesis, University of Groningen, Groningen.

Van der Wissel, A. & Zegers, F. E. (1985). Reading retardation revisited. *British Journal of Developmental Psychology, 3*, 3-19.

Van Yperen, T. A. (1990). *Multi-axiale classificatie van specifieke ontwikkelings-stoornissen: Een studie over as II van het MAC.* Doctoral thesis, Rijksuniversiteit Leiden, Leiden.

Willson, V. L. & Reynolds, C. R. (1984). Another look at evaluating aptitude- achievement discrepancies in the diagnosis of learning disabilities. *The Journal of Special Education, 18*, 477-487.

World Health Organization. (1957). *Manual of the international statistical classification of diseases: Injuries and causes of death* (Rev. ed.) Geneva: World Health Organization.

World Health Organization. (1978). *International classification of diseases* (9th rev.). Geneva: World Health Organization.

World Health Organization (1992). *The ICD-10 classification of mental and behavioural disorders: Clinical descriptions and diagnostic guidelines.* Geneva: World Health Organization.

WILLIAM YULE AND BARBARA MAUGHAN

# CRITERIA FOR RESEARCH AND CLINICAL PRACTICE: A CRITICAL DISCUSSION

## INTRODUCTION

Rispens and Van Yperen (this volume) have put a strong case for improving on current classificatory systems of Specific Developmental Disorders. Their historical overview illustrates how existing classificatory systems have developed largely from a medical perspective and how the details of the resultant systems have not always been informed by concepts from psychology and education. And yet, from whatever disciplinary perspective, there is a need to develop better classificatory systems. The need comes from a wish both to improve educational and clinical practice and to enhance research endeavours. This paper will, therefore, look at both research and clinical criteria for specific developmental disorders.

In some areas of psychology and education, "classification" is seen as an unnecessary and negative activity. It is often assumed that the effects of labelling a disorder are synonymous with labelling a child, and that both sets of effects are always harmful. Inappropriately used, there can of course be damaging consequences of labels, but the positive value of classifications must also be considered. The purposes of developing and employing a proper classificatory scheme are to improve the description of a particular problem so as to lead to better agreed definitions; through this, to lead to better scientific studies in that different researchers can be more certain they are studying the same phenomena; and, running in parallel with these research-oriented needs, to improve the clinical or educational management of the child's condition. As our knowledge of learning disabilities accrues, so classificatory systems will develop and change. The resulting systems have to meet the needs of both the practitioner and the researcher.

Rutter (1965), Rutter and Gould (1985) and Cantwell (1996) have argued the case for better systems of classification over the past thirty years. A good scheme must satisfy many criteria. Disorders must be objectively described and should, wherever possible, be operationally defined. In the field of learning disabilities with its tradition of



*J. Rispens et al. (eds.),*
*Perspectives on the Classification of Specific Developmental Disorders*, 39–57.

educational measurement, one might have thought that at least this criterion would have been easily met; in practice, however, the literature is replete with studies using differing measures and cut-offs, making comparisons between their findings exceedingly difficult. Any categorization of disorders should be just that - a classification of *disorders* and not of the people who present with them. The label is of the problem, not the person. The definitions should be clear enough that different research and clinical workers should be able to agree on their application, and issues of reliability and validity are paramount. So far as possible, the classification should carry implications about the course and natural history of the disorder, for its prognosis and, ultimately, for its aetiology.

There is agreement that for many disorders an aetiologically based system will be the eventual aim, but that until processes are better understood and pathognomonic indices are identified, one has to make do with a system based on phenomenology. As far as learning disabilities are concerned, the existence of measures of educational performance, as well as of some of the underlying processes assumed to affect educational attainment, should have made the development of objective definitions easier. However, when it comes to the classification of *specific* learning disabilities, a number of conceptual difficulties arise. As most of our own work has been concerned with reading disabilities, we will use examples from that field to raise more general issues.

Three basic distinctions have to be made in the differential diagnosis of low scholastic achievement (Rutter, 1974). First, there must be a differentiation according to the type of scholastic skill involved (reading, spelling, mathematics, writing). Secondly, failure to acquire educational skills must be differentiated from a later loss of those skills, or a later failure to make scholastic progress. Thirdly, most clinical and research studies have distinguished between children with specific difficulties in particular academic skills, discrepant from their general abilities, and those for whom poor reading, spelling or mathematical attainment forms part of a wider pattern of intellectual difficulties. Children have been taken as showing specific under-achievement if their performance is discrepant from expectations based on both age (or grade) and IQ. Such a concept of specific underachievement is central to current definitions of learning disabilities in both ICD-10 (World Health Organization [WHO], 1992) and DSM-IV (American Psychiatric Association [APA], 1994) diagnostic criteria. It is also, however, the issue that has generated most heated debate. Most concerns have centred on the appropriateness and utility of an IQ-discrepant definition, so we will begin by briefly examining these.

## THE USE OF IQ SCORES IN DEFINING SPECIFIC READING DISABILITIES

Over the years and even contemporaneously, some have questioned the appropriateness of using IQ as a benchmark for assessing reading problems, objecting to what they see as a "capacity" notion of IQ (Siegel, 1988, 1989), perpetuating the misunderstanding articulated by Burt in the 30s and 40s (Burt, 1937; Crane, 1959). IQ does not reflect capacity; many children read above the level predicted from their IQ (Rogers, 1983; Yule, Rutter, Berger & Thompson, 1974), and lower-ability children can sometimes maintain the same levels of progress in reading as their more able peers (Share, McGee & Silva, 1989). The use of a test of general intelligence to predict reading (or any other academic skill) is a convenient way of predicting the specific skills from the general, and carries no claims that IQ causes or constrains reading ability. The procedure is purely empirical, and stands or falls by its utility. The central question is whether underachievers form a distinct - and possibly qualitatively different - group from other poor readers.

Even when research workers and clinicians argue against the use of IQ scores to predict reading scores, they often use an arbitrary cut-off point on IQ tests to eliminate children from studies of learning disability. Here, the aim may be a rather different one, of excluding children whose academic problems are strongly associated with - and possibly attributable to - other conditions. It is well documented, for example, that the lower the IQ, especially below IQ 50, the greater the prevalence of physical and biological abnormalities found in children. It is also found that the lower the IQ, the greater the prevalence of psychiatric disorders. Given both these findings, it may seem reasonable to exclude from study children whose associated, comorbid disorders may account for or be strongly related to their learning disability. But how is the cut-off point to be determined? A cut-off point of IQ 70 will exclude 2.5% of children from studies; a cut-off point of IQ 90 - quite frequently applied in studies of reading disabilities - rules out 25% of children. Such seemingly sensible decisions greatly affect the subjects selected for study. From a research perspective, they render comparisons between studies difficult and sometimes impossible. Applied in educational and clinical practice, they also affect which children are eligible for additional help within school systems.

## IMPLICATIONS OF DIFFERING DEFINITIONS

Before getting into more technical matters, let us consider the research and practical consequences of the definitions used. Let us take a very old example, slightly adapted from Phillips (1961). The hypothetical problem posed is all too real: there are many more children with additional needs in reading than there are specialist services to meet those needs. Let us say that in one school, teachers have identified five children each of whom they consider would benefit from additional, individual, remedial tuition. The problem is, which child should get the additional help? Should it be Child A because s/he is the brightest or Child E because s/he has the least going for him/her?

TABLE 1

Measures of underachievement

| CHILD | IQ | RQ | DIFF. IQ-RQ | 100 x RQ / IQ | PAYNE JONES | PRED. RQ | PRED-OBS |
|---|---|---|---|---|---|---|---|
| A | 140 | 100 | 40 | 71 | 2.99 | 124 | 24 |
| B | 120 | 88 | 32 | 73 | 2.38 | 112 | 24 |
| C | 100 | 76 | 24 | 76 | 1.79 | 100 | 24 |
| D | 80 | 64 | 16 | 80 | 1.20 | 80 | 24 |
| E | 60 | 52 | 8 | 87 | 0.59 | 76 | 24 |

Predicted RQ = 40 + 0.6 x IQ (Adapted from C. Phillips, 1961)

Table 1 shows standard IQ and reading scores for each child, together with a number of different methods of assessing reading-IQ discrepancies. Comparing these figures highlights all sorts of value judgements and assumptions about who is most deserving. The various ways of comparing the scores indicate that Child A has the largest absolute discrepancy between ability and attainment, whereas the use of a regression (prediction) equation indicates that all five are equally deserving. The point to make here is that different definitions will identify different children, and may have significant consequences for those children's education. That alone is sufficient reason for clinicians and educators to be clear about the ways that different definitions work.

From a group, rather than an individual perspective, Figure 1 is familiar. It shows the simple scattergram of the relationship between IQ and reading scores. Assuming the usual correlation of about +0.6 between the two measures, then the line AOB reflects that correlation. If we are interested in stüdying or intervening with a group of poor readers, then we can ignore the variation on IQ and merely select some point on the vertical axis below the mean to identify poor readers. The choice point is purely arbitrary. In this example, a point 2 SD below the mean is selected so that all children lying below the line FDG are regarded as poor readers. Imposing an IQ cut-off, at say an IQ of 90, restricts the group considerably.

FIGURE 1

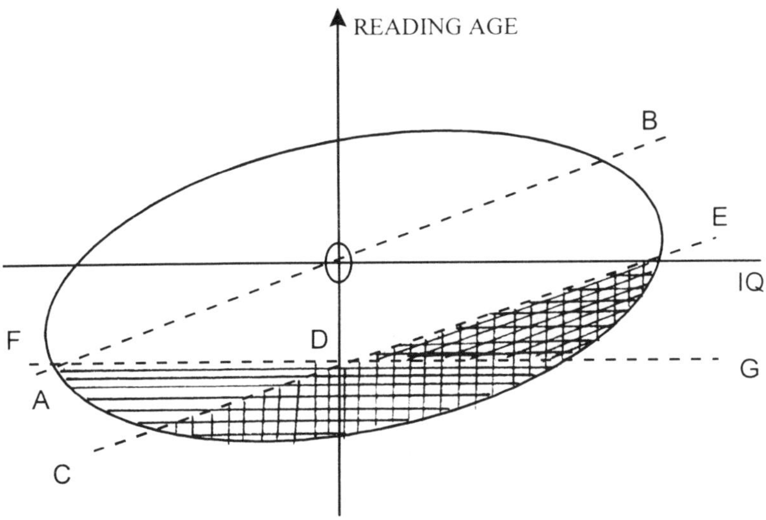


Retarded readers lie below line CDE
Backward readers lie below line FDG

A third strategy is to take a regression-based definition. The line CDE is the line below which children scoring more than two standard errors of prediction below their predicted level of reading are to be found. As Figure 1 demonstrates, there is considerable overlap between the children identified in all three ways. But equally important for the purposes of the present discussion, these different approaches to defining reading difficulties will identify different children. Unless there is a better level of agreement among researchers, and between researchers and clinicians, then studies of children with poor reading skills will continue to yield contradictory results for no other reason than that different types of problems are being studied.

## MEASURING UNDERACHIEVEMENT

If definitions of specific learning disabilities are to include the concept of underachievement, a series of more complex measurement issues arises. Underachievement is a matter of degree, and we need to ask what should be the expected level attainment for any child, and what constitutes achievement significantly below that level.

Clearly, these questions can only be posed in the context of particular educational systems and cultures. When reading was confined to monks in the monasteries, then not reading was the norm for the population. Without good, universal education, the distinctions made here are of limited relevance. But throughout this century in countries where there is a tradition of providing at least some elementary education for all children, then people have been aware of wide individual differences in the rate at which children learn to read. As soon as formal tests of attainment were developed, people have considered the difference between tested reading age and actual chronological age (or grade level). This difference (sometimes expressed as a ratio of RA:CA, which is mathematically equivalent) examines degrees of general backwardness in reading. But where is the cut-off point to be placed to identify those who are severely underfunctioning? Clearly being one year behind at age 7 years is much more serious than being one year behind at age 14 years (Applebee, 1971; Lyle & Goyen, 1969), so some authorities introduced arbitrary sliding scales.

Accomplishment quotients - the ratio of attainment age to mental age - were fashionable many years ago, and, despite serious criticisms on statistical grounds (Crane, 1959; Thorndike, 1963; Yule, 1979), reappear in recent literature (Erikson, 1975; Finucci, Isaacs, Whitehouse, & Childs, 1982). Since IQ and achievement are not perfectly correlated, it is inevitable that children who are well above average on one measure will be less superior on the second, and vice versa, assuming that the correlation is linear. Thus, indices such as achievement ratios or learning quotients will overestimate the number of highly intelligent children with specific reading difficulties.

The most appropriate way to avoid the distorting influence of the regression effect is to use some kind of regression (i.e., prediction) equation in which achievement is predicted on the basis of the observed correlations between educational attainment, age and IQ (Angoff, 1971; Thorndike, 1963). This approach has now been widely applied in reading research (Berger, Yule, & Rutter, 1975; Rutter, Tizard, & Whitmore, 1970; Share & Silva, 1986; Shaywitz, Escobar, Shaywitz, Fletcher, & Makuch, 1992; Yule, Gold, & Busch, 1981; Yule, Lansdown, & Urbanowicz, 1982). It enables both the calculation of the degree of the child's underachievement in reading and an estimate of the expected frequency of different degrees of underachievement.

The decision on what cut-off point to use for a clinically significant degree of specific reading retardation remains necessarily somewhat arbitrary, and any difference or discrepancy score is inherently unreliable, as it can inflate the errors of measurement making up each separate score. This is a very important methodological point. The only way to be sure that a discrepancy score reflects a true difference between the scores is to use a very extreme difference. Follow-up studies have demonstrated empirically that when one uses a cut-off point of at least two standard errors of prediction (not standard deviations as DSM-IV has it) then such identified children have a very persistent disability that constitutes a real handicap (Maughan, Gray, & Rutter, 1985; Rutter, Tizard, Yule, Graham, & Whitmore, 1976; Yule, 1973).

These differing approaches to assessment and identification are not merely theoretical niceties. As we have shown, they can have very real practical implications because different definitions identify different children. Many of the apparent disagreements in the research literature may stem from researchers unwittingly studying different types of reading difficulty as a result of applying different criteria. For example, a common problem is that of relaxing the stringency of the cut-off point in order to boost the numbers of children identified as poor readers. To achieve adequate power for statistical comparisons, it is understandable that researchers want to work with large enough groups of children in the hope they may identify true differences between their poor readers and their controls. When an extreme discrepancy score fails to yield large enough numbers, all too often they relax the cut-off point. Then they are surprised that they fail to replicate the findings of studies where a more extreme cut-off point was employed. What is being argued here is that by relaxing the cut-off point, they then include children whose identification is unreliable and so the additional error variance may mask true differences.

It is heartening to see that the Psychological Corporation, the publisher of the Wechsler intelligence scales, has now recognised the utility of the prediction approach to identifying children who are underachieving in reading. In introducing their new reading and spelling tests - The Wechsler Objective Reading Dimensions (Rust, Golombek, & Trickey, 1993) - they provide data whereby Wechsler IQ scores can be used to predict reading and spelling scores at different age levels. This will inevitably influence practitioners and make such data more readily available for future research. It is only to be hoped that those who use these methods have some appreciation of the methodological problems raised above.

## SOME EMPIRICAL FINDINGS

Notwithstanding the many controversies that surround the operationalizing of underachievement in reading, it has been reported in all countries where it has been studied (Aaron & Malatesha Joshi, 1987). Most estimates of the prevalence of severe underachievement in reading fall in the range 3 to 10%, despite variations in writing systems and educational organization (Stevenson et al., 1982). Specific reading problems may be less common in those languages such as Italian, which have much more regular orthographies than English (Lindgren, DeRenzi, & Richman, 1985).

The Isle of Wight studies of 30 years ago were among the first systematic, epidemiological studies to examine many of these issues (Berger et al., 1975; Rutter et al., 1970; Rutter & Yule, 1975). In five large samples, IQ-discrepant reading difficulties - Specific Reading Retardation (SRR) in the Isle of Wight terminology - were found to occur more frequently than would have been expected had poor readers simply formed the bottom of the normal curve on reading skills (Yule et al., 1974). Van der Wissel and Zegers (1985) argued that some of the excess of SRRs could have been due to floor and ceiling effects on group tests. Other population studies have reported similar bimodality in the distribution of underachievement in reading (Dobbins & Tafa, 1992; Stevenson, 1988), while yet others have not replicated the finding (Rodgers, 1983; Shaywitz et al., 1992). Different measures, different sampling and, above all, different and usually less stringent cut-off points in defining SRR can account for some of these differences in findings. What is required are true replication studies.

But the question of whether there is an excess or not does not in itself invalidate the concept of underachievement. If an excess exists, it adds to the value of the concept, but other tests of the utility of the concept are equally if not more important. Differentiable subgroups of reading difficulties should show different patterns of correlates; differences in prognosis; differences in response to intervention; and possibly differences in functional impairment in reading and related cognitive skills. Behavioural genetic studies should also be crucial in establishing whether there are meaningful ways of sub-classifying poor readers.

## *Correlates*

The original Isle of Wight studies of 9 to 10 year olds (Rutter & Yule, 1975) reported a series of differences between retarded readers and those showing reading problems as part of a more general pattern of low attainment (Generally Reading Backwardness, or GRB, in the Isle of Wight terminology): (1) children with SRR were much more likely to be boys (a ratio of 3 or 4 to 1) whereas the sex distribution of GRB was nearly equal; (2) overt neurological disorders were much more frequent in the GRB group; (3) children with GRB tended to have a wide range of developmental difficulties including motor and praxic abnormalities, whereas SRR was strongly associated only with speech and language impairment; and (4) more of the GRB children came from socially disadvantaged homes. These differences were largely replicated by Silva, McGee, and Williams (1985) in their New Zealand study. Few other studies have examined the same broad range of potential correlates.

Gender differences have been looked at in a number of other putative replication studies. Clinic based studies almost always report an excess of boys. Both Shaywitz, Shaywitz, Fletcher, and Escobar (1990) and Wadsworth, DeFries, Stevenson, Gilger, and Pennington (1992) report an excess of boys in referred groups, but found more balanced gender ratios among their research defined poor readers. Once again, proper comparisons are complicated by definitional differences, especially in terms of severity. It is possible that the excess of boys among underachievers is focused at the extremes of the distribution of underachievement. Cases of this level of severity will find their ways to clinics, but large general population samples may be needed to identify a significant number for study. Lowering the severity of the cut-off point will allow more girls into the samples and may disguise the gender difference.

Studies of differences between underachieving and generally poor readers in relation to other skills thought to be important in reading are only just being published, and, as yet, the findings are inconsistent (Stanovich, 1994). Elliott (1989) found that GRB and SRR children showed very different patterns of subscores on the British Ability Scales. Jorm, Share, Maclean, and Matthews (1986a) reported that SRR was associated with deficits in phonological processing, whereas Ellis and Large (1987) found relatively normal phonological skills but disabilities in visual processing. Fredman and Stevenson (1988) found significant differences between the two broad groups of poor readers in phonological, whole-word reading skills on both regular and irregular words, but the differences were no longer statistically significant when reading age and IQ were further controlled.

### *Follow-up studies*

Follow-up and treatment studies do not help much in that few studies using the underachievement versus "garden variety" of poor reading have been reported. The outcome of both SRR and GRB groups is poor (Yule, 1985). Despite their higher intelligence, the original group of SRR on the Isle of Wight made significantly *less* progress in reading and spelling between the ages of 10 and 14 years than the children with GRB. They did make more progress on mathematics. However, a parallel follow up-study of the more socially disadvantaged poor readers in an inner London borough failed to find significant differences in progress between backward and retarded readers (Maughan, Hagell, Rutter, & Yule, 1994). The meaning of the disorder may thus be somewhat different in different social and cultural contexts.

### *Genetic influences*

Plomin and Rende (1991) have described an exciting new technique designed to test how far extreme scores on a distribution reflect discrete disorders or the extremes of the normal range. The results in its first application to the study of reading disability are not conclusive (DeFries, Fulker, & LaBuda, 1987), but the findings are consistent with the existence of a distinct group of severe underachievers.

Plomin (1991) suggests that mild, common disorders may represent the extreme of normal continua, but that severe, rare problems may be aetiologically distinct. These differential patterns may reflect either greater genetic influences on severe conditions, as in the case of schizophrenia, or lesser genetic influences on severe conditions, as in severe mental retardation which appears less heritable than variations in the normal IQ range.

Genetic studies have also begun to examine which components of the reading process are most likely to be subject to genetic influence, concluding so far that there are markedly different patterns of heritability in phonological and orthographic skills (Olson, Wise, Conners, Rack, & Fulker, 1989; Olson, Rack, Conners, DeFries, & Fulker, 1991; Stevenson, 1991). Stevenson (1991) argues that there may be different genetic mechanisms, each contributing to different aspects of reading. One, reflecting general genetic effects shared with IQ, may contribute to orthographic skills, while a second, more modular and specific pathway, may provide links with phonological processing.

Other behavioural genetic studies will also help to identify sub-types of reading (and other learning) disabilities. In relation to reading, familial risk is known to be higher among parents of affected boys than of affected girls (Vogler, DeFries, & Decker, 1985). While most examples of poor reading seem best accounted for by heterogeneity, with polygenic inheritance in some families (Finucci, Guthrie, Childs, Abbey, & Childs, 1976), there are indications of single gene effects in some cases. Smith, Pennington, Kimberling, and Ing (1990) report evidence of an autosomal dominant form of reading disability, with linkage to chromosome 15, in some 15-20% of the families they studied.

The implication of all this genetic work is that in the very near future, some types of reading difficulties will have identifiable genotypes. It remains to be seen whether these will form meaningful large groups with distinct behavioural phenotypes, let alone whether these phenotypes will match on to the underachievement/low-end-of-continuum distinction. These, however, are among the types of test that need to be applied to refine classifications in the future.

### *Reading Difficulties and Psychiatric Problems*

Many learning disabled children show behaviour problems in the classroom (McKinney, 1989) which is not surprising, but they also show an excess of other more severe psychiatric problems. In particular, while backward readers show both emotional and conduct problems (Jorm, Share, Matthews, & Maclean, 1986b; Kellam, Brown, Rubin, & Ensminger, 1983; Richman, Stevenson, & Graham, 1982), children with SRR show a particular excess of conduct disorder, at least in the middle years of schooling (Rutter et al., 1970). In very recent years, there has been increased interest in this co-morbidity and it is now recognised that there may be developmental changes in the nature of the association over time.

Rutter et al. (1970) set out the three main broad hypotheses that might account for the reading-behaviour problem links. Firstly, the behaviour problems might be primary, and give rise to reading difficulties by interfering with a child's learning. Secondly, reading problems might be primary, and lead, through lowered self esteem or frustration, to the expression of behaviour disorder. Thirdly, both sets of difficulties might share common roots in organic, temperamental or environmental adversities. Some combination of these models, including reciprocal as well as unidirectional influences, may prove the most likely picture in practice.

Longitudinal studies have provided evidence on these issues. Studies beginning early in childhood show that both sets of problems, or precursors to them, are often evident by the time children start school, well before the time they are exposed to a formal curriculum (McMichael, 1979; McGee, Share, Moffitt, Williams, & Silva, 1988). These findings argue for a number of shared risk factors such as low social class (Offord & Poushinsky, 1981); maternal depression (Richman et al., 1982); speech and language deficits (Silva, 1987) and neurodevelopmental immaturity (Beitchman, 1985). Singly or in combination, such factors may be important for some groups of children.

If shared risk factors account for at least some of the links in early childhood, reciprocal effects may be important at later stages. Poor readers show increased behaviour problems across the primary school years (McGee et al., 1988), and it is likely that difficult behaviour in the classroom has an effect on progress in academic achievement (Fergusson & Horwood, 1992; Rowe & Rowe, 1992).

While the debate about how best to define reading problems has raged, so too have the debates about defining psychiatric problems. One effect has been a greater awareness of the effects of inattention and hyperactivity. Thus, more recent studies, while generally supporting the existence of a link between reading disorder and externalizing behaviours, also implicate inattentive, overactive behaviours in young children and the emergence of conduct problems rather later (Hinshaw, 1992). Thus, the pattern of relationship between reading disorder and psychiatric disorder may change across the years. In one of the Australian studies (Jorm et al., 1986a), it was found that GRBs had a history of inattentiveness and overactivity, whereas SRRs did not, suggesting two different pathways to the co-morbidity.

In adolescence, one can ask whether reading difficulties make it more likely that the earlier behaviour problems will persist, and whether they increase the vulnerability to the emergence of new disorders. The evidence on the first point seems clear. The Isle of Wight, inner London and Dunedin follow-up studies all found that reading problems play little if any role in the persistence of psychiatric disorders after middle childhood (McGee, Feehan, Williams, & Anderson, 1992; Maughan et al., 1985; Rutter et al., 1976). Findings are less clear with respect to the question of the link to new disorders. There was a trend towards higher rates of *juvenile* offending in both behaviourally deviant and nondeviant poor readers, suggesting some increased risk associated with reading problems in inner London (Maughan et al., 1985), but no such elevated rates in *adult* criminality have been found among previously poor readers (Maughan, Pickles, Hagell, Rutter, & Yule, 1996). This suggests that any increases in poor readers' delinquency in their teens may reflect relatively time-limited reactions or vulnerabilities, rather than ongoing deviant tendencies.

The picture in early adulthood is generally reasonably positive, both from clinic based follow-ups (Bruck, 1985) and population studies (Maughan et al., 1996). There was a tendency within the latter study for male poor readers to have an excess of social problems as opposed to psychiatric ones. But even these varied according to the circumstances in which the men found themselves. Many of the problems evident in the school years may be avoidable in adult environments that are supportive or present a limited range of challenges, and where the persisting reading difficulties are of less importance.

## SPELLING, WRITING AND ARITHMETIC

We began by saying that learning disabilities have to be differentiated according to the skills involved. All the methodological problems that have been examined in relation to reading apply equally to disabilities in spelling, handwriting, arithmetic and other mathematical skills, and to developmental problems such as clumsiness. These will be discussed elsewhere in this volume. For present purposes, we will comment on only a few salient issues in relation to these other skills.

In DSM-IV, problems in spelling, handwriting and grammatical expression are all classified together as features of Disorders of Written Expression. In ICD-10, difficulties in expressive writing do not appear in the main classifications of academic skills disorders, but can be recorded among other Disorders of Scholastic Skills. Spelling is closely correlated with reading but is not identical with it. Spelling problems can occur on their own and may have a different pattern of heritability.

However, much less is known reliably of the prevalence, antecedents, course, correlates or outcome of specific spelling disorders isolated from reading problems. We have summarized some recent developments elsewhere (Maughan & Yule, 1994).

Problems with number have been even less systematically studied. Here, it must be recognized that there is little agreement as to how to categorise different types of numerical and/or mathematical problems. Does one look only at a child's ability to perform the basic arithmetical operations (addition, subtraction, multiplication, division) or at performance on tests of higher order concepts such as algebra, geometry, trigonometry or calculus? There may be very different cognitive processes, subserved by different neuropsychological mechanisms, underlying these different functions. Some are predominantly verbal and some are spatial. It is not unknown for some children to perform well in basic arithmetic only to fail badly at mathematics.

It has long been claimed clinically that difficulties in calculation are related to anxiety in children (Lansdown, 1978). An interesting and important question is whether arithmetic difficulties are related to an increase in psychiatric problems and, if so, whether they are differentially related to neurotic, anxiety disorders as opposed to conduct disorders. This was examined in a series of studies by Rourke and Fuerst (1991) who concluded that children with good reading and spelling relative to their scores on arithmetic showed much more clinically significant psychopathology than did those who show poor reading and spelling relative to their arithmetic. The former group - in a sense those with specific deficits in arithmetic - showed much more anxiety and other internalized psychopathology. Unfortunately, in a preliminary secondary analysis of some of our own data sets, we have as yet been unable to replicate these findings (Pouretemad, Chadwick, & Yule, 1995).

## CLINICAL CRITERIA

At the lowest level, the clinical implications of all this work are that whenever a child presents at a specialist service for investigation, both psychological and educational factors must be considered along with medical and family influences. In other words, a holistic approach is needed and this requires an interdisciplinary approach. The exact way this will need to be organised will differ across different countries and educational systems. As more countries adopt national curriculums with supposedly standardised assessments at key stages in the child's educational career, it may be possible to rely on the results of such routine assessments. However, we suspect that they will never fully substitute for having children assessed individually.

Perhaps one should consider the results of school assessments as being systematic screening for major problems. Indeed, there are a number of instances of developing useful preschool screening instruments and certainly if society is serious about wanting to improve children's reading and spelling attainment, then more systematic screening by the age of 7 should be supported.

And this is one aspect of the whole definitions debate that too often receives too little consideration. We have been at pains to point out that definitions matter. They matter in the sense of who is identified. And this carries resource implications. In the UK and the USA there are instances where apparently well intentioned legislation that aimed at improving input to children with special educational needs gets totally undermined when local education authorities determine at a local level where cut-off points are to be placed. As noted, DSM and ICD both are moving towards an acceptance of a discrepancy model for defining poor reading. This is quite legitimate for some purposes, but it is not meant to deny that children with severe problems in attainment (i.e. severe GRBs) do not also need extra help at school. It would be scandalous were education authorities to use the ICD and DSM classifications to regulate access to additional resources for such children.

The argument has also been put forward by researchers and educationalists that bright children who have specific reading or spelling difficulties, and yet may be reading at chronological age level, should not be considered as having any reading problem. This argument fails to address the emotional responses of such children to their handicapping condition. It may be that in fully comprehensive schooling where children of all levels of attainment are educated together, then the performance of bright underachievers does not stand out. But in systems of selective secondary education, such children may not have access to advanced levels of instruction, thereby exacerbating their frustrations. Taken holistically, such children are socially handicapped by their specific learning disabilities.

As experimental, cognitive studies of children with specific learning difficulties continue and as research workers and educators and clinicians pool their observations more closely, then we will see an increase in the number of specific procedures that will aim to identify strengths and weaknesses that are causally relevant to educational attainment. In turn, these measures may provide new criteria by which to identify children with specific learning disabilities. In the meantime, there is a great deal of hard work needed to test out the existing hypotheses in relation to reading disorders and extend these into the study of other learning disabilities.

## REFERENCES


Aaron P. & Malatesha Joshi R. (1987). *Reading and writing disorders in different orthographic systems.* Dordrecht: Kluwer.

American Psychiatric Association. (1994). *Diagnostic and statistical manual of mental disorders* (4th ed.). Washington, DC: American Psychiatric Association.

Angoff, W. H. (1971). Scales, norms and equivalent scores. In R. L. Thorndike (Ed.), *Educational measurement* (2nd ed.). Washington, DC: American Council on Education.

Applebee, A. N. (1971). Research in reading retardation: Two critical problems. *Journal of Child Psychology and Psychiatry, 12*, 91-113.

Beitchman, J. H. (1985). Speech and language impairment and psychiatric risk: Toward a model of neurodevelopmental immaturity. *Psychiatric Clinics of North America, 8*, 721-735.

Berger, M., Yule, W., & Rutter, M. (1975). Attainment and adjustment in two geographical areas II: The prevalence of specific reading retardation. *British Journal of Psychiatry, 126*, 510-519.

Bruck, M. (1985). The adult functioning of children with specific learning disability: A follow-up study. In I. Sigel (Ed.), *Advances in applied developmental psychology* (pp. 91-129). Norwood, NJ: Ablex.

Burt, C. (1937). *The backward child* (3rd ed., 1950). London: University of London Press.

Cantwell, D. P. (1996). Classification of child and adolescent psychopathology. *Journal of Child Psychology and Psychiatry, 37*, 3-12.

Crane, A. R. (1959). An historical and critical account of the accomplishment quotient idea. *British Journal of Educational Psychology, 29*, 252-259.

DeFries, J. C., Fulker, D. W., & LaBuda, M. C. (1987). Evidence for a genetic aetiology in reading disability of twins. *Nature, 329*, 537-539.

Dobbins, D. A. & Tafa, E. (1992). The 'stability' of identification of underachieving readers over different measures of intelligence and reading. *British Journal of Educational Psychology, 61*, 155-163.

Elliott, C. D. (1989). Cognitive profiles of learning disabled children. *British Journal of Developmental Psychology, 7*, 171-178.

Ellis, N. C. & Large, B. (1987). The development of reading: As you seek so shall you find. *British Journal of Psychology, 78*, 1-28.

Erickson, M. T. (1975). The Z-score discrepancy method for identifying reading-disabled children. *Journal of Learning Disabilities, 8*, 308-312.

Fergusson, D. M. & Horwood, L. J. (1992). Attention deficit and reading achievement. *Journal of Child Psychology and Psychiatry, 33*, 375-385.

Finucci, J. M., Guthrie, J. T., Childs, A. C., Abbey, H., & Childs, B. (1976). The genetics of specific reading disability. *Annals of Human Genetics, 40*, 1-23.

Finucci, J. M., Isaacs, S. D., Whitehouse, C. C., & Childs, B. (1982). A quantitative index of reading disability for use in family studies. *Developmental Medicine and Child Neurology 24*, 733-744.

Fredman, G. & Stevenson, J. (1988). Reading processes in specific reading retarded and reading backward 13 year olds. *British Journal of Developmental Psychology, 6*, 67-108.

Hinshaw, S. P. (1992). Externalizing behaviour problems and academic underachievement in childhood and adolescence: Causal relationships and underlying mechanisms. *Psychological Bulletin, 111*, 127-155.

Jorm, A., Share, D., Maclean, R., & Matthews, R. (1986a). Cognitive factors at school entry predictive of specific reading retardation and general reading backwardness: A research note. *Journal of Child Psychology and Psychiatry, 27*, 45-54.

Jorm, A. F., Share, D. L., Matthews, R., & Maclean, R. (1986b). Behaviour problems in specific reading retarded and general reading backward children: A longitudinal study. *Journal of Child Psychology and Psychiatry, 27*, 33-43.

Kellam, S. G., Brown, C. H., Rubin, B. R., & Ensminger, M. E. (1983). Paths leading to teenage psychiatric symptoms and substance use: Developmental epidemiological studies in Woodlawn. In S. B. Guze, F. J. Earls, & J. E. Barratt (Eds), *Childhood psychopathology and development* (pp. 17-51). New York: Raven Press.

Lansdown, R. (1978). Retardation in mathematics: A consideration of multifactorial determination. *Journal of Child Psychology and Psychiatry, 19*, 181-185.

Lindgren, S. D., DeRenzi, E., & Richman, L. C. (1985). Cross-national comparisons of developmental dyslexia in Italy and the United States. *Child Development, 56*, 1404-1417.

Lyle, J. C. & Goyen, J. (1969). Performance of retarded readers on the WISC and educational tests. *Journal of Abnormal Psychology, 74*, 105-112.

Maughan, B., Gray, G., & Rutter, M. (1985). Reading retardation and antisocial behaviour: A follow-up into employment. *Journal of Child Psychology and Psychiatry, 26*, 741-758.

Maughan, B., Hagell, A., Rutter, M., & Yule, W. (1994). Poor readers in secondary school. *Reading and Writing: An Interdisciplinary Journal, 6*, 125-150.

Maughan, B., Pickles, A., Hagell, A., Rutter, M. & Yule, W. (1996). Reading problems and antisocial behaviour: Developmental trends in comorbidity. *Journal of Child Psychology and Psychiatry, 37*, 405-418.

Maughan, B. & Yule, W. (1994). Reading and other learning disabilities. In M. Rutter, E. Taylor, & L. Hersov (Eds.), *Child and adolescent psychiatry: Modern approaches* (3rd ed., pp. 647-665). Oxford: Blackwell.

McGee, R., Feehan, M., Williams, S., & Anderson, J. (1992). DSM-III disorders from age 11 to age 15 years. *Journal of the American Academy of Child and Adolescent Psychiatry, 31*, 50- 59.

McGee, R., Share, D., Moffitt, T. E., Williams, S., & Silva, P. A. (1988). Reading disability, behaviour problems and juvenile delinquency. In D. H. Saklofske & S. B. G. Eysenck (Eds.), *Individual differences in children and adolescents: International perspectives* (pp. 158-172). London: Hodder and Stoughton.

McKinney, J. D. (1989). Longitudinal research on the behavioural characteristics of children with learning disabilities. *Journal of Learning Disabilities, 22*, 141-150.

McMichael, P. (1979). The hen or the egg? Which came first -- antisocial emotional disorder or reading disability? *British Journal of Educational Psychology, 49*, 226-235.

Offord, D. R. & Poushinsky, M. F. (1981). School performance IQ and female delinquency. *International Journal of Social Psychiatry, 21*, 267-283.

Olson, R. K., Rack, J. P., Conners, F. A., DeFries, J. C., & Fulker, D. W. (1991). Genetic etiology of individual differences in reading disability. In L. V. Feagans, E. J. Short & L. J. Meltzer (Eds.), *Subtypes of Learning Disabilities* (pp. 113-135). Hillsdale, NJ: Lawrence Erlbaum.

Olson, R. K., Wise, B. W., Conners, F., Rack, J., & Fulker, D. (1989). Specific deficits in component reading and language skills: Genetic and environmental influences. *Journal of Learning Disabilities, 22*, 339-349.

Phillips, C. J. (1961). On comparing scores from tests of attainment with scores from tests of ability in order to obtain indices of retardation by differences or ratios. Unpublished dissertation, University of Birmingham.

Plomin, R. (1991). A behavioural genetic approach to learning disabilities and their subtypes. In L. V. Feagans, E. J. Short, & L. J. Meltzer (Eds.), *Subtypes of learning disabilities* (pp. 83-111). Hillsdale, NJ: Lawrence Erlbaum.

Plomin, R. & Rende, R. (1991). Human behavioural genetics. *Annual Review of Psychology 1991, 42*, 161-190.

Pouretemad, H. R., Chadwick, O., & Yule, W. (1995). *Behavioural and emotional correlates of underachievement in arithmetic.* Unpublished manuscript, University of London, Institute of Psychiatry.

Richman, N., Stevenson, J., & Graham, P. J. (1982). *Pre-school to school: A behavioural study*. London: Academic Press.

Rodgers, B. (1983). The identification and prevalence of specific reading retardation. *British Journal of Educational Psychology, 53*, 369-373.

Rourke, B. P. & Fuerst, D. R. (1991). *Learning disabilities and psychosocial functioning: A neuropsychological perspective*. New York: Guilford Press.

Rowe, K. J. & Rowe, K. S. (1992). The relationship between inattentiveness in the classroom and reading achievement (part B): An exploratory study. *Journal of the American Academy of Child and Adolescent Psychiatry, 31*, 357-368.

Rust, J., Golombek, S., & Trickey, G. (1993). *WORD: Wechsler Objective Reading Dimensions Manual*. Sidcup: The Psychological Corporation Ltd.

Rutter, M. (1965). Classification and categorization in child psychiatry. *Journal of Child Psychology and Psychiatry, 6*, 71-83.

Rutter, M. (1974). Emotional disorder and educational underachievement. *Archives of Disease in Childhood, 49*, 249-256.

Rutter, M. & Gould, M. (1985). Classification. In M. Rutter & L. Hersov (Eds.), *Child and adolescent psychiatry: Modern approaches* (2nd ed., pp. 304-331). Oxford: Blackwell Scientific Publications.

Rutter, M., Tizard, J., & Whitmore, K. (Eds.) (1970). *Education, health and behaviour*. London: Longman and Green.

Rutter, M., Tizard, J., Yule, W., Graham, P., & Whitmore, K. (1976). Isle of Wight studies 1964-1974. *Psychological Medicine, 6*, 313-332.

Rutter, M. & Yule, W. (1975). The concept of specific reading retardation. *Journal of Child Psychology and Psychiatry, 125*, 181-197.

Share, D. L. & Silva, P. A. (1986). The stability and classification of specific reading retardation: A longitudinal study from age 7 to 11. *British Journal of Educational Psychology, 56*, 32-39.

Share, D. L., McGee, R., & Silva, P. A. (1989). IQ and reading progress: A test of the capacity notion of IQ. *Journal of the American Academy of Child and Adolescent Psychiatry 28*, 97-100.

Shaywitz, S. E., Escobar, M. D., Shaywitz, B. A., Fletcher, J. M., & Makuch, R. (1992). Evidence that dyslexia may represent the lower tail of a normal distribution of reading ability. *The New England Journal of Medicine, 326*, 145-150.

Shaywitz, S. E., Shaywitz, B. A., Fletcher, J. M., & Escobar, M. D. (1990). Prevalence of reading disability in boys and girls: Results of the Connecticut longitudinal study. *Journal of the American Medical Association, 264*, 998-1002.

Siegel, L. S. (1988). Evidence that IQ scores are irrelevant to the definition and analysis of reading disability. *Canadian Journal of Psychology, 42*, 201-215.

Siegel, L. S. (1989). IQ is irrelevant to the definition of learning disabilities. *Journal of Learning Disabilities, 22*, 469-478.

Silva, P. A. (1987). Epidemiology, longitudinal course, and some associated factors: An update. In W. Yule & M. Rutter (Eds.), *Language Development and Disorders* (pp. 1-15). Oxford: MacKeith.

Silva, P. A., McGee, R., & Williams, S. (1985). Some characteristics of 9-year-old boys with general reading backwardness or specific reading retardation. *Journal of Child Psychology and Psychiatry, 26*, 407-421.

Smith, S. D., Pennington, B. F., Kimberling, W. J., & Ing, P. S. (1990). Familial dyslexia: Use of genetic linkage data to define subtypes. *Journal of the American Academy of Child and Adolescent Psychiatry, 29*, 204-213.

Stanovich, K. E. (1994). Annotation: Does dyslexia exist? *Journal of Child Psychology and Psychiatry, 35*, 579-595.

Stevenson, H. W., Stigler, J. W., Lucker, G. W., Lee, S. Y., Hsu, C-C., & Kitamura, S. (1982). Reading disabilities: The case of Chinese, Japanese, and English. *Child Development, 33*, 1164-1181.

Stevenson, J. (1988). Which aspects of reading ability show a "hump" in their distribution? *Applied Cognitive Psychology, 2*, 77-85.

Stevenson, J. (1991). Which aspects of processing text mediate genetic effects? *Reading and Writing: An Interdisciplinary Journal, 3*, 249-269.

Thorndike, R. L. (1963). *The concepts of over- and under-achievement* New York: Columbia University, Teachers College.

Van der Wissel, A. & Zegers, F. E. (1985). Reading retardation revisited. *British Journal of Developmental Psychology, 3*, 3-19.

Vogler, G. P., DeFries, J. C., & Decker, S. N. (1985). Family history as an indicator of risk for reading disability. *Journal of Learning Disabilities, 18*, 419-421.

Wadsworth, S. J., DeFries, J. C., Stevenson, J., Gilger, J. W., & Pennington, B. F. (1992). Gender ratios among reading-disabled children and their siblings as a function of parental impairment. *Journal of Child Psychology and Psychiatry, 33*, 1229-1239.

World Health Organization. (1992). *The ICD-10 classification of mental and behavioural disorders. Clinical Descriptions and Diagnostic Guidelines*. Geneva: World Health Organization.

Yule, W. (1973). Differential prognosis of reading backwardness and specific reading retardation. *British Journal of Educational Psychology, 43*, 244-248.

Yule, W. (1979). *Correlates of reading retardation among junior school children: An epidemiological study*. Unpublished PhD Thesis, University of London.

Yule, W. (1985). Comments on Van der Wissel and Zegers: Reading retardation revisited. *British Journal of Developmental Psychology, 3*, 11-13.

Yule, W., Gold, R. D., & Busch, C. (1981). WISC-R correlates of academic attainment at 16 1/2 years. *British Journal of Educational Psychology, 51*, 237-240.

Yule, W., Lansdown, R., & Urbanowicz, M. (1982). Predicting educational attainment from WISC-R in a primary school sample. *British Journal of Clinical Psychology, 21*, 43-46.

Yule, W., Rutter, M., Berger, M., & Thompson, J. (1974). Over-and underachievement in reading: Distribution in the general population. *British Journal of Educational Psychology, 44*, 1-12.

# SECTION 2

# SPECIFIC DEVELOPMENTAL READING DISORDERS

JAN RISPENS

# THE VALIDITY OF THE CATEGORY OF SPECIFIC DEVELOPMENTAL READING DISORDER

## INTRODUCTION

The first descriptions of children who failed to learn to read in the absence of intellectual or sensory impairments appeared at the turn of the century (Hinshelwood, 1917). Since then, specific developmental reading disorder has been gradually recognized as a separate clinical entity. Various terms, such as word blindness (Orton, 1937), dyslexia (Money, 1962), specific reading retardation (Rutter & Yule, 1975), learning disability (Kirk, 1962), have been used to denote this disorder, that has been included in successive versions of DSM and ICD. In DSM-IV (American Psychiatric Association [APA], 1994) the disorder is called Reading Disorder and it is part of the section of 'Learning Disorders', while in ICD-10 (World Health Organization [WHO], 1992) Specific reading disorder is one of the subcategories of the section 'Specific developmental disorders of scholastic skills'. Throughout this chapter I will use the term Specific reading disorder (SRD), and we treat this term as synonymous with concepts such as dyslexia or learning disabilities.

Although a generally accepted definition is not available, most descriptions of the disorder share two common elements, namely the concepts of discrepancy and exclusion. **Discrepancy** pertains to the difference between observed and expected reading performance. The relevance of this concept for the description of dyslexia has generally been accepted, both in research and clinical practice (Stanovich, 1992). It is the key element in virtually all definitions of specific reading disorders. For example, the first criterion of the DSM-IV description of Reading Disorder reads: "The essential feature of Reading Disorder is reading achievement (....) that falls substantially below that expected given the individual's chronological age, measured intelligence, and age-appropriate education (Criterion A)." (APA, 1994, p. 48).

**Exclusion,** implying an enumeration of factors that are not the cause of the disorder, is another common element in descriptions of dyslexia. Specific reading disability, then, is generally characterized



*J. Rispens et al. (eds.),*
*Perspectives on the Classification of Specific Developmental Disorders,* 61–82.

as reading performance that lags behind expected performance, given the child's intellectual capacity, while the disorder is not attributable to a lack of schooling, or to sensory or other neurological impairments. For example, ICD-10 (WHO, 1992, p. 245) describes Specific reading disorder as follows: "The main feature of this disorder is a specific and significant impairment in the development of reading skills, which is not solely accounted for by mental age, visual acuity problems, or inadequate schooling".

This description assumes that SRD constitutes a separate category within the larger group of poor readers. Specific reading disorder refers to underachievement, namely poor performance that cannot be accounted for in terms of low intelligence, sensory deficits, or poor schooling. The assumption is that underachievement differs from backwardness in reading or low-achievement that may be due to factors such as limited intelligence or poor educational background. Sometimes backwardness in reading (BR) is called the 'garden-variety' of poor reading (Gough & Tunmer, 1986).

SRD has become a popular classification in clinical child psychology and psychiatry practice, well known to the general public. However, from its inception, the scientific status of the concept and its relevance for clinical practice has been doubted (Stanovich, 1994). The debate circles around two issues that are particularly problematic. First, the technicalities of the classification cause many problems that have not been solved to date. For example, there is no consensus about the standardization of the diagnostic procedure. Part of these difficulties stem from the fact that the operationaliza-tion of the concept of a discrepancy is beset with problems (Shaw, Cullen, McGuire, & Brinckerhoff, 1995).

Second, the validity of the concept of specific reading disorder is debated. A number of studies failed to demonstrate that SRD may be distinguished from the garden-variety type of poor reading (Fletcher, Francis, Rourke, Shaywitz, & Shaywitz, 1992; Fletcher et al., 1994; Pennington, Gilger, Olson, & DeFries, 1992; Siegel, 1992; Stanovich & Siegel, 1994; Ysseldyke, Algozzine, Shinn, & McGue, 1982). Hence, some researchers conclude that the distinction between SRD and BR types of poor reading is not appropriate (Shaywitz, Fletcher, Holahan, & Shaywitz, 1992). They argue that reading disability simply represents the lower end of the distribution of reading scores and that there is no reason to distinguish between various types of poor reading.

In this chapter I summarize the empirical literature on the validity of the concept of SRD. In the first section I discuss the results of a number of validity studies. Our conclusion is that empirical support in favour of the distinction between SRD and backwardness in reading is not convincing. However, the outcomes of these studies do not allow final conclusions regarding the validity of the concept of SRD.

In the concluding section I try to answer the question how to proceed with the concept of specific reading disorder. I briefly discuss the problems inherent in the use of discrepancy based definitions of the disorder, since several authors argue that this notion of a discrepancy is the main obstacle to an improved definition of SRD.

## EMPIRICAL STUDIES OF THE VALIDITY OF THE CONCEPT OF SPECIFIC READING DISORDER

### *Introduction*

The issue of the validity of the concept of SRD has been the subject of an ongoing debate. The conclusion of many reviews (e.g.Benton, 1978; Hooper & Willis, 1989; Keogh, 1986; Stanovich, 1994) is that both the construct validity and the descriptive validity of the category are far from satisfactory. For example, although empirical data are relatively scarce, there is some evidence that the stability of the classification over time is not high. Jorm, Share, MacLean, and Matthews (1986) reported in their longitudinal study that only 6 of the 25 children classified as SRD in grade 1, obtained the same classification in grade 2. Similarly, Shaywitz, Escobar, Shaywitz, Fletcher, and Makuch (1992) found that only 28 percent of the children classified as SRD in grade 1, received the same classification in grade 3. However, Dobbins and Tafa (1986) presented data that suggest a fair stability of underachieving readers.

Heterogeneity is another impediment to the validity of the categories of a classification system. The descriptive validity of a diagnostic category depends on homogeneity in behavioural attributes and course of the disorder (Volkmar, 1991). There is ample empirical evidence that the category of SRD does not meet this criterion. One explanation might be that the category consists of several subtypes (Feagans & McKinney, 1991). Unfortunately, research in this area has not resulted in a generally accepted subdivision into a number of subtypes. Therefore, the contribution of subtype research to improving the validity of the category, is limited (Snowling, 1991).

Comorbidity is another well known factor that affects both the reliability and the validity of classifications of childhood disorders (Rutter, 1989). This also applies to the category of SRD. Much attention, both in research and in clinical practice, has been paid to co-occurrence of SRD and attentional and behavioural problems (Cantwell & Baker, 1991; Gilger, Pennington, & DeFries, 1992) and to the relationship of SRD with language problems (Catts, 1993; Vellutino, 1979).

One might argue that SRD is no exception to the general rule that the validity of most categories of a classification system of childhood psychiatric disorders is not satisfactory (Cantwell, 1996). In other words, one might expect the kind of conclusions about the validity of the category of SRD I just mentioned. However, in the case of SRD there is reason for extra concern since there is doubt about the very concept of specific underachievement. Several recent studies failed to demonstrate that children classified as SRD differ from the garden-variety type of poor reading. Based on the outcomes of these studies, one may even ask whether SRD exists. In this section we summarize these studies in order to see whether the conclusion of some researchers that SRD simply represents the lower end of the distribution of reading scores and does not constitute a separate clinical entity, is warranted.

I start my analysis with a brief description of the Isle of Wight data (Rutter & Yule, 1973, 1975; Yule, 1973; Yule, Rutter, Berger, & Thompson, 1974). This study provided, for the first time, empirical evidence for the validity of the distinction between backward readers (the garden-variety type of poor reading) and (specific) reading retardation or underachievers.

I already noted that the concept of SRD originated from clinical practice. At the beginning of this century clinicians published case studies, demonstrating that children with reading problems despite normal (or even above average) intelligence differ from backward readers, whose poor performance may be due to a lack of capacities or to poor educational backgrounds. In the decades that followed this notion was further elaborated. Studies appeared about the aetiology of the disorder (Orton, 1937), about familial backgrounds (Hermann, 1959), and about the typical error pattern of SRD (Rawson, 1968). An intriguing problem, that caused much debate, pertained to the validity of the distinction between SRD and other types of poor reading. Unfortunately, most empirical studies conducted in the Sixties addressing this issue, suffered from the use of inadequate statistical techniques, or relied exclusively on clinical data (Fransella & Gerver, 1965). In the Isle of Wight study epidemiological data were used and statistically appropriate ways of defining underachievement and backwardness in reading were applied. Therefore, the study is considered especially relevant to the issue of validity of SRD. It has contributed significantly to the acceptance of SRD as a separate disorder. I start our analysis with a brief description of this landmark study. Then I summarize more recent validity studies in order to see whether the conclusions of Rutter and Yule about the distinction of SRD and backwardness in reading still hold.

## *The Isle of Wight Study*

In the Isle of Wight Study a two-step sampling procedure was applied (Yule et al. 1974). First, reading performance and intelligence of three age groups (9-years-olds, 10-years-olds and 11-years-olds), representing the general population of that age group, was measured. Each group consisted of about 1100 children. The nine- and ten-years-olds were followed until they were about 14 years old. The proportion of under- and overachievers was computed. Under- and overachievement was defined as: reading performance below or above expected reading performance as predicted from IQ by means of a regression equation. In each age group the differences between actual and predicted reading scores were plotted. In all samples there was an overrepresentation of under-achievers at the extreme of the distribution. This 'hump' may be interpreted as an indication of the existence of a subgroup in the distribution.

In the second step children likely to have reading difficulties were tested individually. The group of poor readers was divided into a group of 'backward readers', based on the criterion of a reading accuracy or comprehension score of 2 years 4 months below their chronological age, and a group labelled 'specific reading retardation'. The criterion here was: a reading score of 2 years 4 months below the score predicted on the basis of age and IQ (Yule, 1973), which implies a significant discrepancy (at the 5% percent level) between observed and expected performance. The total group of poor readers consisted of 155 backward readers and 86 retarded readers. There was a considerable overlap, since 76 children of the group of backward readers belonged to both groups. These children were removed from further analysis, which implied a group comparison. This comparison yielded interesting results.

First, the sex distribution in the specific reading retarded group differed considerably: the ratio of boys to girls was 3.3 to 1, compared with 1.3 to 1 in the group of backward readers. Second, both groups differed regarding the presence of neurological disorders, of motor and praxic abnormalities, as well as in speech and language features, and in prognosis (Rutter & Yule, 1975; Yule, 1973). There was no influence of social class.

An interesting feature of the Isle of Wight study is that it introduced a psychometrically adequate procedure to measure a discrepancy that takes regression into account. Regression pertains to the fact that if there is no perfect correlation between two measures (such IQ and reading), the children who are superior on one measure, will obtain a somewhat lower score on the other. As a consequence, they may be labelled 'discrepant' due to this statistical artefact.

Although the Isle of Wight data contributed considerably to the recognition of SRD as a separate clinical entity, different from general backwardness in reading, the conclusions of the study also have met critical appraisal. I briefly summarize a number of these studies.

### *a. The Problem of the 'Hump'*

It is generally assumed that a specific (for example: a bimodal) type of frequency distribution of a variable serving as a marker of symptomatology of a disorder, points to the existence of subtypes. Hence, Rutter and Yule (1975) interpreted their finding in the Isle of Wight study that underachievers were overrepresented in the distribution of residuals (differences between observed and expected scores on a reading test) as an argument in favour of the existence of two subtypes of poor readers, namely specific reading retarded children and backward readers.

Their finding has been replicated in a limited number of investigations. For example, Stevenson (1988) investigated the performance of groups of 7-, 11- and 13-year-old children on tests of reading, spelling and maths. He found an overrepresentation at the lower end of the distribution at 11 and 13 years, both in reading and spelling, but not in maths. At 7 years no hump was found.

However, other researchers have expressed doubt regarding the existence and the meaning of a hump. Rodgers (1983) made some cautionary remarks. He suggested that skewedness of the distribution of both reading scores and residuals in some of the groups of the Isle of Wight study might be responsible for the overrepresentation of underachievers. His own data seemed to confirm his doubt about the existence of a hump. In a large group of children (n = 8461) no difference between predicted and observed number of children with a discrepancy was found. Similarly, Van der Wissel and Zegers (1985) argued, based on data from a computer simulation, that non-normality of a distribution of residuals may be a statistical artefact, caused by ceiling effects of reading tests. Since in the Isle of Wight study these ceiling effects were present, the hump might be an artefact. In the Dunedin study (McGee,Williams, Share, Anderson, & Silva, 1986; Share, McGee, McKenzie, Williams, & Silva, 1987) no evidence for bimodality was found. Hence, the number of children with specific reading disorder corresponded with the expected number. Similarly, S. E. Shaywitz et al. (1992) found in their longitudinal data (n= 414; followed as a cohort from grade 1 through grade 6) no overrepresentation in the lower end of the distribution. The application of various cut-off levels (-2 or -1,5 standard deviation of estimation) yielded the same results. The data fitted into a normal-distribution model. Therefore, S. E. Shaywitz et al. (1992) conclude that dyslexia simply represents the lower end of the distribution of reading scores.

Based on these studies I conclude that a hump in the distribution of discrepancy scores in the age range from 7 to 10 years is not very likely, although it was present in the Isle of Wight data. However, this is no reason to doubt the validity of the distinction between backward readers and SRD, since bimodality is a sufficient but not a necessary condition for the presence of subtypes (Everitt, 1981; Pennington et al., 1992). Everitt mentions two examples demonstrating that unimodality does not exclude the presence of subtypes, namely the case of not well separated means of subtypes, or subtypes that are present in widely different proportions. As we will argue later on, specific reading disorder and backwardness in reading may constitute an example of subtypes with not well separated means. Therefore, the conclusion of S. E. Shaywitz et al. (1992) that the absence of bimodality implies that dyslexia is not a discrete entity, may be premature.

### *b. Prognosis, Sex Ratio and Other Correlates*

The Rutter and Yule (1975) study demonstrated that specific reading retardation (SRD) and backward readers (BR) differed with respect sex ratio, prognosis, presence of neurological disorders and language problems, which supports the validity of the classification.

These findings have been replicated to a certain extent in other longitudinal studies. The difference in sex ratio has found support. For example, both Silva, McGee, and Williams (1985) and Jorm et al. (1986) found a much higher sex ratio difference in the SRD groups, although these differences were not statistically significant. The sex ratios in the SRD and BR groups were about 7:1 and 2,5:1 respectively. Shaywitz, Shaywitz, Fletcher, and Escobar (1990) found much smaller differences in prevalence between boys and girls in a SRD group. Therefore, although the data about sex ratios are not completely in agreement, we conclude that there is a clear preponderance of boys in the case of SRD, as found by Rutter and Yule.

Silva et al. (1985) found, in accordance with the Isle of Wight data, that their BR group had more neurological abnormalities than the SRD group, but their SRD group did not show delays in language development. Pennington et al. (1992) and Fletcher et al. (1992) reported that children in their SRD groups had more language deficits, compared to the BR group. Fredman and Stevenson (1988) concluded, based on epidemiological data from a study about the genetics of reading disability, that their SRD and BR groups differed in sex-ratio, educational profile and spelling difficulties in the same way as in the Rutter and Yule study. Unfortunately, in most studies pertaining to the relationship between reading disability and other disorders such as ADHD, conduct disorder, and language disorders or language delays, no attention has been paid to the SRD and BR distinction. Therefore, data about differences in neurological and language problems are relatively scarce. Nevertheless, Rutter and Yule's finding that both groups differ has received support.

Rutter and Yule's finding regarding differential progress in reading was not replicated in the Dunedin study of Silva et al. (1985). Their groups did not show differences in progress, neither in reading nor in arithmetic. Maughan, Hagell, Rutter and Yule (1994), found in their follow up study of poor readers in secondary education that all children who lag behind in reading performance in middle childhood still have considerable reading problems in secondary education.

The studies mentioned thus far do not allow definite conclusions regarding the validity of the category of SRD. Some of the findings of Rutter and Yule have been replicated, and in other cases the outcomes are mixed. Therefore, the validity of the distinction may be disputed to a certain extent. More data are needed for a final judgement about this issue.

## OTHER EVIDENCE PERTAINING TO THE VALIDITY OF THE CATEGORY OF SRD

### *Introduction*

Rutter and Yule (1975) observed that although SRD and BR may be separated in a psychometrically adequate way, this does not necessarily imply that they also differ in a psychologically meaningful way. For example, one might ask whether the distinction makes sense if a comparison demonstrates that both groups apply the same reading strategies, and that they do not differ in their type of reading errors. And what is the usefulness of the distinction if there is no clear differential progress, and finally, if both groups do not differ on cognitive or other tasks that are (causally) related to reading performance? The answer might be, probably, that if there are no such differences, the distinction may be meaningless.

These issues have been addressed in a number of recent studies, comparing groups of SRD and BR children on tasks that are closely related to reading. The aim of several of these studies was not only to compare both groups, but also to test a hypothesis regarding the cause of the reading disorder. A clear example is Stanovich's so-called phonological-core variable-difference model (e.g. Stanovich 1993; Stanovich & Siegel, 1994). This model assumes that SRD and BR children share a phonological deficit as a cause of their reading problems, which constitutes the phonological core of the reading disorder. Both groups differ with respect to a number of cognitive processes that are related to reading, which represents the 'variable-differences' aspect of this model. The model is based on the assumption that by definition the SRD group has a higher aptitude level compared to the BR group, since BR implies poor reading in accordance with mental capacities. Therefore, the SRD group will perform better on reading related cognitive and memory tasks. The model predicts, if the distinction makes sense, differences between both groups in the domain of cognition and memory, but about equal (relatively poor) performance on phonological tasks. Poor reading of the BR group may be understood in terms of a developmental lag, i.e. slow progress, compared to normal readers, while poor performance of the SRD group represents a specific, isolated (cognitive) deficit. Hence, a study of the validity of the distinction also implies a test of this hypothesis of differences in aetiology.

Various studies about the validity of the SRD and BR distinction have been undertaken during the last years. Before we summarize their results, a remark must be made about the methodology of comparing groups. Two paradigms are in use. The first implies comparing SRD and BR groups of the same age and about the same reading level. In this design control groups of normal reading children of the same age are also used. This design does not allow inferences about possible causes of poor performance in reading, since one cannot exclude the possibility that a characteristic irregular cognitive profile or a specific deficit is a consequence (and not the cause) of poor reading. Another method implies the so-called reading-level match design. Here children of the same reading level but of different chronological ages are compared, for example younger normal readers with older SRD children, matched on reading level. The assumption is that if good and poor readers differ only in their rate of progress and not in their skill pattern or cognitive profile, the comparison should reveal no specific deficits in the profile of the poor readers, i.e. tasks on which the older (poor) readers perform poorly, compared to the younger normal readers. Although there are some pitfalls (Jackson & Butterfield, 1989), this design clearly has the advantage that it enables identification of specific deficits of SRD or BR groups. In some studies both designs are combined.

## *Data from Recent Studies*

Fredman and Stevenson (1988) compared SRD and BR groups regarding their use of reading strategies. Their sample consisted of 101 children (mean age 13 years; 4 months) who where part of a larger group of 285 pairs of twins. SRD was defined as 2 years (2 standard errors of prediction) or more below the predicted level. As in the Rutter and Yule studies, predictions were based on a multiple regression equation including Full Scale WISC IQ and age. BR was defined as reading performance two years or more below the mean reading age of the original twin sample. Dependent variables in this study were scores on several lists of regular, irregular and non-words. Interestingly, the comparisons were made in two ways. First, both groups were compared, controlling for IQ, which implies a mental-age control design, and second, the comparison was made in a reading-age match design with IQ as a covariate, which implies control for both IQ and reading level.

In the mental-age control condition both groups differed on all word lists, with the SRD group performing worse than the BR group. In other words, differences in performance are not due to the differences in intelligence between both groups. However, in the IQ and reading age control condition, there were no differences between the SRD and BR group. This implies that differences in the two groups in ability to read nonwords are a function of differences in reading level. Therefore, Fredman and Stevenson (1988) suggest that both groups do not differ in their reading strategy. The only relevant factor is the difference in level of reading.

Several other studies seem to support this conclusion. Siegel (1992) compared SRD, BR and normal reading children (n=1657; aged 7 to 16) on a variety of measures, including both standardized tests and experimental tasks encompassing reading, spelling, phonological processing, language and memory. She found on the majority of tests no differences between SRD and BR groups. Her conclusion is rather straightforward: "Therefore, there does not seem to be any reason to differentiate between individuals with dyslexia and poor readers" (Siegel, 1992, p. 627). Some caution is needed in the interpretation of her results since Siegel applied a relatively small discrepancy of only 1 s.d. between IQ score and reading score as the criterion to classify SRD.

Pennington et al. (1992) compared a group of SRD (IQ discrepant) readers with a group of BR (age discrepant) readers and a group of children who were both IQ and age discrepant. Unfortunately a less stringent discrepancy criterion was used, compared to the Isle of Wight study. The three groups were compared in different domains, including heritability and sex ratio. All children had IQ's of 90 or more. Not much evidence in favour of the external validity of the SRD and BR distinction was found. For example, both groups had nearly identical group heritabilities. As in the Isle of Wight study, the SRD group had more specific language deficits. Analysis of the various cognitive tests revealed different ability patterns, but group membership did not account for much variance. Therefore, the authors conclude that there is no reason to assume different etiologies for both groups. Differences between groups can be accounted for by differences in environmental risk factors (SRD children are in a better position here) and the presence of more specific deficits in the case of BR.

Fletcher et al. (1994) compared several groups of poor reading children. Unfortunately, their SRD and BR classification criteria are not completely in line with those applied in the studies I just mentioned. The comparison involved a great number of reading related cognitive and linguistic abilities, such as verbal and non-verbal short-term memory, speech production, word finding and word naming. Although their findings might not be completely comparable to the SRD and BR distinction as it was found in the Isle of Wight study, it is interesting to note that they failed to demonstrate substantial differences between their groups of poor reading children.

In a complicated study, Stanovich and Siegel (1994) tested several hypotheses pertaining to profiles of reading subskills of poor reading children. A comparison of SRD and BR children was part of this study. Three groups of children (SRD, BR and controls) were compared in a reading-level match design. I will not go into the details of the design and the outcome of the study. Suffice it to note their conclusion regarding the SRD and BR comparison: they found no significant differences between both groups.

However, a few studies did find differences between SRD and BR groups. Aaron, Kuchta and Grapenthin (1988) compared children with word recognition problems, but normal listening comprehension, who were labelled dyslexic, with children who performed poorly both in word recognition and listening comprehension, and normal readers. They found significant differences in oral reading errors, spelling and effect of context on reading between the groups of poor readers. Therefore, they concluded that dyslexia is different from other forms of poor reading. Unfortuna-tely they used an unusual procedure to define and measure a discrepancy. Hence, their results are incomparable to the outcome of the studies I reviewed thus far.

Badian (1994) compared SRD, BR and normal groups aged 6 to 10 years, on scores on nine different measures of reading related tasks such as phonological awareness and phonological recoding. She found that SRD and BR groups, matched on word recognition and age, differed in two of these nine measures. Since these measures tap skills that are highly relevant to word reading she concludes that "...reading disability or dyslexia is a separate entity from garden-variety poor reading (....)" (Badian, 1994, p. 61). However, as she admits, it is also possible to conclude from her data that both groups are more similar than dissimilar.

In another study (Badian, 1996) six to seven years-old SRD, BR and normal readers, were compared to three groups of children of eight to ten years old, classified in the same way, on measures of phonological processing, lexical retrieval (e.g. naming skills) and orthographic skills. This study demonstrated an age effect: at a younger age no difference was found between the SRD and BR group, while in the group of eight to ten years old the garden- variety children outperformed the SRD group on the measures of phonological processing. Therefore, Badian concludes that the SR and garden-variety (BR) distinction is not relevant at a younger age, but makes sense after a number of years of reading instruction.

Wolf (1986) criticized the conclusion of Seidenberg, Bruck, Fornarolo, and Backman (1985) that their investigation into word recognition processes of SRD and BR readers yielded no differences between both groups. They compared three groups of children, poor readers (the BR group) classified as such because they read below the 40th percentile of a standardized reading test, disabled readers (the SRD group), classified on the basis of exclusion and discrepancy, and a control group of normal readers. Unfortunately, their criteria differ from those applied in most other studies. For example, in most cases the cut-off for the classification of poor readers is the 25th percentile.

Seidenberg et al. (1985) found that the differences between SRD and BR groups were relatively small. Both groups were more similar than dissimilar, and both groups differed from the control group. For example, the mean of number of vowel and consonant errors (in the case of a list of regular words) was 2.4 for the SRD group, 1.2 for the BR group and 0.3 for the good readers.

Wolf argues that Seidenberg et al. have dismissed incorrectly several differences between both groups as insufficient to allow differentiation. For example, both groups differ on such measures as longer reading latencies, or more substitution errors in the pronunciation of consonants. Wolf suggests that these errors point to a real difference.

In their reply Seidenberg, Bruck, Fornarolo, and Backman (1986) state that the performance of their dyslexics did not reveal impaired processes, not seen in the BR group. There were quantative differences, but also a considerable overlap between the SRD and BR groups. However, both groups differed significantly from normal readers. Both groups had the same pattern of differences, compared to the normal reading controls. Hence, the conclusion of no difference seems warranted.

In another study (Wolf & Obregón, 1992), no difference between garden-variety poor readers and a SRD group was found on a rapid naming test. However, the authors conclude that although both groups perform poorly compared to a control group, they differ in the underlying cause of poor performance. For that reason both groups must be distinguished.

Ysseldyke et al. (1982) compared a sample of children classified as SRD with a group of poor performing children, comparable to BR children, on a great number of cognitive and academic tests. They concluded that a differential diagnosis, distinguishing SRD and BR groups, was hardly possible. Therefore, they concluded that the distinction between both groups does not make much sense.

However, in a recent re-analysis of the data of this study, Kavale, Fuchs, and Scruggs (1994) argue that at a closer look a distinction can be made: the performance of the SRD children is much lower, compared to the BR group. This must reflect a qualitatively different level of performance.

## *Conclusion*

In this section I reviewed several studies comparing SRD and BR groups of poor readers on reading related measures. My analysis may be summarized as follows.

a. Various studies failed to demonstrate substantial differences between SRD and BR with respect to reading related tasks. SBR and BR groups seem to be more similar than dissimilar, compared to normal readers, in their use of reading strategies. However, there are some studies that replicated several aspects of the Isle of Wight findings. For that reason a 'no difference' conclusion might be too rash.

b. In most studies the general pattern is the same: SRD's have more or less the same IQ as the normal controls, while the IQ's of the BR group is significantly lower. The BR group occupies the middle position regarding scores on reading and reading related measures, with the SRD group at the bottom. In other words, SRD differ from BR groups in that they have more serious reading problems.

c. SRD and BR groups manifest the same problems in the domain of phonological abilities. Therefore, it seems safe to assume that at least part of their reading problems stem from the same source, namely inadequate phonological skills. Nearly all studies failed to demonstrate that impairments of SRD readers in the domain of reading are different from those of BR readers.

d. In most studies no significant differences between the cognitive profiles of SRD and BR readers have been found. When groups are controlled for IQ and reading level, most differences tend to disappear.

e. SRD and BR groups tend to differ regarding sex ratio and behavioural correlates such as the presence of neurological disorders and language deficits, which may point to different etiologies.

In sum, there is no unequivocal empirical support for the validity of the category of SRD. On the contrary, most studies dit not replicate the Isle of Wight finding that both groups differ. Some caution is needed, since most studies are not completely comparable with the original Isle of Wight study. I will not go into details, but point briefly to two aspects. Most studies applied less stringent classification criteria. It may be that in the Isle of Wight study the more 'pure' cases have been selected. Another difference pertains to the way the problem of overlap has been handled. Overlap implies that children may be classified as both SRD and BR. In the Isle of Wight study the overlap was excluded. In the validity studies we discussed this procedure has not been followed. This is another reason why I assume that the Isle of Wight study contained more 'typical' cases of SRD and BR.

Despite these objections, nearly all studies point to a 'no difference' position, and for that reason doubts about the validity of the SRD and BR distinction seem warranted.

## HOW TO PROCEED WITH THE CATEGORY OF SPECIFIC READING DISORDER

How to proceed with the category of specific reading disorder, given the disappointing results of the validity studies? Broadly speaking, the answers to this question fall into three different categories.

First, a number of researchers (for example Fletcher, 1992; Siegel, 1992; S. A. Shaywitz et al., 1992) argue that the SRD and BR distinction cannot be defended. Their conclusion is that only one category of reading disabilities, including both SRD and BR poor readers, based on the notion of low achievement, should be recognized. In other words, they suggest that we abandon the distinction, since the validity studies I briefly summarized clearly point into the direction of 'no difference'. This answer has the advantage of being straightforward. However, from a clinical point of view it may be hard to accept, since most clinicians agree about their experience that SRD and BR readers differ.

An interesting consequence of this position is that a number of poor reading children who perform significantly below their expected level and who are labelled 'discrepant', will not be classified as reading disabled if their poor performance is not significantly below the average score of their age group. In other words, children who are underachievers but not low-achievers will not be classified, and will probably not receive special treatment in order to improve their relatively poor performance. Interestingly, these are the children that constitute the 'pure' cases of SRD in various studies.

Second, there are those who stress the importance of the clinical notion from which the concept of SRD originated, namely that underachievers are to be distinguished from low-achievers. Some argue that there is evidence that both groups need different treatment (Kavale, 1995). They admit that it is difficult to reliably distinguish both groups, due to the shortcomings of the definitions and diagnostic criteria that are in use at this moment. For that reason they conclude that we should strive for a renewed definition of SRD. They suggest that we need a process-oriented description of the disorder, which implies that the definition should point to underlying cognitive processes or skills that are causally related to reading. Their implicit suggestion is that there are processes in which SRD and BR readers may differ.

Unfortunately, our body of knowledge regarding those processes and skills is very weak. The notion that SRD and BR differ in underlying causes of poor performance has a long history. For example, in 1970 Critchley concluded in his review of half a century of research: "The arguments in favour of a specific type of developmental dyslexia occurring in the midst of but nosologically apart from the *olla podrida* of bad readers, may be said to rest upon four premises. These compromise: persistence into adulthood; the peculiar and specific nature of the errors in reading and writing; the familial incidence of the defect; and the frequent association with other symbol-defects" (Critchley, 1970, p. 11). In the previous section I demonstrated that recent research has demonstrated that these factors are irrelevant for the distinction between both groups. As a consequence, there is no clear evidence which processes or skills might be suitable candidates to distinguish between SRD and BR. Much is to be expected from the type of search for specificity as described in the next chapter of Remschmidt, SchulteKörne, and Hennighausen.

Third, a less far reaching solution implies a critical look at the concept of discrepancy, that plays such an important role in the definition of SRD. Various researchers argue that the lack of validity may be caused by the inadequacy of this criterion to distinguish both groups. Classifying children as discrepant, and hence as SRD, implies a procedure to measure both expected and observed reading performance, and to evaluate whether the observed reading score lags significantly behind the expected score. There is a growing tendency, both in research and in clinical practice, to apply a regression based procedure. A multiple regression equation avoids statistical artefacts such as regression (Reynolds, 1984). Usually, age, IQ, reading score and the correlation between IQ and the reading test that has been used to measure the observed reading performance are included in the equation.

There are many objections towards this procedure. For example, the regression procedure I described is sensitive to test reliabilities (Macmann, Barnett, Lombard, Belton-Kocher, & Sharpe, 1989), it may be influenced by the type of test that is used (Evans, 1992), and it implies the relatively arbitrary choice of cut-off points to measure the severity of a discrepancy which influences the number of children that are classified (Rispens & Van Yperen, 1990).

A much discussed problem pertains to the role of IQ in the classification procedure. For example, in criterion A of the DSM-IV description of specific reading disorder, the expected level of reading is defined as: performance according to chronological age and measured intelligence (APA, 1994, p. 42). However, the role of IQ as diagnostic criterion is much debated (Siegel, 1989). It is conceivable that the IQ of poor readers may be influenced negatively by their reading difficulties. As a consequence, the use of IQ underestimates the cognitive abilities of these children, who may be excluded from a classification as SRD. Another reason is that it is uncertain whether a verbal or a non-verbal intelligence test should be used.

Some argue that a discrepancy is the end-product of a development leading to poor reading, that is caused by some underlying process, for example a specific cognitive deficit (Shaw et al., 1994; Stanovich, 1993). Therefore, we should strive towards a definition of SRD in which those processes or skills are mentioned, instead of relying on a criterion that refers to IQ, which is a very global and unspecific index for cognitive capacities.

Finally, the concept of discrepancy does not necessarily refer to poor reading. Hence, some very bright, underachievers are classified 'discrepant' even if their reading performance is not significantly below the average score of their age group. In other words: they are not 'poor readers'. In order to avoid this situation, recent definitions of SRD (APA, 1994; Dykman & Ackerman, 1992) suggest a two step classification procedure, in which SRD implies both poor reading performance and a discrepancy, as implied in all definitions of SRD. A consequence is a large overlap (of more than fifty percent) between the SRD and BR groups, since many BR readers also read below their expected level.

From this brief analysis I conclude that the notion of IQ-discrepancy is an inadequate criterion to distinguish between SRD and BR poor readers. The traditional description of specific reading disorder needs further clarification, in which an alternative operationalization of the concept of discrepancy is applied. Unfortunately, as in the case of the suggestion of a process-oriented definition, it is not easy to find suitable alternatives.

My first suggestion that may be helpful to purify the concept of SRD, is to distinguish between a research and a clinical version of the definition of SRD and its diagnostic criteria. For research purposes, aiming at the search for factors that distinguish SRD from BR, very strict criteria are needed. For example, if the concept of discrepancy will remain in use, a severe (at least at the 5 percent level of significance) discrepancy is needed, in order to select 'pure', prototypical cases. Exclusion criteria should be applied, and it would be interesting to test other forms of discrepancy, for example a discrepancy between listening and reading achievement. For practical purposes less stringent criteria may be applied, in order to avoid false negatives, which may exclude children from a treatment they need.

Second, we should strive towards an improved definition. There is no doubt that in the end a description is preferable that indicates which cognitive processes or underlying abilities are causally related to SRD. In other words, the definition should specify what is meant by 'specific'. However, since SRD is a heterogeneous category, it is highly improbable that only one factor will be responsible for the condition. For that reason, research should accept not only the existence of subtypes, but be aware of all kinds of mixed forms. Research should aim at finding and describing a limited number of more or less prototypical cases, representing those subtypes. We should accept that probably many children belong to a mixed category.

## REFERENCES

Aaron, P. G., Kuchta, S., & Grapenthin, C. T. (1988). Is there a thing called dyslexia? *Annals of Dyslexia, 37,* 109-125.

American Psychiatric Association. (1994). *Diagnostic and statistical manual of mental disorders* (4th ed.) Washington DC: APA.

Badian, N. A. (1994). Do dyslexic and other poor readers differ in reading-related cognitive skills? *Reading and Writing: An Interdisciplinary Journal, 6,* 45-63.

Badian, N. A. (1996). Dyslexia: A validation of the concept at two age levels. *Journal of Learning Disabilities, 29,* 102-112.

Benton, A. L. (1978). Some conclusions about dyslexia. In A. L. Benton & D. Pearl (Eds.) *Dyslexia: An appraisal of current knowledge* (pp. 451-527). New York: Oxford University Press.

Cantwell, D. P. (1996). Classification in child and adolescent psychopathology. *Journal of Child Psychology and Psychiatry, 37,* 1-13.

Cantwell, D. P. & Baker, L. (1991). Association between attention deficit hyper-activity disorder and learning disorders. *Journal of Learning Disabilities, 24,* 88-94.

Catts, H. W. (1993). The relationship between speech-language impairments and reading disability. *Journal of Speech and Hearing Research, 36,* 948-958.

Critchley, M. (1970). *Developmental dyslexia.* London: Heinemann.

Dobbins, A. & Tafa, E. (1990). The 'stability' of identification of underachieving readers over different measures of intelligence and reading. *British Journal of Educational Psychology, 61,* 155-163.

Dykman, R. A. & Ackerman, P. T. (1992). Diagnosing dyslexia: IQ regression plus cut-points. *Journal of Learning Disabilities, 25,* 574-576.

Evans, L. D. L. (1992). Severe does not always imply significant: Bias of a regression discrepancy model. *Journal of Special Education, 26,* 57-67.

Everitt, B. S. (1981). Bimodality and the nature of depression. *British Journal of Psychiatry, 138,* 336-339.

Feagans, L. V. & McKinney, J. D. (1991). Subtypes of learning disabilities: A review. In L. V. Feagans, E.J. Short, & L. J. Meltzer (Eds.), *Subtypes of learning disabilities: Theoretical perspectives and research* (pp. 3-33). Hillsdale, NJ: Erlbaum.

Fletcher, J. M. (1992). The validity of distinguishing children with language and learning disabilities according to discrepancies with IQ: Introduction to the special series. *Journal of Learning Disabilities, 25,* 546-548.

Fletcher, J. M., Francis, D. J., Rourke, B. P., Shaywitz, S. E., & Shaywitz, B. E. (1992). Validity of discrepancy-based definitions of reading disabilities. *Journal of Learning Disabilities, 25,* 555-561.

Fletcher, J. M., Shaywitz, S. E., Shankweiler, D. P., Katz, L., Liberman, I. Y., Stuebing, K. K., Francis, D. J., Fowler, A. E., & Shaywitz, B. A. (1994). Cognitive profiles of reading disability: Comparisons of discrepancy and low achievement definitions. *Journal of Educational Psychology, 86,* 6-23.

Fransella, F. & Gerver, D. (1965). Multiple regression equations for predictive reading age from chronological age and WISC verbal IQ. *British Journal of Educational Psychology, 35,* 86-89.

Fredman, G. & Stevenson, J. (1988). Reading processes in specific reading retarded and reading backward 13-years-olds. *British Journal of Developmental Psychology, 1,* 329-342.

Gilger, J. W., Pennington, B. F., & DeFries, J. C. (1992). A twin study of the aetiology of comorbidity: Attention-deficit hyperactivity disorder and dyslexia. *Journal of the American Academy of Child and Adolescent Psychiatry, 31,* 343-349.

Gough, P. B. & Tunmer, W. E. (1986). Decoding, reading and reading disability. *Remedial and Special Education, 7,* 6-10.

Hermann, K. (1959). *Reading disability: A medical study of word-blindness and related handicaps.* Copenhagen: Munksgaard.

Hinshelwood, J. (1917). *Congenital word blindness.* London: Lewis.

Hooper, S. R. & Willis, W. G. (1989). Historical foundations and definitional issues. In S. R. Hooper & W. G. Willis (Eds.), *Learning disability subtyping* (pp. 3-18). New York: Springer.

Jackson, N. E. & Butterfield, E. C. (1989). Reading-level-match designs: Myths and reality. *Journal of Reading Behaviour, 21,* 387-412.

Jorm, A. F., Share, D. L., Maclean, R., & Matthews, R (1986). Cognitive factors at school entry predictive of specific reading retardation and general reading backwardness: A research note. *Journal of Child Psychology and Psychiatry, 27,* 45-54.

Kavale, K. A. (1995). Setting the record straight on learning disability and low achievement: The tortuous path of ideology. *Learning Disabilities: Research and Practice, 10,* 145-152.

Kavale, K. A., Fuchs, D., & Scruggs, T. E. (1994). Setting the record straight on learning disability and low achievement: Implications for policymaking. *Learning Disabilities Research and Practice, 9,* 70-77.

Keogh, B. K. (1986). A marker system for describing learning-disabilities samples. In S. J. Ceci (Ed.), *Handbook of cognitive, social, and neuropsychological aspects of learning disabilities* (Vol 1, pp. 55-81). Hillsdale, NJ: Erlbaum.

Kirk, S. A. (1962). *Education of exceptional children.* New York: Grune & Stratton.

Macmann, G. M., Barnett, D. W., Lombard, T. J., Belton-Kocher, E., & Sharpe, M. N. (1989). On the actuarial classification of children: Fundamental studies of classification agreement. *Journal of Special Education, 23,* 127-149.

Maughan, B., Hagell, A., Rutter, M., & Yule, W. (1994). Poor readers in secondary school. *Reading and Writing: An Interdisciplinary Journal, 6,* 125-150.

McGee, R., Williams, S., Share, D. L., Anderson, J., & Silva, P. A. (1986). The relationship between specific reading retardation, general reading backwardness and behavioural problems in a large sample of Dunedin boys: A longitudinal study from five to eleven years. *Journal of Child Psychology and Psychiatry, 27,* 597-610.

Money, J. (1962). A post-conference review. In J. Money (Ed.), *Reading disability: Progress and research needs in dyslexia* (pp. 9-33). Baltimore: John Hopkins Press.

Orton, S. T. (1937). *Reading, writing and speech problems in children.* New York: Norton.

Pennington, B. F., Gilger, J. W., Olson, K. R., & DeFries, J. C. (1992). External validity of age versus IQ discrepant definitions of reading disability: Lessons from a twin study. *Journal of Learning Disabilities, 25,* 562-573.

Reynolds, C. R. (1984). Critical measurement issue in learning disabilities. *Journal of Special Education, 18,* 451-476.

Rawson, M. B. (1968). *Developmental language disability.* Baltimore: John Hopkins Press.

Rispens, J. & Van Yperen, T. A. (1990). The identification of specific reading disorders: Measuring a severe discrepancy. In G. T. Pavlides (Ed.), *Perspectives on dyslexia* (Vol. 2, pp. 17-42.) New York: Wiley.

Rodgers, B. (1983). The identification and prevalence of specific reading retardation. *British Journal of Educational Psychology, 53,* 369-373.

Rutter, M. (1989). Isle of Wight Revisited: Twenty-five years of child psychiatric epidemiology. *Journal of the American Academy of Child and Adolescent Psychiatry, 29,* 633-653.

Rutter, M. & Yule, W. (1973). Specific reading retardation. In L. Mann & D. A. Sabatino (Eds.), *The first review of special education* (pp. 1-51). Philadelphia: JSE Press.

Rutter, M., & Yule, W. (1975). The concepts of specific reading retardation. *Journal of Child Psychology and Psychiatry, 16,* 181-197.

Seidenberg, M. S., Bruck, M., Fornarolo, G., & Backman, J. (1985). Word recognition processes of poor and disabled readers: Do they necessarily differ? *Applied Psycholinguistics, 6,* 161-180.

Seidenberg, M. S., Bruck, M., Fornarolo, G., & Backman, J. (1986). Who is dyslexic? Reply to Wolf. *Applied Psycholinguistics, 7,* 77-84.

Share, D. L., McGee, R., McKenzie, D., Williams, S., & Silva, P. (1987). Further evidence relating to the distinction between specific reading retardation and general reading backwardness. *British Journal of Developmental Psychology, 5,* 35-44.

Share, D. L. & Silva, P. A. (1986). The stability and classification of specific reading retardation: A longitudinal study from age 7 to age 11. *British Journal of Educational Psychology, 56,* 32-39.

Shaw, S. F., Cullen, J. P., McGuire, J. M., & Brinckerhoff, L. C. (1995). Operationalizing a definition of learning disabilities. *Journal of Learning Disabilities, 28,* 586-597.

Shaywitz, S. E., Escobar, M. D., Shaywitz, B. A., Fletcher, J. M., & Makuch, R. (1992). Distribution and temporal stability of dyslexia in an epidemiological sample of 414 children followed longitudinal. *New England Journal of Medicine, 326,* 145-150.

Shaywitz, B. A., Fletcher, J. M., Holahan, J. M., & Shaywitz, S. E. (1992). Discrepancy compared to low achievement definitions of reading disability: Results from the Connecticut longitudinal study. *Journal of Learning Disabilities, 25,* 639-648.

Shaywitz, S. E., Shaywitz, B. A., Fletcher, J. M., & Escobar, M. D. (1990). Prevalence of reading disability in boys and girls: Results of the Connecticut longitudinal study. *Journal of the American Medical Association, 264,* 998-1002.

Siegel, L. S. (1989). IQ is irrelevant to the definition of learning disabilities. *Journal of Learning Disabilities, 22,* 469-478, 486.

Siegel, L. S. (1992). An evaluation of the discrepancy definition of dyslexia. *Journal of Learning Disabilities, 25,* 618-629.

Silva, P. A., McGee, R., & Williams, S. M. (1985). Some characteristics of 9-year-old boys with general reading backwardness or specific reading retardation. *Journal of Child Psychology and Psychiatry, 26,* 407-421.

Snowling, M. J. (1991). Developmental reading disorder. *Journal of Child Psychology and Psychiatry, 32,* 49-79.

Stanovich, K. E. (1992). Developmental reading disorder. In S. R. Hooper, G. W. Hynd, & R. E. Mattison (Eds.) *Developmental disorders: Diagnostic criteria and clinical assessment* (pp. 173-209). Hillsdale, NJ: Erlbaum.

Stanovich, K. E. (1993). A model for studies of reading disability. *Developmental Review, 13,* 225-245.

Stanovich, K. E. (1994). Does dyslexia exist? *Journal of Child Psychology and Psychiatry, 35,* 579-597.

Stanovich, K. E. & Siegel, L. S. (1994). Phenotypic performance profile of children with reading disabilities: A regression-based test of the phonological-core variable-difference model. *Journal of Educational Psychology, 86,* 24-53.

Stevenson, J. (1988). Which aspects of reading disability show a 'hump' in their distribution? *Applied Cognitive Psychology, 2,* 77-85.

Van der Wissel, A. & Zegers, F. E. (1985), Reading retardation revisited. *British Journal of Developmental Psychology, 3,* 3-19.

Vellutino, F. R. (1979). *Dyslexia: Theory and research.* Cambridge, MA: MIT Press.

Volkmar, F. R. (1991). Classification in child and adolescent psychiatry: Principles and issues. In M. Lewis (Ed.), *Child and adolescent psychiatry: A comprehensive textbook* (pp. 415-422). Baltimore: Williams & Williams.

Wolf, M. (1986). The question of essential differences in developmental dyslexia: A response to Seidenberg, Bruck, Fornarolo, and Backman. *Applied Psycholinguistics, 7,* 69-76.

Wolf, M. & Obregón, M. (1992). Early naming deficits, developmental dyslexia, and a specific deficit hypothesis. *Brain and Language, 42,* 219-247.

World Health Organization. (1992). *The ICD-10 classification of mental and behavioural disorders: Clinical descriptions and diagnostic guidelines.* Geneva: World Health Organization.

Ysseldyke, J. E., Algozzine, B., Shinn, M. R., & McGue, M. (1982). Similarities and differences between low achievers and students classified learning disabled. *Journal of Special Education, 16,* 73-85.

Yule, W. (1973). Differential prognosis of reading backwardness and specific reading retardation. *British Journal of Educational Psychology, 43,* 244-249.

Yule, W., Rutter, M., Berger, M., & Thompson, J. (1974). Over- and underachievement in reading: Distribution in the general population. *British Journal of Educational Psychology, 44,* 1-12.

HELMUT REMSCHMIDT, GERD SCHULTE-KÖRNE,
AND KLAUS HENNIGHAUSEN

# WHAT IS SPECIFIC ABOUT THE SPECIFIC READING DISORDER?

## INTRODUCTION

The term specific reading and/or spelling disorder (synonym: "dyslexia; "developmental dyslexia") is used to characterize disorders in which the main feature is a serious impairment in the development of reading or spelling skills which is not explicable in terms of general intellectual retardation or inadequate schooling. First descriptions were given by Berkhan (1885, 1886), Hinshelwood (1904) and Morgan (1896).

TABLE 1

| Classification of specific reading/and spelling disorder |
|---|
| Specific delays in development (MAS-ICD-9) (1976) |
| * Specific reading retardation |
| Specific developmental disorders (DSM-III) (1980) |
| * Developmental reading disorder |
| Developmental disorders (DSM-III-R) (1987) |
| * Developmental reading disorder |
| * Developmental expressive writing disorder |
| Disorders of psychological development (ICD-10) (1992) |
| * Specific reading disorder |
| * Specific spelling disorder |
| Learning disorders (DSM-IV) (1994) |
| * Reading disorder |
| * Disorder of written expression |

Table 1 gives an overview of recent classification of specific reading- and spelling disorders. As the table demonstrates, the terminology has changed from ICD-9 to ICD-10 and from DSM-III to DSM-IV. Whereas the older classification systems (ICD-9 and



*J. Rispens et al. (eds.),*
*Perspectives on the Classification of Specific Developmental Disorders,* 83–104.

DSM-III) classify specific reading disorder under the heading of Specific Delays in Development (ICD-9) and Specific Developmental Disorders (DSM-III), the new versions of both systems use more general headlines, namely Disorders of Psychological Development (ICD-10) and Learning Disorders (DSM-IV). However, within the ICD-10 system, there is still the notion of specific reading disorders and specific spelling disorder, whereas the aspect of specificity has been omitted in DSM-IV, which distinguishes only between "reading disorder" and "disorder of written expression", the heading for both being Learning Disorders. Does this development reflect progress of our knowledge, or has it simply to do with the fact that modern classification systems try to exclude aetiological implications as far as possible? This raises the question of specificity. Specificity means that the disorder in question can clearly be distinguished from other reading and spelling disorders. Specific means a reading and/or spelling disorder in the absence of general intellectual impairments and in the absence of difficulties in other academic areas. Further, specificity can be looked upon in terms of qualitative and quantitative differences. A narrow definition of the term "specificity" would include qualitative rather than quantitative differences with other disorders.

## POSSIBLE INDICATORS OF SPECIFICITY

The specific characteristics of "specific reading and spelling disorder" can be sought in different fields: symptomatology, comorbidity, social context, morphological factors, information processing, neurophysiological aspects, genetic factors, and longterm course.

### *Symptomatology*

The symptomatology of specific reading disorder depends largely on the definition and the sample. In the Isle of Wight-Study, Rutter and Yule (1975) found that children who had a reading achievement below age revealed more neuropsychological symptoms than children who showed a discrepancy between observed reading and predicted reading based on age and IQ. Denckla (1978) proposed a distinction between reading disorder with additional symptoms such as hyperactivity and neurological signs (dyslexia plus) and reading disorder without any additional symptoms (dyslexia pure).

Another problem, widely discussed with regard to specific reading and spelling disorder, is the question whether these children makc specific spelling errors which allow one to differentiate them from children with other reading disorders. Several studies have shown that children with specific reading and spelling disorders do not produce quantitatively different errors when compared with normal children or children with a reduced intelligence level, although there are qualitative differences between normal spellers and specific spelling disabled children. The spelling errors of dyslexics are more frequently dysphonetic (Boder, 1973; Fox & Routh, 1983; Lennox & Siegel, 1993; Whiting & Jarrico, 1980). However, frequency and types of errors change with regard to the process of learning and the difficulty of the tasks (Grissemann, 1974).

As far as sex distribution is concerned, there is a clear dominance of boys in clinical studies (3:1 or 2:1) (Finucci & Childs, 1981), whereas some epidemiological studies found no significant differences in prevalence of specific reading disability in research-identified boys compared with girls (Flynn & Rahbar, 1994; Shaywitz, Shaywitz, Fletcher, & Escobar, 1990), depending on the diagnostic criteria used.

## *Comorbidity*

As Rutter and Yule (1975) discovered in the Isle of Wight Studies, children with specific reading disorder differ from those with reading backwardness in several areas: specific reading disorder is more frequent in boys, and children with this condition show less neurological disorders than children with reading backwardness. Finally, reading difficulties in general (probably irrespective of the kind of reading disorder) are associated with other psychiatric problems and boys with severe reading problems do appear to be at risk for later conduct disorders (Lewis, Hitch, & Walker, 1994).

## *Social Context*

In clinical samples, there seems to be no correlation between specific reading disorder and social class. In a total clinical population comprising more than 3.000 patients, we found approximately 30% of all patients with the diagnosis of "specific developmental disorders". As far as specific reading and spelling disorder is concerned, there was no correlation with social class, but this did not apply for specific developmental language disorder or motor retardation. These disorders did reveal a clear relation with social class (Remschmidt, 1987).

### *Morphological Correlates and Brain Function*

Galaburda and co-workers (Galaburda & Kemper, 1979; Galaburda, Sherman, Rosen, Aboitiz, & Geschwind, 1985; Humphreys, Kaufmann, & Galaburda, 1990) described neuropathological results after studying the brains of five male and three female dyslexics. They obtained the following results: there was a symmetry instead of asymmetry of the planum temporale; they found several cortical anomalies in the form of ectopias and structural dysplasias mainly in the perisylvian regions of the left brain. According to Galaburda (1985), these anomalies occur in regions that are relevant for speech and language and represent neurodevelopmental disturbances within the fetal period. According to Geschwind (1985), the anatomic anomalies are very close to the gyrus angularis which is looked upon as a kind of "reading centre". According to the model of Masland (1981), there is an area near the gyrus angularis which is responsible for the integration of visual patterns and phonological perceptions.

Computerized Tomography (CT) studies and Magnetic Resonance Imaging (MRI) studies demonstrate that there are deviations in brain morphology in dyslexic subjects. However, one has to take into consideration that the diagnostic criteria for sample selection and the methods outlining the planum temporale (Steinmetz & Galaburda, 1991) were very different between the studies. Nevertheless, there is a detectable tendency towards a higher proportion of dyslexics who do not develop classical brain asymmetry as normals do. A majority of them reveal a significantly smaller left planum temporale than normal subjects. Some of the investigators have tried to correlate the size of the planum temporale on both sides with verbal IQ. Hier, LeMay, Rosenberger, and Perlo (1978) found that dyslexics with a greater right than left parieto-occipital region had a significantly reduced verbal IQ.

Tables 2 and 3 show the main results of CT and MRI studies of dyslexics and the morphological substrates found so far.

TABLE 2

Dyslexia and deviations in brain morphology (CT studies)

| Study | N/Age | Results |
|---|---|---|
| Hier, LeMay, Rosenberger, & Perlo (1978) | 24 dyslexics (mean age 25). Diagnostic criterium of dyslexia was a performance on Gray Oral Reading Test less than 5th grade or two-grade level delay in reading. | 10 dyslexics had a wider right than left parieto-occipital region, 6 dyslexics had approximately symmetrical and 8 dyslexics had a wider left than right parieto-occipital region. The dyslexics with a right greater than left p.o.-region had in comparison to the other examined dyslexics a significant reduced VIQ. |
| Haslam, Dalby Johns, & Rademaker (1981) | 26 dyslexics (mean age 11 years). Diagnostic criteria of dyslexia were a reading performance at least 2 years behind the expected level and WISC-R FIQ >80. | 12 dyslexics showed a normal occipital asymmetry, 11 dyslexics showed symmetric hemispheres, 3 dyslexics with reversed occipital asymmetry. |

The new technique of positron emission tomography (PET) opens the possibility to investigate dyslexics in a functional way and during a more or less specific task. The results of two recent studies are demonstrated in Table 4.

Whereas Gross-Glenn et al. (1991) did not find interhemispheric differences for temporal or parietal lobes between the two groups (dyslexics and controls), the study by Rumsey et al. (1992) showed clearly that during a rhyme-detection task dyslexics showed less activation in two left temporo-parietal regions than controls. Higher verbal IQs of dyslexics were associated with greater left parietal activation. Studies of this type can give us more insight into basic processes going on during reading or, in more general terms, processing of verbal information.

TABLE 3

Dyslexia and deviations in brain morphology (MRI studies)

| Study | N/Age/Diagnostic criteria | Results |
|---|---|---|
| Larsen, Hoien, Lundberg, & Odegaard (1990) | 19 dyslexics, 18 age-, intelligence- and SES-matched control adolescents. Diagnostic criteria were poor word recognition and an IQ in the normal range. | 70% of dyslexics showed a symmetry of the planum, 70% of controls showed a greater left planum temporale. Association of abnormal symmetry of planum with phonological deficits. |
| Hynd, Semrud-Clikeman, Lorys, Novey, & Eliopulos (1990) | 10 dyslexics, 10 children with a ADD/H, 10 normal and age- and sex-matched controls (age range for all groups 9-11 years). Diagnostic criteria for dyslexia were a reading achievement ≥20 standard score points below FSIQ on Word Attack and Passage Comprehension subtests of the Woodcock Reading Mastery Tests-Revised (WRMT-R), a FSIQ ≥85, and a positive family history for learning problems. | Dyslexics had a significantly smaller left planum temporale than the normal subjects. 70% of the ADD/H and normal children had the expected left greater than right pattern of the plana asymmetry, while only 10% of dyslexic children did. |
| Leonard et al. (1993) | 9 dyslexics, 12 controls, 10 unaffected relatives of dyslexic probands (age range 6-63 years). Diagnosis of dyslexics was based on a clinical inter-view, family history, and the results of phonological decoding tests. | Interhemispheric asymmetries: regardless of group, all subjects demonstrated a leftward asymmetry in the temporal bank and rightward asymmetry in the parietal bank of the planum. Intrahemispheric asymmetries: a significantly larger proportion of the right planum was shifted from the temporal to the parietal bank. |

TABLE 4

Dyslexia and deviations in brain morphology (PET studies)

| Study | N/Age/Diagnostic criteria | Task | Results |
|---|---|---|---|
| Gross-Glenn et al. (1991) | 11 dyslexics (mean age 30), 14 controls (mean age 27). Diagnostic criteria were a childhood history of severe reading and spelling problems, a family history of reading and spelling difficulties, and an IQ in the normal range. | Word reading | For the occipital lobe (lingual lobule) the regional metabolic values were nearly equal for the dyslexics, for controls there were left greater than right hemisphere values. (Possibly the higher lingual activity shown by dyslexics reflect inefficient visual word-form processing.) No group or interhemispheric differences for temporal or parietal lobes. |
| Rumsay et al. (1992) | 14 dyslexics (mean age 27), 14 matched (IQ, handedness, SES) controls (mean age 26 years). Diagnostic criteria were VIQ or PIQ from the WAIS-R ≥89, the DSM-III-R criteria for developmental reading disorder and the Finucci criteria for severe dyslexic adults. | Rhyme detection task | Dyslexics showed significantly less activation than controls in two left-tempo-parietal regions (left parietal and left middle temporal regions) by rhyme detection. Higher VIQs of dyslexics were associated with greater left parietal activation. |

## *Information Processing*

The hypothesis that in children with specific reading disorder the integration of visually presented information and language processing is dysfunctional, was tested in a group of 30 dyslexic boys who met the Denckla (1978) criterion of "dyslexia pure", i.e. a severe spelling disability in the absence of other behavioural problems or neurological dysfunctions (e.g. hyperactivity, motor abnormalities) and 28 control subjects matched for sex, age, and

WISC-R performance IQ. The subjects had to compare two strings consisting of five letters which differed in one letter. They had to mark the different letter within a certain amount of time. The presentation time was continuously and automatically adjusted to the individual performance level by a computer program. EEGs were recorded during rest conditions, and at different levels of performance during twenty minutes. The main results, which have since been replicated in two studies, were: (1) Dyslexic children processed visually presented letter strings more slowly than controls; (2) their processing speed showed neither more variability nor a decline over the period of twenty minutes, and there was no deficit in sustained attention; (3) increasing cognitive activation and performance speed resulted in the EEG in an attenuation of the relative power in the alpha band in both groups, but dyslexics showed a faster attenuation even at low performance levels; and (4) the dyslexic group did not reveal specific abnormal EEG features when the task difficulty was adjusted individually (Remschmidt & Warnke, 1992).

The significant delay in visual information processing in dyslexics corresponds with the results found by other authors. We found also a significant between-group difference in simple visuomotoric reaction time, with dyslexics on the average showing a delay of 28 msec. The main deficit seems to be the delay in the translation or integration of visually recognized verbal letter strings into a speech code. The other interesting result was the increase of EEG activity in the dyslexic group in relation to the level of visual information processing. At a low performance level in discriminative reading of matched letter strings, there was a maximum of brain electrical activity in the dyslexic group. This result corresponds with findings by Martinius (1976), who found the higher electrocortical activity in dyslexic children compared to groups with attention deficit disorder and controls.

## *Neurophysiological Aspects*

Visually evoked potentials (VEP) have been employed in numerous studies to examine whether deficits in visual information processing are present in the genesis of developmental dyslexia. Although most of these studies found significant differences between dyslexics and normal controls, the variety of the discriminating features does not account for a unique defect in the visual pathway. Conners (1971) reported an attenuation of a negative component peaking about 200 msec after stimulus over the left parietal region in dyslexic children and a positive correlation between reading ability and the amplitude of this component. Attempts to replicate these findings led to inconsistent results (Preston, Guthrie, & Childs, 1974; Sobotka & May, 1977; Symann-Louett, Gascon, Matsumiya, & Lombroso, 1977; Weber & Omenn, 1977). Unequal recording procedures and stimulus conditions may account for these contradictory results. Symann-Louett et al. (1977) pointed out that it is arbitrary to measure latencies or amplitudes of components which do not seem to be equivalent in dyslexics and controls.

In later studies mainly higher cortical functions of visual information processing such as selective visual attention (Holcomb, Ackerman, & Dykman, 1985), probe event related potentials during reading (Johnstone et al, 1984), semantic priming (Jones & Michie, 1986), letter and word discrimination (Taylor & Keenan, 1990), learning and memory (Brandeis, Vitacco, & Steinhausen, 1994; Stelmack, Saxe, Hondy-Cullum, Campbell, & Armitage, 1988), spatial orienting (Harter, Anllo-Vento, & Wood, 1989) and slow brain potentials related to different cognitive tasks (Landwehrmeyer, Gerling, & Wallesch, 1990) were explored. Basic features of visual processing again came into the centre of attention by works of Lehmkuhle, Garzia, Turner, Hash, and Baro (1993), Livingstone, Rosen, Drislane, and Galaburda (1991) and May, Lovegrove, Martin, and Nelson (1991) who applied pattern reversal visual evoked potentials and found an impaired processing of rapid changing patterns with low spatial frequency and low contrast. They suggest that in dyslexics the fast subdivision of the visual pathway (i.e. the magnocellular system) may be defective. This hypothesis has been supported by anatomical findings (Livingstone et al., 1991).

In a recent study (Hennighausen, Remschmidt, & Warnke, 1994), we investigated pattern reversal with visually evoked potentials (VEP) in a group of 16 boys with developmental dyslexia and 17 controls matched for sex, age, and intelligence. We found wave form differences between the groups over the left hemisphere in the pilot and replication study. This abnormality is characterized by a lower negative amplitude deflection in the visually evoked potential 160-190 msec after stimulus presentation (N1 component) at the left central region. Only 44% of the dyslexics showed a N1 component in comparison to more than 80% of the controls. The lack of this component was most prominent in dyslexics whose spelling scores were more than 1.5 standard deviations below their intelligence score (IQ-discrepant dyslexics).

It is arguable that the N1 component really disappears or, because of an increased latency, sums up in later components. In contradiction to Symann-Louett et al. (1977), who observed simular differences, we did not see a more complex shape of the visual evoked potential after 200 msec in the dyslexic group.

The question has to be answered why the N1 component is absent more frequently in IQ-discrepant dyslexics. All dyslexics had low scores on the spelling test and at this low level the test cannot differentiate sufficiently between the more or less reading disabled. Therefore the difference between IQ and spelling score might contain more information than spelling score alone. In this case the IQ-discrepant dyslexics should be considered as the more severe dyslexics and an aberrant VEP is related to the severity of dyslexia. However, there is another and probably more interesting explanation. Dyslexics with an aberrant VEP had significantly higher scores on the WISC-R verbal IQ than dyslexics without an aberrant VEP, and did not deviate from the controls. It can be hypothesised that this subgroup has normal verbal abilities and unaffected language functions but impaired visual information processing, while in the other subgroup dyslexia is associated with reduced verbal abilities. Since performance IQ was used as matching sample criterion and a full scale IQ consists of both verbal and performance scores, the higher verbal abilities of the aberrant VEP subgroup will lead to a larger difference between full scale IQ and spelling score.

Another essential question is how and at which level visual information processing is disturbed in a subgroup of dyslexic children. Evidence from recent studies suggest that earlier components of visually evoked potentials between 70 and 170 msec after stimulus are delayed in dyslexics over the occipital areas and under certain stimulus conditions (Lehmkuhl et al., 1993; Livingstone et al., 1991). Variations of the stimuli revealed that patterns with low spatial frequency, low contrast and rapid onset led to increased latencies of VEP components in dyslexics. These patterns are supposed to be processed by a subdivision of the visual pathway that is called the magnocellular system. Moreover, Livingstone et al. reported anatomical abnormalities in the magnocellular layers of the lateral geniculate nucleus, but not in the parvocellular layers (which are presumed to be the complementary subsystem in the visual pathway).

Our results, of course, do not prove a direct correlation of left central brain electrical anomalies in VEP and structural anomalies in the same area of the brain. Nevertheless, the assumption is supported that at least in a subgroup of developmental dyslexics there is a dysfunction in those areas of the brain which are involved in the basic processing of visual information, and one component of this dysfunction could be a primary delay in processing visually presented stimuli.

## *Genetic Factors*

### *Family Studies*

Since the first descriptions, it was evident that dyslexia runs in families (Fisher, 1905; Hinshelwood, 1907; Thomas 1905). The first family studies contributed important observations about reading disability as problems in letter-naming, variation of the severity of the disorder in different family members, a relatively good efficiency in arithmetics in contrast to reading disability, and persistence of the spelling disorder in adulthood. Also, the connection between a familial pattern of dyslexia and a disorder in the acquisition of language was described (Orton, 1930) and replicated (Eustis, 1947).

Further observations from family studies were that a transmission of reading disability occurs across two or more generations and that the recurrence rate among first-degree relatives is between 30% to 70% irrespective of the chosen diagnostic criteria and sample ascertainment strategies (Finucci, Guthrie, Childs, Abbey, & Childs, 1976; Hallgren, 1950; Gilger, Pennington, & DeFries, 1991; Pennington et al., 1991; Vogler, DeFries, & Decker, 1985; Wolff & Melngailis, 1994; Zahalkova, Vrzal, & Klobouka, 1972). The familial aggregation was mainly found for reading and spelling, whereas the phenotype definition is based on the reading ability only. Analyses of single and extended German families showed a familial aggregation of spelling disability too (Schulte-Körne & Remschmidt, 1994). In a further study (Schulte-Körne, Deimel, Müller, Gutenbrunner, & Remschmidt, in press), we examined the familial aggregation of spelling disability in a sample of 32 probands. The diagnostic criteria were regression based IQ discrepancy and low achievement. The discrepancy between actual and expected spelling ability predicted based on IQ or age was one standard deviation or more. We found 52.3 % to 61.9% (depending on the chosen diagnostic criteria) affected siblings and 26% to 34% affected parents. A reason for the lower rate of affected parents could be the effect of compensation. Compensation means that adult spelling ability is improved during childhood, e.g. by remediation and tutoring at school. Affected children no longer fulfil the diagnostic criteria for spelling disability examined as an adult but severe spelling difficulties were reported during school. Regarding this compensation effect, we found 54% affected adults, including compensated adults (Schulte-Körne et al., 1996).

As genetic models for reading and spelling disability, an autosomal-dominant as well as a polygenic/multifactorial inheritance model were discussed. Recent segregation analyses of 204 families provided evidence for sex-influenced, additive or dominant transmission under the assumption of a prevalence of 7.5% and a male-to-female ratio of 1.8:1 in three or four samples (Pennington et al., 1991). Results obtained from the fourth sample provided evidence for a polygenetic model.

As a contribution to specificity, molecularbiological abnormalities associated with dyslexia could be a further step towards understanding the biological aetiology of dyslexia. We examined a family in which dyslexics had a retarded speech development and a balanced translocation (1;2) (Froster, Schulte-Körne, Hebebrand, & Remschmidt, 1993). All affected family members were severely spelling disabled, i.e. their actual spelling achievement was two standard deviations below the expected level given the child's grade. Interestingly, the affected family members had a severe expressive language disorder too. This coincidence suggests that genes important for dyslexia and/or retarded speech development might be linked to chromosome 1p22 and/or 2q31. Perhaps these candidate gene regions will be of special interest for a subtype of reading and spelling disability which is characterized by deficits in the language domain as well.

Results of linkage analyses support the existence of different candidate gene regions for reading and spelling disability. Smith, Kimberling, Pennington, and Lubs (1983) reported a linkage of reading disability to a region near the centromere of chromosome 15. Rabin, Wen, Hepburn, and Lubs (1993) reanalysed these pedigrees, which contributed to a great extent to the high lode score, and found no evidence for a linkage between reading disability and DNA markers on the proximal region of the short arm of chromosome 15. However, Rabin et al. (1993) found a loose linkage with protein marker Rh (1p34-p36) with reading disability. These results suggest that there might be loci on chromosome 1 which contribute to the reading and spelling phenotype.

Recently, Cardon et al. (1994) found a linkage of reading and spelling disability to quantitative trait loci on chromosome 6 (6p21.3) in a family sample. A replication of this result with a twin sample (Cardon et al., 1994) confirms the strong linkage results.

Moreover, when only the severely affected twins and siblings from these two samples are considered, the evidence for a QTL on chromosome 6 becomes even stronger. These results indicate that different chromosome regions could be of major interest in the further genetic analysis of reading and spelling disability. Also, different mutations might contribute to different phenotypes of reading and/or spelling disability.

### *Twin Studies*

Naturally, familial aggregation does not necessarily imply genetic transmission, since families also share the same environment and culture. The best experimental design to differentiate between genetic and environmental influences on reading and/or spelling disorders is provided by twin studies. The early twin studies (Bakwin, 1973; Hallgren, 1950; Hermann, 1956; Norrie, 1954) reported very high concordance rates which varied between 83 and 100 for monozygotic twins and between 29 and 35 in dizygotic twins. They were, however, criticized for several methodological shortcomings as regards the sample selection, the definition of reading disability, absence of controls for the cognitive level, and inadequate methods for determining zygosity. However, recent twin studies show clearly that there is a genetic factor. These studies looked for different functions such as spelling, word recognition, phonological and orthographic coding. A large-scale London twin study found a heritability for spelling of 0.75 after controlling for the individual differences in IQ (Stevenson, Graham, Fredman, & McLoughlin, 1987), and only a modest proportion of the variance in reading was explained by genetic effects. Another study by Gillis, DeFries, and Fulker (1992) found a high heritability for reading in a sample of reading disabled twin pairs ($h^2$ g = .78) and for a non-reading disabled control sample ($h^2$ g = .74).

Naturally, heritability for reading and spelling varies depending on the psychometric tests used and on different samples. Stevenson (1991) found a significantly higher heritability for spelling only (IQ-adjusted), while Olson, Wise, Conners, Rack, and Fulker (1989) found a high heritability for phonological coding which accounted for most of the heritable variance in the word recognition deficits. Orthographic coding was not found to be heritable and accounted for much of the environmental variance in the word recognition deficit. A question in terms of specificity is whether there are differences in heritability of reading deficits for individuals with higher versus lower IQs. Rack and Olson (1993) found that reading disabled children with high IQs had a word recognition deficit that was more heritable than subjects with lower IQs.

Two conclusions can be drawn. Firstly, that there is a genetic basis for reading and spelling ability; secondly, that different functions, such as phonological coding, which contribute to the overall ability of reading disorder or spelling disability, have to be examined instead of the very broad categories that have been used so far. Additionally, as shown by the twin studies, part of the variance in reading and spelling is due to environmental effects.

### *Long-term Course and Longitudinal Studies*

Longitudinal and follow-up studies indicate that dyslexia often persists into adulthood (Bruck, 1985; Finucci, Gottfredson, & Childs, 1985; LaBuda & DeFries, 1988; Maughan, 1995). The aim of follow-up studies is to determine whether the same pattern of deficits (word recognition, phonological awareness) persists into adulthood. If the same deficits are also found in adults, this would provide some evidence in support of the specificity hypothesis. Basically, there are two designs for studying the developmental lag or the specific deficit hypothesis:

- First, the children can be classified as dyslexic on the basis of childhood test performance and studied as a follow-up sample.
- Second, a sample of adults with known histories of childhood dyslexia can be examined.

The developmental aspects of specific deficits can only be examined by a follow-up design. As far as adult poor readers are concerned, the comparison with an age-matched control group as well as the comparison with reading level-matched young readers could give further information about a specific deficit. If adult dyslexics perform worse than both comparison groups, this result would imply that their deficits are not merely understandable as a developmental delay, but rather as the reflection of a persistent and specific deficit.

The analysis of recent longitudinal studies do not give a clear answer to the question of specificity. Bruck (1990) compared college students with a childhood diagnosis of reading disability with two control groups (an age-matched normal reading college students group and a second group of reading level-matched grade six children). She demonstrated that the word recognition deficits of dyslexics persist into adulthood. In comparison with the grade six reading level-matched children, the dyslexic adults were substantially slower in word recognition, but they made the same number of errors. A second important result of this study concerned the knowledge of spelling-sound correspondence. The dyslexics relied to a higher degree on this knowledge than did the age-matched controls and the reading level-matched children. The two control groups recognized highly familiar words more on the basis of visual-orthographic properties in contrast to the dyslexics who predominantly used their inadequate knowledge of spelling-sound correspondence for the recognition of highly familiar words. This result underlines the notion that adults who were diagnosed as dyslexic in childhood did not acquire an adequate knowledge of the correspondence between spelling and sound.

In a second study, Bruck (1992) examined the hypothesis of a specific deficit of phonological awareness by administering three different tasks: a syllable counting task, a phoneme counting and phoneme deletion task. All items were non-words and presented auditorally. In the first task, the dyslexics' performance was poorer than that of the age-matched adults, but equal to grade 2 and grade 3 children. The dyslexics' performance in the second and third task was poorer than that of the age-matched adults and the grade 3 children, but equal to the grade 2 children. There were also significant correlations between the phonological awareness measures and verbal intelligence. The data of this study support the idea that the role of a phonological awareness deficit might be a specific core symptom of dyslexia. Dyslexics do not acquire appropriate levels of phoneme awareness, regardless of their age or their reading levels. With regard to their processing strategy, dyslexics seem to continue with a strategy of word recognition, namely the spelling-sound correspondence, which is typical for beginning readers.

If one relates these results with the other important results from longitudinal studies, namely the high persistence of poor reading performance (Finucci et al., 1985; Scarborough, 1984), it could very well be that the phonological awareness deficit is one of the key variables characteristic for reading disability in general and for the persistence of this disorder in particular.

## CONCLUSIONS

If we come back to the initial question of this paper, we find that several possible indicators of specificity do not contribute much to the specificity issue. Children with specific reading or spelling disorder are not characterized by a clear symptomatology that could distinguish them from other kinds of reading and spelling disabilities. In addition, the sex distribution with a dominance of the male sex is not as impressive as was thought to be for many years. As far as comorbidity and social class are concerned, there are not many arguments in favour of the specificity hypothesis. Though some studies found that specific reading disorder is not correlated with lower social class, in contrast to specific language disorder and motor retardation.

Morphological correlates and several variables of brain dysfunction show, however, some patterns that might be specific for probands with specific reading disorder. Computerized tomography, MRI, and PET studies allow the conclusion that a high proportion of individuals with specific reading disorders do not show the classical functional asymmetry of the brain. They do seem to be less activated than controls in the left temporo-parietal regions. This finding is also in line with some studies on information processing and visually evoked potentials. As far as information processing of verbal material is concerned, dyslexics reveal a delayed pattern of information processing, show increased cognitive activation during reading performance, and are also characterized by a significant difference in comparison to a control group in simple visuo-motor reaction time. There are also interesting results in visually evoked potentials that might be looked upon as characteristic for at least a subgroup of children with specific reading disorder. Only a small proportion of dyslexics show a negative component of VEP between 110 and 115 msec after a stimulus onset in comparison to more than 80% of controls. The lack of this component was most prominent in those dyslexics whose spelling scores were more than 1.5 standard deviations below their intelligence score.

Family studies and twin studies demonstrate a strong genetic factor for specific reading and spelling disorder. It is, however, very difficult to compare the different studies, because they use different definitions and different samples. There is evidence that several candidate gene regions are associated with specific reading and spelling disorder. Although gene(s) defect(s) causing dyslexia or a specific subtype have not yet been identified, the isolation of a gene and the examination of the gene function could lead to an important understanding of the neuropathology of dyslexia.

Finally, studies on long-term course of specific reading disorder demonstrate a high persistence and give rise to the notion that a phonological awareness deficit might be a core symptom of specific reading disorder. It seems that dyslexics continue a processing strategy of word recognition which is typical for beginning readers. In other words, they are not able to develop other strategies that are based primarily on visual orthographic properties. This persistence of a basic deficit draws our attention to structural and functional studies in dyslexic children and adults, in order to detect different basic deficits that may be responsible for their lifelong poor achievement in reading and spelling.

We assumed that it is quite difficult to find specific deficits in dyslexics because the children considered as specific reading and spelling disordered might constitute a heterogeneous population consisting of different subtypes. Each subtype seemed to be homogeneous, e.g. dysphonetic vs. phonetic subtype regarding spelling errors, but the number of subtypes seems unclear.

Probably, for each subtype a different deficit factor can be postulated. For a visual-deficient subtype temporal processing deficits in the occipital lobe may be essential, for a phonological subtype, deficits in the temporo-parietal lobe may play an important role.

Genetic studies support this assumption of heterogeneity. However, no clear association of a specific dyslexic subtype with a genetic marker in a candidate region has been reported.

Finally, the specific reading and spelling disorder could represent the phenotype of different aetiologies. In that case, the attempt to find specific deficits in a population of many different subject samples of reading and spelling disabled children would be pointless.

Alternatively, the examination of specific subtypes could give further insight in to how the specific reading and spelling disorder develops. Therefore genetic analyses (family studies, linkage analyses) and neuro-imaging (MRT, CT) could make a major contribution to understanding how specific the deficits in specific reading and spelling disorders are.

## REFERENCES

American Psychiatric Association. (1980). *Diagnostic and statistical manual of mental disorders* (3rd. ed.). Washington, DC: APA.

American Psychiatric Association. (1987). *Diagnostic and statistical manual of mental disorders* (3rd. ed., rev.). Washington, DC: APA.

American Psychiatric Association. (1994). *Diagnostic and statistical manual of mental disorders* (4th. ed.). Washington, DC: APA.

Bakwin, H. (1973). Reading disability in twins. *Developmental Medicine and Child Neurology, 15*, 184-187.

Berkhan, O. (1885). Über die Schriftsprache bei Halbidioten und ihre Ähnlichkeit mit dem Stammeln. *Archiv für Psychiatry, 16*, 78-86.

Berkhan, O. (1886). Über die Störung der Schriftsprache bei Halbidioten und ihre Ähnlichkeit mit dem Sprachgebrechen, 2. Stammeln und Stottern. *Archiv für Psychiatry, 17*, 897-900.

Boder, E. (1973). Developmental dyslexia: A diagnostic approach based on three atypical reading spelling patterns. *Developmental Medicine and Child Neurology, 15*, 663-687.

Brandeis, D., Vitacco, D., & Steinhausen, H. C. (1994). Mapping brain electric micro-states in dyslexic children during reading. *Acta Paedopsychiatrica, 56*, 239-247.

Bruck, M. (1985). The adult functioning of children with specific learning disabilities. In I. Siegel (Ed.), *Advances in applied developmental psychology* (pp. 91-120). Norwood: Ablex.

Bruck, M. (1990). Word-recognition scales of adults with childhood diagnoses of dyslexia. *Developmental Psychology, 26*, 439-454.

Bruck, M. (1992). Persistence of dyslexics' phonological awareness deficits. *Developmental Psychology, 28*, 874-886.

Cardon, L. R., Smith, S. D., Fulker, D. W., Kimberling, W. J., Pennington, B. F., & DeFries, J. C. (1994). Quantitative trait locus for reading disability on chromosome 6. *Science, 226*, 276-279.

Conners, C. K. (1971). Cortical visual evoked response in children with learning-disorders. *Psychophysiology, 7*, 418-428.

Denckla, M. B. (1978). Critical review of "Electroencephalographic and neuro-physiological studies in dyslexia". In A. Benton & D. Pearl (Eds.), *An appraisal of current knowledge* (pp. 241-249). New York: Oxford University Press.

Eustis, R. S. (1947). The primary aetiology of specific language disorders. *Journal of Pediatrics, 31*, 448-455.

Finucci, J. M. & Childs, A. L. (1981). Are there really more dyslexic boys than girls? In A. Ansara, N. Geschwind, A. Galaburda, M. Albert, & N. Gartell (Eds.), *Sex differences in dyslexia* (pp. 1-9). Touson: The Orton Dyslexia Society.

Finucci, J. M., Guthrie, J. T., Childs, A. L., Abbey, H., & Childs, B. (1976). The genetics of specific reading disability. *Annual Review of Human Genetics, 40*, 1-23.

Finucci, J. M., Gottfredson, L. S., & Childs, B. (1985). A follow-up study of dyslexic boys. *Annals of Dyslexia, 35*, 117-136.

Fisher, I. (1905). Case of congenital word-blindness (inability to learn to read). *Ophthalmic Review, 24*, 315-318.

Flynn, J. M. & Rahbar, M. H. (1994). Prevalence of reading failure in boys compared with girls. *Psychology in the Schools, 31*, 66-71.

Fox, B. & Routh, D. K. (1983). Reading disability, phonemic analysis, and dysphonetic spelling: A follow-up study. *Journal of Clinical Child Psychology, 12*, 28-32.

Froster, U., Schulte-Körne, G., Hebebrand, J., & Remschmidt, H. (1993). Co-segregation of balanced translocation (1;2) with retarded speech development and dyslexia. *Lancet, 342*, 178-179.

Galaburda, A. M. (1985). Developmental dyslexia: A review of biological interactions. *Annals of Dyslexia, 35*, 21-33.

Galaburda, A. M. & Kemper, T. L. (1979). Cytoarchitectonic abnormalities in developmental dyslexia: A case study. *Annals of Neurology, 6*, 94-100.

Galaburda, A. M., Sherman, G. F., Rosen, G. D., Aboitiz, F., & Geschwind, N. (1985). Developmental dyslexia: Four consecutive patients with cortical anomalies. *Annals of Neurology, 18*, 222-233.

Geschwind, N. (1985). Biological foundations of reading. In F. H. Duffy & N. Geschwind (Eds.), *Dyslexia: A neuroscientific approach to clinical evaluation* (pp. 197-211). Boston: Little Brown.

Gilger, J. W., Pennington, B. F., & DeFries, J. C. (1991). Risk for reading disability as a function of parental history in three family studies. *Reading and Writing, 3*, 205-217.

Gillis, J. J., DeFries, J. C., & Fulker, D. W. (1992). Confirmatory factor analysis of reading and mathematics performance: A twin study. *Acta Genetica Med. Gemellol, 41*, 287-300.

Grissemann, H. (1974). *Die Legasthenie als Deutungsschwäche*. Bern: Huber.

Gross-Glenn, K., Duara, R., Barker, W. W., Loewenstein, D., Chang, J. Y., Yoshii, F., Apicella, A. M., Pascal, S., Boothe, T., Sevush, S., Jallad, B. J., Novoa, L., & Lubs, H. A. (1991). Positron emission tomographic studies during serial word-reading by normal and dyslexic adults. *Journal of Clinical and Experimental Neuropsychology, 13*, 531-544.

Hallgren, B. (1950). Specific dyslexia: A clinical and genetic study. *Acta Psychiatrica et Neurologica Scandinavica (Suppl. 65)*.

Harter, M. R., Anllo-Vento, L., & Wood, F. B. (1989). Event-related potentials, spatial orienting and reading disabilities. *Psychophysiology, 26*, 404-421.

Haslam, R. H., Dalby, J. T., Johns, R. D., & Rademaker, A. W. (1981). Cerebral asymmetry in developmental dyslexia. *Archives of Neurology, 38*, 679-682.

Hennighausen, K., Remschmidt, H., & Warnke, A. (1994). Visually evoked potentials in boys with developmental dyslexia. *European Child and Adolescent Psychiatry, 3*, 72-81.

Hermann, K. (1956). Congenital word-blindness. *Acta Psychiatrica et Neurologica Scandinavica (Suppl. 103)*, 1-138.

Hier, D. B., LeMay, M., Rosenberger, P. B., & Perlo, V. P. (1978). Developmental dyslexia: Evidence for a subgroup with reversal cerebral asymmetry. *Archives of Neurology, 35*, 90-92.

Hinshelwood, J. (1904). A kind of congenital word-blindness. *British Medical Journal, 2*, 1303-1304.

Hinshelwood, J. (1907). Four cases of congenital word-blindness occurring in the same family. *British Medical Journal, 2*, 1229-1232.

Holcomb, P. J., Ackerman, P. T., & Dykman, R. A. (1985). Cognitive event-related potentials in attention and reading deficits. *Psychophysiology, 22*, 656-667.

Humphreys, P., Kaufmann, W. E., & Galaburda, A. M. (1990). Developmental dyslexia in women: Neuropathological findings in three patients. *Annals of Neurology, 28*, 727-738.

Hynd, G. W., Semrud-Clikeman, M., Lorys, A. R., Novey, E. S., & Eliopulos, D. (1990). Brain morphology in developmental dyslexia and attention deficit disorder/hyperactivity. *Archives of Neurology, 47*, 919-926.

Johnstone, J., Galin, D., Fein, G., Yingling, C., Herron, J., & Marcus, M. (1984). Regional brain activity in dyslexic and control children during reading test: Visual probe event-related potentials. *Brain and Language, 21*, 233-254.

Jones, A. & Michie, P. T. (1986). Reading disability and cerebral lateralisation. In W. C. McCallum, R. Zappoli, & F. Denoth (Eds.), *Electroencephalography and clinical neurophysiology: Supplement Vol. 38. Cerebral psychophysiology: Studies in event-related potentials* (pp. 323-325). Amsterdam: Elsevier Science Publishers.

LaBuda, M. & DeFries, J. C. (1988). Cognitive abilities in children with reading disabilities and controls: A follow-up study. *Journal of Learning Disabilities, 21*, 562-566.

Landwehrmeyer, B., Gerling, J., & Wallesch, C. W. (1990). Patterns of taskrelated slow brain potentials. *Archives of Neurology, 47*, 791-797.

Larsen, J. P., Hoien, T., Lundberg, I., & Odegaard, H. (1990). MRI evaluation of the size and symmetry of the planum temporale in adolescents with developmental dyslexia. *Brain and Language, 39*, 289-310.

Lehmkuhle, S., Garzia, R. P., Turner, L., Hash, T., & Baro, J. A. (1993). A defective visual pathway in children with reading disability. *New England Journal of Medicine, 328*, 989-996.

Lennox, C. & Siegel, L. (1993). Visual and phonological spelling errors in subtypes of children with learning disabilities. *Applied Psycholinguistics, 14*, 473-488.

Leonard, C. M., Voeller, K. S., Lombardino, L. J., Morris, M. K., Hynd, G. W., Alexander, A. W., Andersen, H. G., Garofalakis, M., Honeyman, J. C., Mao, J., Agee, F., & Staab, E. V. (1993). Anomalous cerebral structure in dyslexia revealed with magnetic resonance imaging. *Archives of Neurology, 50*, 461-469.

Lewis, C., Hitch, G. J., & Walker, P. (1994). The prevalence of specific arithmetic difficulties and specific reading difficulties in 9- to 10- year old boys and girls. *Journal of Child Psychology and Psychiatry, 35*, 283-292.

Livingstone, M. S., Rosen, G. D., Drislane, & Galaburda, A. M. (1991). Physiological and anatomical evidence for a magnocellular defect in developmental dyslexia. *Proceedings of the National Academy of Science, USA, 88*, 7943-7947.

Martinius, J. (1976). Untersuchungen zur zentralen Aktivierung bei leistungsschwachen und gesunden Kindern. In G. Nissen, & F. Specht (Eds.), *Psychische Gesundheit und Schule* (pp. 117-124). Neuwied: Luchterhand.

Masland, R. L. (1981). Neurological aspects of dyslexia. In G. Th. Pavlidis & T. R. Miles (Eds.), *Dyslexia research and its implications to education* (pp. 35-36). New York: Wiley.

Maughan, B. (1995). Annotation: Long-term outcomes of developmental reading problems. *Journal of Child Psychology and Psychiatry, 36*, 357-371.

May, J. G., Lovegrove, W. J., Martin, F., & Nelson, P. (1991). Pattern-elicited visual evoked potentials in good and poor readers. *Clinical Vision Science, 6*, 131-136.

Morgan, W. P. (1896). A case of congenital word-blindness. *British Medical Journal, 2*, 1378.

Norrie, E. (1954). Ordblindhednes (Dyslexiens) aregang. *Laesepaedagogen, 2*, 61.

Olson, R. K., Wise, B., Conners, F., Rack, J. C., & Fulker, D. W. (1989). Specific deficits in component reading and language skills: Genetic and environmental influences. *Journal of Learning Disabilities, 22*, 339-349.

Orton, S. T. (1930). Familial occurrence of disorders in the acquisition of languages. *Eugenics, 3*, 140-147.

Pennington, B. F., Gilger, J., Pauls, D., Smith, S. A., Smith, S. D., & DeFries, J. C. (1991). Evidence for a major gene transmission in developmental dyslexia. *Journal of the American Medical Association, 18*, 1527-1534.

Preston, M. S., Guthrie, J. T., & Childs, B. (1974). Visual evoked responses (VERs) in normal and disabled readers. *Psychophysiology, 11*, 452-457.

Rabin, M., Wen, X. L., Hepburn, M., & Lubs, H. A. (1993). Suggestive linkage of developmental dyslexia to chromosome 1p34-p36. *Lancet, 342*, 178.

Rack, J. P. & Olson, R. K. (1993). Phonological deficits, IQ, and individual differences in reading disability: Genetic and environmental influences. *Developmental Review, 13*, 269-278.

Remschmidt, H. (1987). Was sind Teilleistungsschwächen? *Monatsschrift für Kinderheilkunde, 135*, 290-296.

Remschmidt, H. & Warnke, A. (1992). Visual information processing and cerebral activation in dyslexic boys: Quantitative EEG analysis during discrimination reading tasks. *European Child and Adolescent Psychiatry, 1*, 42-53.

Rumsey, J. M., Andreason, P., Zametkin, A. J., Aquino, T., King, C., Hamburger, S. D., Picus, A., Rapoport, J. L., & Cohen, R. M. (1992). Failure to activate the left temporoparietal cortex in dyslexia. *Archives of Neurology, 49*, 527-534.

Rutter, M.. Shaffer, D., & Sturge, C. (1976). *A guide to a multi-axial classification scheme for psychiatric disorders in childhood and adolescence.* Institute of Psychiatry, London.

Rutter, M. & Yule, W. (1975). The concept of specific reading retardation. *Journal of Child Psychology and Psychiatry, 16*, 181-197.

Scarborough, H. S. (1984). Continuity between childhood dyslexia and adult reading. *British Journal of Psychology, 75*, 329-348.

Schulte-Körne, G. & Remschmidt, H. (1994). Genetic aspects of dyslexia. In F. Poustka (Ed.), *Basic approaches to genetics in developmental psychiatry* (pp. 163-173). Berlin: Quintessenz Verlag.

Schulte-Körne, G., Deimel, W., Müller, K., Gutenbrunner, C., & Remschmidt, H. (1996). Familial aggregation of spelling disability. *Journal of Child Psychology and Psychiatry, 37*, 817-823.

Shaywitz, S. E., Shaywitz, B. A., Fletcher, J. M., & Escobar, M. D. (1990). Prevalence of reading disability in boys and girls: Results of the Conneticut longitudinal study. *Journal of the American Medical Association, 264*, 9981002.

Smith, S. D., Kimberling, W. J., Pennington, B. F., & Lubs, H. A. (1983). Specific reading disability: Identification of an inherited form through linkage analysis. *Science, 219*, 1345-1348.

Sobotka, K. R. & May, J. G. (1977). Visual evoked potentials and reaction time in normal and dyslexic children. *Psychophysiology, 14*, 18-24.

Steinmetz, S. E. & Galaburda, A. M. (1991). Planum temporale asymmetry: In vivo morphometry affords a new perspective for neuro-behavioural research. *Reading and Writing, 3*, 331-343.

Stelmack, R. M., Saxe, B. J., Hondy-Cullum, N., Campbell, K. B., & Armitage, R. (1988). Recognition memory for words and event-related potentials: A comparison of normal and disabled readers. *Journal of Clinical and Experimental Neuropsychology, 10*, 185-200.

Stevenson, J. (1991). Which aspects of processing text mediate genetic effects? *Reading and Writing, 3*, 249-169.

Stevenson, J., Graham, P., Fredman, G., & McLoughlin, V. (1987). A twin study of genetic influences on reading and spelling ability and disability. *Journal of Child Psychology and Psychiatry, 28*, 229-247.

Symann-Louett, N., Gascon, G. G., Matsumiya, Y., & Lombroso, C.T. (1977). Wave form difference in visual evoked responses between normal and reading disabled children. *Neurology, 27*, 156-159.

Taylor, M. J. & Keenan, N. K. (1990). Event-related potentials to visual and language stimuli in normal and dyslexic children. *Psychophysiology, 27*, 318-327.

Thomas, C. I. (1905). Congenital word-blindness and its treatment. *Ophthalmoscope, 3*, 380-385.

Vogler, G. P., DeFries, J. C., & Decker, S. N. (1985). Family history as an indicator of risk for reading disability. *Journal of Learning Disabilities, 18*, 419-421.

Weber, B. A. & Omenn, G. S. (1977). Auditory and visual evoked responses in children with familial reading disabilities. *Journal of Learning Disabilities, 10*, 32-37.

Whiting, S. A. & Jarrico, S. (1980). Spelling patterns of normal readers. *Journal of Learning Disabilities, 13*, 45-47.

Wolff, P. H. & Melngailis, L. (1994). Family patterns of developmental dyslexia: Clinical findings. *American Journal of Medical Genetics (Neuropsychiatry Genetics), 54*, 122-131.

World Health Organization. (1992). *The ICD-10 classification of mental and behavioural disorders: Clinical descriptions and diagnostic guidelines*. Geneva: World Health Organization.

Zahalkova, M., Vrzal, V., & Klobouka, E. (1972). Genetic investigations in dyslexia. *Journal of Medical Genetics, 9*, 48-52.22

KEITH E. STANOVICH AND LINDA S. SIEGEL

# THE ROLE OF IQ IN THE DIAGNOSIS OF READING DISORDERS:

# THE QUEST FOR A SUBTYPE BASED ON APTITUDE/ACHIEVEMENT DISCREPANCY

## INTRODUCTION

In the history of the reading field, the quest to identify subtypes of reading disability has been as enticing as it has been futile. There is enormous face validity to the idea that poor readers differ among themselves in the way they have become poor readers and in the cognitive underpinnings of their disability. Yet the field has failed to progress beyond step one in defining separable groups of disabled readers - that is, subgroups who are behaviourally, genetically, and physiologically different from other poor readers.

One reason is that in the early history of the field the definition of reading disability or dyslexia was tied to the notion of aptitude/achievement discrepancy (Ceci, 1986; Reynolds, 1985; Shepard, 1980; Siegel, 1989; Stanovich, 1991a, 1993b; see Rispens, this volume). One might have thought that researchers would have begun with the broadest and most theoretically neutral definition of reading disability - reading performance below some specified level on some well-known and psychometrically sound test - and then proceeded to investigate whether there were poor readers with differing cognitive profiles within this broader group. What happened instead was that the discrepancy notion became so quickly reified in practice that researchers often culled so-called garden-variety poor readers (see Gough & Tunmer, 1986) from their samples in order to attain "purer groups", thus precluding the critical comparison of poor readers with and without aptitude/achievement discrepancy.

As a result, for many years, most investigations of reading disabilities provided no information on the field's foundational assumption about subtypes: that degree of discrepancy from IQ was meaningful in the sense that the reading difficulties of the reading disabled child with IQ discrepancy were aetiologically and neurologically distinct from those characterizing the reading disabled child without IQ discrepancy. Rutter and Yule's (1975) ground-breaking



*J. Rispens et al. (eds.),*
*Perspectives on the Classification of Specific Developmental Disorders,* 105–136.

investigation of differences between discrepant and garden-variety children stood alone for over a decade before being joined by other investigations (Fletcher et al., 1989; Fletcher, Francis, Rourke, Shaywitz, & Shaywitz, 1992; Fletcher et al., 1994; Jorm, Share, Maclean, & Matthews, 1986; Pennington, Gilger, Olson, & DeFries, 1992; B. A. Shaywitz, Fletcher, Holahan, & Shaywitz, 1992; Siegel, 1988, 1989, 1992; Stanovich & Siegel, 1994).

Much attention has focused on the issue of whether there is a statistically discernible "hump" in the lower tail of the distribution of reading ability. Rutter and Yule (1975) found evidence for such a hump (see also Stevenson, 1988), but others have not (Rodgers, 1983; S. E. Shaywitz, Escobar, Shaywitz, Fletcher, & Makugh, 1992). Resolving the "hump issue", however, will not give the definitive answer to the distinct aetiology question because, even if such a hump is not found, "a few aetiologically distinct factors, plus noise, can give rise to a normal phenotypic distribution" (Pennington et al., 1992, p. 563).

Genetic epidemiology provides a sounder basis for establishing distinct causation for some cases of reading disability. Here the evidence is more definitive. In several samples, Pennington, Gilger, et al. (1991) found evidence for sex-limited, autosomal additive or dominant transmission of reading disability, although there is evidence for genetic heterogeneity (see Pennington, 1990; Smith, Kimberling, & Pennington, 1991; Stevenson, 1992a). Cardon and colleagues (Cardon et al., 1994) recently reported a quantitative trait locus for reading disability on chromosome 6.

Additionally, twin studies have also consistently indicated a moderate heritability for the group deficit in reading ability displayed by the twin probands - as well as significant genetic covariance between the group deficit and phonological coding and awareness skills (DeFries, Fulker, & LaBuda, 1987; Olson, Wise, Conners, Rack, & Fulker, 1989; Pennington et al., 1992; Stevenson, 1992a, 1992b). Pennington, Van Orden, Kirson, and Haith (1991) summarize the evidence: "These behaviour genetic analyses are consistent with the view that the heritable component in dyslexia at the written language level is in phonological coding and the heritable precursor to this deficit in phonological coding is a deficit in phoneme awareness" (p. 183).

Further evidence that reading disability might have distinct aetiology comes from neuro-anatomical studies (see Hynd, Marshall, & Gonzalez, 1991 and Hynd, Marshall, & Semrud-Clikeman, 1991 for reviews). For example, both post mortem and in-vivo studies have indicated that atypical brain symmetries are associated with reading disability (Galaburda, 1991; Galaburda, Sherman, Rosen, Aboitz, & Geschwind, 1985; Larsen, Hoien, Lundberg, & Odegaard, 1990; Steinmetz & Galaburda, 1991). Larsen et al. (1990) found that the atypical symmetry was directly associated with the phonological coding deficit that is the primary phenotypic indicator of reading disability (see below). Additional cortical anomalies have been identified in other studies reviewed by Hynd, Marshall, and Gonzales (1991) and Galaburda (1994; see also Semrud-Clikeman, Hynd, Novey, & Eliopulos, 1991).

Thus, there is some support for a distinct aetiology for at least some cases of reading disability. Reading difficulty appears to be moderately heritable. At least some cases of reading difficulty appear to be genetically influenced. Some cases also appear to be associated with distinct neuro-anatomical anomalies. All of these findings provide a foundation for a principled concept of subtypes of dyslexia, but they are not - in and of themselves - enough to justify using discrepancy measurement as a first pass method of identifying poor reader subtypes. There is still one critical link missing in the chain of evidence. Specifically, there was, until quite recently, little evidence that degree of IQ reading discrepancy was differentially related to the primary phenotypic indicators of dyslexia.

## AN ANALYTIC METHOD FOR EXAMINING THE PROCESSING PROFILES OF READING DISABLED CHILDREN

One way to address the question of whether reading disabled children (however defined) are different from nondisabled children in developmental sequence is by examining cognitive profiles in a reading-level match design. The reading-level (RL) match design is one in which an older group of reading disabled children is compared with a younger group of nondisabled children who are matched on reading level (Backman, Mamen, & Ferguson, 1984; Bisanz, Das, & Mancini, 1984; Bradley & Bryant, 1978; Guthrie, 1973; Snowling, 1980). In the mid-1980s this design underwent a dramatic increase in popularity because it is more selective than the traditional chronological age (CA) match design in isolating processing differences between reading disabled and nondisabled children. When reading disabled children are compared with CA controls, it is well known that they display significant differences on a multiplicity of tasks (vocabulary, syntactic knowledge, metalinguistic awareness, verbal short-term memory, inferential comprehension, semantic memory, and verbal fluency form only a partial list; see Share & Stanovich, 1995; Siegel, 1993; Siegel & Ryan, 1988; Stanovich, 1986a, 1992; Stanovich & Cunningham, 1991; Vellutino & Scanlon, 1987), thereby reducing the diagnosticity of any single difference (Bryant & Goswami, 1986; Goswami & Bryant, 1989). A particular difference in a CA design is thus open to an unusually large number of alternative explanations (Bryant & Goswami, 1986), including the very real possibility that the processing difference is the result of the different reading experiences of the two groups (Stanovich, 1986b, 1993a). In contrast, the number of tasks on which reading disabled children display deficits relative to RL controls is much smaller. Additionally, any differences that are observed cannot be the result of differences in reading ability between the groups because the design eliminates such differences.

Nevertheless, viewed as a diagnostic tool to test whether a particular variable is causally linked to reading disability - in other words, when viewed as a sort of quasi-experiment - the RL design is fraught with methodological and statistical complications (Goswami & Bryant, 1989; Jackson & Butterfield, 1989). For example, regression artifacts are particularly prone to obscure inferences about single variables (see Jackson & Butterfield, 1989). The previous focus on the design as a kind of quasi-experimental method to test a causal hypothesis about a single variable (e.g. Backman et al., 1984; Bradley & Bryant, 1978; Bryant & Goswami, 1986) seems to have been misplaced (see Jackson & Butterfield, 1989). However, as a context for the comparison of cognitive profiles in a multivariate study, the design can still be of great utility (e.g. Bowey, Cain, & Ryan, 1992; Olson, Wise, Conners, & Rack, 1990; Siegel & Ryan, 1988; Stanovich, Nathan, & Zolman, 1988; Vellutino & Scanlon, 1987, 1989). For example, it provides one way to operationalize the question of whether readers progressing at different rates are going through the same developmental stages. If they are, then relationships among cognitive subskills should be the same for older disabled readers as they are for younger nondisabled readers at the same reading level. Any imbalance in cognitive subskills that appears when the two groups are compared is an indication that they must be reaching their similar levels of reading skills in different ways. Provided there is independent evidence from other types of designs indicating that the skills examined in the multivariate profile are indeed linked to reading ability, then mismatched cognitive profiles in an RL study are an empirical indication that the developmental paths by which the two groups came to their similar reading levels must be different. Note that this outcome is agnostic regarding the issue of what might be the cause of the different developmental paths - of which there may be many alternative explanations.

However, there remain obstacles to using the RL design for even the more modest purpose proposed here. It is difficult for many investigators to procure enough matched subjects at any one age level to insure a powerful statistical test. This forces many investigators to collapse subjects across rather wide age ranges (e.g. Snowling, Stackhouse, & Rack, 1986), introducing possibly confounding variability. Problems with subject procurement have precluded most investigators from examining RL matches at more than one reading level (see Bisanz et al., 1984; Siegel & Ryan, 1988; Szeszulski & Manis, 1987, for exceptions) and almost never have investigators included both IQ-discrepant and nondiscrepant poor readers in reading-level studies. The latter is a particularly important missing dimension in investigations of reading disability.

Recently, we introduced an analytic logic that removes many of the statistical artifacts of matched-groups RL designs and that allows investigators to use subjects over a wide range of reading levels while still attaining the empirical comparison that is the desired result of the traditional RL design (see Stanovich & Siegel, 1994). Our solution was to reconceptualize the entire logic of the RL design into the continuous framework of regression analysis. Other investigators have suggested reformulating RL designs within a continuous framework (Bryant & Goswami, 1986; Jackson & Butterfield, 1989; Mamen, Ferguson, & Backman, 1986), but, to our knowledge, no investigation has used the procedure described here.

The analyses to be presented will utilize an amalgamated data base consisting of data from children who participated in several previously published studies and data from new, unpublished studies. The total amalgamated sample consisted of over 1500 children, aged 7 to 16 years. Some of the children were from schools in southern Ontario and were tested in their schools. Others came to a psycho-educational assessment clinic in order to participate in studies of reading-related cognitive processes. The participants were predominantly middle class and less than 2% were non Caucasian. All were being educated in English, and had English as their major language. Children with neurological problems, English as a second language, severe behavioural deficits, and sensory deficits were excluded from the sample.

From this sample, we selected all children who were reading at grade levels 1 through 5 on the Wide Range Achievement Test.

These 907 children were classified into one of three categories: not reading disabled (NRD) if their percentile score on the WRAT was ≥ 30; reading disabled discrepant (RD-D) if their percentile score on the WRAT was ≤ 25 and their IQ was > 90; and reading disabled not discrepant (RD-N) if their percentile score on the WRAT was ≤ 25 and their IQ was ≤ 90. This classification procedure - an absolute IQ cut-off - is of course the simplest possible procedure for defining discrepancy. However, different methods of discrepancy definition - for example, standard-score discrepancy or regression discrepancy procedures - can easily be incorporated into the analysis and, in this case, result in exactly the same pattern of findings (see below). One advantage of this analytic method is that it is easily adapted in order to accommodate different methods of discrepancy measurement.

Table 1 displays the mean WRAT percentile score, IQ, and age in months for each of the three groups at each of the five WRAT reading levels. From the Table it is clear that the NRD group is performing nearly average for their age whereas the RD-D and RD-N are both performing substantially below expectation for their chronological age (roughly around the 10th percentile). The NRD and RD-D groups have near normal IQs that are substantially higher than those of the RD-N group which averages slightly below 80. The RD-D and RD-N groups are over two years older than the NRD groups matched to them on reading-level.

The analytic strategy proceeds as follows: for each criterion variable, the performance of all three groups across all five reading levels is examined together in one simultaneous regression equation in which WRAT grade level and two contrasts are entered as predictors. The analysis begins by partialling from the criterion variable the linear trend of WRAT reading level and all significant higher-order trends. Entering WRAT reading grade level removes all of the variance in the criterion variable that is associated with overall reading level - a procedure that simulates, statistically, the RL matching procedure. After the variance associated with WRAT reading level is extracted, two contrasts are entered simultaneously into the regression equation: one contrast capturing the reading disabled versus nondisabled comparison and the other the RD-D versus RD-N comparison. The coding for the former contrast is +1 for RD-N and RD-D children and -1 for NRD children. A positive beta weight for this contrast indicates that the reading disabled children outperform the nondisabled children on the variable when the effects of WRAT Reading level and the other contrast are partialed. A significant negative beta weight is analogous to a deficit in the more traditional matched-group RL design.

The second contrast reflects the comparison between nondiscrepant and discrepant disabled readers. The coding for this contrast is +1 for the RD-N group, -1 for the RD-D group, and 0 for the NRD children. A positive beta weight for this contrast indicates that the RD-N children outperform the RD-D children on the variable in question when the effects of reading level and the other contrast are partialed.

TABLE 1

Mean WRAT reading percentile, IQ, and age for the samples of nondisabled (NRD) children, reading disabled children with IQ discrepancy (RD-D) and reading disabled children without IQ discrepancy (RD-N) as a function of reading grade level on the WRAT.

| Variable | NRD | RD-D | RD-N |
|---|---|---|---|
| **WRAT percentile** | | | |
| Reading Grade Level 1 | 40.7 (3) | 5.0 (85) | 5.5 (28) |
| Reading Grade Level 2 | 47.0 (56) | 10.2 (114) | 6.8 (49) |
| Reading Grade Level 3 | 52.8 (89) | 14.8 (66) | 11.1 (49) |
| Reading Grade Level 4 | 55.9 (134) | 14.1 (50) | 9.6 (24) |
| Reading Grade Level 5 | 61.4 (117) | 15.3 (26) | 12.3 (17) |
| **IQ score** | | | |
| Reading Grade Level 1 | 106.7 (3) | 106.5 (85) | 73.3 (28) |
| Reading Grade Level 2 | 104.2 (56) | 107.0 (114) | 78.9 (49) |
| Reading Grade Level 3 | 102.8 (89) | 102.6 (66) | 79.2 (49) |
| Reading Grade Level 4 | 105.2 (134) | 101.8 (50) | 76.5 (24) |
| Reading Grade Level 5 | 104.7 (117) | 104.3 (26) | 81.4 (17) |
| **Age in months** | | | |
| Reading Grade Level 1 | 91.7 (3) | 98.0 (85) | 101.1 (28) |
| Reading Grade Level 2 | 91.0 (56) | 112.5 (114) | 121.1 (49) |
| Reading Grade Level 3 | 102.5 (89) | 130.5 (66) | 139.1 (49) |
| Reading Grade Level 4 | 112.3 (134) | 147.1 (50) | 157.5 (24) |
| Reading Grade Level 5 | 120.5 (117) | 158.5 (26) | 168.4 (17) |

Note: The number of subjects in each group is indicated in parentheses.

Results consistent with a developmental lag model of reading acquisition would be indicated by a significant beta weight for WRAT Reading level but not for either of the contrasts. This would be an indication that overall reading level is associated with performance on the criterion variable, but not how quickly the subject attained that reading level (the RD-D and RD-N versus NRD contrast) nor by the level of intelligence of the poor reading groups (RD-D versus RD-N). Such a pattern is consistent with the prediction of the developmental lag model that subject classification should be irrelevant once the reading level of the subject is taken into account.

Conversely, if either of the contrasts is significant in the simultaneous equation from which WRAT Reading level has been partialed, then this would falsify the prediction of the developmental lag model by indicating that the criterion variable is associated with something more than reading level alone - in this case, either how quickly the subject attained that reading level (RD-D and RD-N versus NRD), the level of intelligence of the poor reading groups (RD-D versus RD-N), or both.

This continuous, regression-based equivalent of the reading level design has several advantages as an analytic strategy. First, the logistical advantage of allowing subjects to be collapsed across several reading levels because there is no necessity to create a matched group at each reading level to be examined. Second, increased representativeness of the samples because case-by-case matching of subgroups on reading level is not required. Third, freedom from the regression confounds that plague the traditional matched extreme-groups RL design. Previous investigations utilizing the reading-level design have been precluded from employing the discrepant/nondiscrepant criterion in part because the selection requirements of an additional category often prohibitively increase the number of matched subjects that the investigator must procure from a single grade level. This analytic strategy allows the investigator to more easily embed a comparison between RD-D and RD-N children into their reading-level designs. In our methodology, the comparison between RD-D and RD-N children is simply created by analyzing the independent contribution of an additional vector that is entered into the regression equation along with the basic contrast between reading disabled and nondisabled children.

## ILLUSTRATING THE METHOD: ARITHMETIC PERFORMANCE

In order to demonstrate the logic of the analytic technique, we will examine a criterion variable on which we might expect both contrasts to be significant. The variable is performance on the Arithmetic subtest of the Wide Range Achievement Test. Table 2 displays the mean WRAT Arithmetic grade equivalent scores for each of the three groups at each of the five WRAT reading levels. It can be seen that there is a tendency for the older RD-D and RD-N groups at each of the reading levels to outperform the younger NRD group on arithmetic. Furthermore, there is a slight tendency for the RD-D group to outperform the lower-IQ RD-N group.

TABLE 2

WRAT arithmetic grade level means for the samples of nondisabled (NRD) children, reading disabled children with IQ discrepancy (RD-D) and reading disabled children without IQ discrepancy (RD-N) as a function of reading grade level on the WRAT.

| Variable | NRD | RD-D | RD-N |
|---|---|---|---|
| **Arithmetic grade level (WRAT)** | | | |
| Reading Grade Level 1<br>(22) | 1.7 (3) | 1.8 (81) | 1 . 5 |
| Reading Grade Level 2<br>(34) | 2.1 (42) | 2.8 (91) | 2 . 2 |
| Reading Grade Level 3<br>(33) | 2.7 (67) | 3.8 (42) | 3 . 5 |
| Reading Grade Level 4<br>(17) | 3.3 (80) | 4.4 (43) | 3 . 4 |
| Reading Grade Level 5<br>(14) | 3.7 (74) | 4.9 (24) | 4 . 4 |

Both of these tendencies are reflected in the results of the regression analysis conducted on the WRAT arithmetic scores. The linear component of WRAT reading level attained a multiple R of .572 when entered as the first predictor. There was also a significant quadratic trend ($F(1, 664) = 13.1$, $p < .001$) which raised the multiple R to .583. Although WRAT Reading grade level accounted for most of the explained variance in WRAT Arithmetic scores, both contrasts had significant beta weights when entered simultaneously after WRAT Reading level. The positive sign on the beta weight for the RD versus NRD contrast (.278, $F(1, 662) = 68.8$, $p < .001$) indicates that the older reading disabled children outperformed the younger nondisabled children on arithmetic even when the effect of WRAT Reading level is controlled (as well as the other contrast). The negative sign on RD-N versus RD-D contrast (-.124, $F(1, 662) = 16.28$, $p < .001$) indicates that the RD-D children outperformed the RD-N children when the effects of

WRAT Reading levels (and the other contrast) are controlled. The latter trend is fairly small in absolute magnitude (accounting for just 1.5% unique variance) but was detected statistically because of the large sample size (N = 667) in this particular analysis.

## PSEUDOWORD READING AND SPELLING

TABLE 3

Regression results for the pseudoword reading and spelling tasks.

| Dependent variable | 1. | 2. | 3. | 4. | 5. |
|---|---|---|---|---|---|
| | | | *Multiple R* | | |
| WRAT grade level | .618** | .807** | .727** | .751* | .751** |
| Quadratic fit | NS | NS | .733** | .802** | .773** |
| | | | *beta weight in final equation* | | |
| RD vs. NRD contrast | -.226** | -.145** | -.175** | -.206** | -.252** |
| RD-N vs. RD-D contrast | .068 | -.033 | -.098** | -.091* | -.044 |
| | | | *unique variance explained* | | |
| RD vs. NRD contrast | .048 | .019 | .023 | .034 | .050 |
| RD-N vs. RD-D contrast | .005 | .001 | .008 | .008 | .002 |
| | | | *F ratio in final equation* | | |
| RD vs. NRD contrast | 13.06 | 9.52 | 26.20 | 19.27 | 26.06 |
| RD-N vs. RD-D contrast | 1.21 | 0.50 | 9.87 | 4.24 | 0.89 |
| | | | *sample size* | | |
| N | 158 | 163 | 497 | 191 | 189 |

Dependent variables:
1 = GFW pseudoword spelling
2 = GFW pseudoword reading
3 = Woodcock Word Attack
4 = experimental pseudowords 1
5 = experimental pseudowords 2

* $p < .05$
** $p < .01$
NS = not significant

We now turn to criterion variables more directly relevant to theories of reading disability. One of the most well replicated findings in reading disability research is that, compared to chronological-age controls, reading disabled children have difficulty pronouncing pseudowords. It has been more difficult to determine whether they display deficits compared to reading-level controls, but the meta-analysis by Rack, Snowling, and Olson (1992) appears to indicate that this is the case. Whether this finding applies to RD-N poor readers as well as RD-D children is less well established. Our battery of tasks contained five measures of pseudoword reading and spelling and the results of the regression analyses conducted on these tasks are displayed in Table 3

Not surprisingly, WRAT reading level was the dominant predictor in all of the analyses. However, in all five of the analyses the RD versus NRD contrast had a significant negative beta weight, indicating that the older reading disabled children underperformed the younger nondisabled children. There was a consistent tendency for the two reading disabled groups to perform less well than the NRD group at all reading levels and on all the tasks. In contrast, there were few systematic differences between the RD-D and RD-N groups. Only two of the RD-N versus RD-D contrasts attained significance (Woodcock Word Attack and experimental pseudowords 1). The negative beta weight on this contrast indicated that the RD-D children outperformed the RD-N children.

However, the beta weight was small in absolute magnitude (-.098 and -.091, respectively), and this contrast accounted for only 0.8% unique variance after the variance explained by WRAT reading level and the other contrast had been extracted. Overall, although there was a consistent tendency for reading disabled children to underperform statistically matched RL-controls on pseudoword tasks, the pseudoword processing differences between reading disabled children with average IQs and those with low IQs were either small or nonexistent.

## FURTHER TESTS OF PHONOLOGICAL CODING SKILL

There were two further tests of phonological coding skill in our battery -the phonological choice task introduced by Olson, Kliegl, Davidson, and Foltz (1985) and the Gates-McKillop pseudoword recognition test. In the former, the subject viewed pairs of pseudowords (e.g. kake-dake, joak-joap) and indicated which pseudoword sounded like a real word when pronounced. In the latter, a nonword such as "wiskate" is read to the child who is then asked to select the correct version of the word from among four printed choices (iskate, wiskay, wiskate, and whestit). These tasks are different from the previous pseudoword tasks in that they do not require overt production of a pronunciation or a spelling. In a sense, these two tasks require less depth of phonological processing. If it is assumed that there is a continuum of tasks that reflect depth of phonological processing and that the deeper the processing, the larger will be the deficits of reading disabled children, then it might be expected that group differences would be smaller on these tasks.

TABLE 4

Regression results for the phonological coding tasks.

| | Dependent variables 1. | 2. |
|---|---|---|
| | *multiple R* | |
| WRAT grade level | .605** | .749** |
| Quadratic fit | NS | .786** |
| Cubic fit | NS | .812** |
| | *beta weight in final equation* | |
| RD vs. NRD contrast | -.066 | -.021 |
| RD-N vs. RD-D contrast | -.014 | -.041 |
| | *unique variance explained* | |
| RD vs. NRD contrast | .005 | .000 |
| RD-N vs. RD-D contrast | .000 | .002 |
| | *F ratio in final equation* | |
| RD vs. NRD contrast | 1.06 | 0.11 |
| RD-N vs. RD-D contrast | 0.06 | 0.44 |
| | *sample size* | |
| N | 209 | 96 |

Dependent variables:
1 = phonological choice task
2 = pseudoword recognition

* p < 05
** p < .01
NS = not significant

As Table 4 indicates, for the phonological choice task, only the linear component of the WRAT scores was statistically significant. When the two contrasts were entered into the regression equation, neither the RD versus NRD contrast (-.066) nor the RD-N versus RD-D contrast (-.014) were statistically significant. Similar results obtained for the pseudoword recognition task. Here, both quadratic and cubic trends of the WRAT reading scores were significant (multiple R = .812). However, when the two contrasts were entered into the regression equation, neither the RD versus NRD contrast

(-.021) nor the RD-N versus RD-D contrast (-.041) were statistically significant. Thus, unlike the case with pseudoword reading, performance level on these two tasks is a function of reading level only and the rate of acquiring a given reading level (or the IQ of the poor reader groups) is not related to performance. In contrast, on pseudo-word reading and spelling tasks where an overt production of the stimulus is required, disabled children display a deficit compared with RL controls. This finding is consistent with the view that the deeper the phonological coding that is required in the task, the larger the deficit displayed by reading disabled children compared to reading- level controls. In neither type of task were there substantial differences in the performance of RD-D and RD-N children.

## TESTS OF ORTHOGRAPHIC CODING SKILL

Some previous research has suggested that reading disabled children are relatively less impaired at orthographic coding than at phonological coding (Frith & Snowling, 1983; Holligan & Johnston, 1988; Olson et al., 1985; Pennington et al., 1986; Rack, 1985; Snowling, 1980). However, it is still unclear whether disabled children display an actual superiority in orthographic processing compared with reading-level controls or whether their impairment in this domain is simply less severe compared to their phonological coding deficit. If pseudoword naming is indicative of a processing subskill that contributes to the ability to recognize words, and if reading disabled children perform more poorly than RL controls on this task, then they must have some other processing superiority that allows them to attain equivalent levels of word recognition. In order to test whether orthographic coding is indeed the compensatory mechanism, we examined performance on three different measures of orthographic coding skill: two spelling recognition measures (one a four alternative task from the PIAT and the other a two alternative choice task modeled on the work of Olson et al., 1985) and a wordlikeness choice task. In the latter task, the subject was shown two nonword strings (e.g. filv-filk, lund-dlun). They are told that neither string looks or sounds like an actual word but that one letter string is more like a word. One member of each pair contains an orthographic sequence that never occurs in English in that particular position in a word (e.g. filv, dlun). The subject's score is the number of times that the nonword without the illegal or low frequency letter string was chosen. Although this task undoubtedly implicates phonological coding to some extent, the coding of frequent and infrequent orthographic sequences in memory should be a substantial contributor to performance.

TABLE 5

Regression results for orthographic coding tasks.

| | Dependent variables 1. | 2. | 3. |
|---|---|---|---|
| | *multiple R* | | |
| WRAT grade level | .775** | .670** | .524** |
| Quadratic fit | NS | .686* | .568** |
| Cubic fit | NS | NS | .591* |
| | *beta weight in final equation* | | |
| RD vs. NRD contrast | .222** | -.121* | .107 |
| RD-N vs. RD-D contrast | .006 | -.021 | .061 |
| | *unique variance explained* | | |
| RD vs. NRD contrast | .041 | .013 | .009 |
| RD-N vs. RD-D contrast | .000 | .000 | .003 |
| | *F ratio in final equation* | | |
| RD vs. NRD contrast | 8.95 | 5.32 | 2.20 |
| RD-N vs. RD-D contrast | 0.01 | 0.14 | 0.83 |
| | *sample size* | | |
| N | 81 | 212 | 164 |

Dependent variables:
1 = spelling recognition (PIAT)
2 = experimental spelling recognition
3 = wordlikeness choice

* $p < .05$
** $p < .01$
NS = not significant

Table 5 displays the results of the regression analyses. Not surprisingly, WRAT Reading grade level was the dominant predictor of performance. In two of the three analyses, the contrast between disabled and nondisabled children displayed a significant regression coefficient. Unlike the analyses of the pseudoword tasks, in two of the three analyses (PIAT spelling recognition and wordlikeness choice), the contrast between disabled and nondisabled children displayed a positive regression coefficient (although only the former was statistically significant) - indicating that disabled subjects perform better than the nondisabled subjects on these two tasks when WRAT Reading grade level is controlled. This coefficient was significantly negative for the experimental spelling recognition task, although small in magnitude (unique variance explained = 1.3%). The word alternatives in this task were all short, highfrequency words. It is possible that, compared to the other two tasks, the two alternative spelling recognition task might not require orthographic representations to be as elaborated and accurate. Nevertheless, collectively, the data from these three tasks indicates that the reading-level deficits of reading disabled children are reduced on orthographic processing tasks.

The contrast between discrepant and nondiscrepant disabled readers did not attain significance in any of the analyses. As was the case with virtually all of the phonological coding tasks, RD-N children performed in a remarkably similar manner to the RD-D children when overall word recognition level was controlled.

## THE SPELLING-SOUND REGULARITY EFFECT

The finding of relative differences in orthographic and phonological coding suggests that perhaps the same relative pattern in processing skills might be demonstrated on different types of English words. For example, it would seem that the so-called spelling-sound regularity effect would provide a converging pattern. Indeed, several theorists (Barron, 1981; Castles & Coltheart, 1993; Manis, Szeszulski, Holt, & Graves, 1990; Olson et al., 1985; Treiman & Hirsh-Pasek, 1985) have suggested that the regularity effect should be an indicator of the differential functioning of phonological and orthographic coding skills. Many investigators have argued that this seems to follow from the classic dual-route model (Barron, 1986; Carr & Pollatsek, 1985; Coltheart, 1978; Humphreys & Evett, 1985) of lexical access:

> The regular words are presumed to be processed by both the phonological and orthographic paths, while the exception words are confined to the orthographic path. In this model, disabled readers should show a smaller regular word advantage because their phonological coding is uniquely deficient (Olson et al., 1985, p. 18). From the perspective of the dual-access model, the regular word advantage may be due to the fact that these words can be read by means of both the phonological and orthographic mechanisms, whereas irregular words can only be correctly pronounced by memorizing a word-specific association between print and pronunciation (i.e. using the orthographic mechanism).... The regularity effect provides an index of subjects' use

> of spelling-to-sound correspondences to pronounce familiar words. If dyslexic children are less able to apply their knowledge of these correspondences, they should show smaller regularity effects than normal readers (Manis et al., 1990, pp. 229-230).

However, the empirical literature is puzzling, because although some studies have found the expected interaction between subject group and spelling-sound regularity (Barron, 1981; Beech & Awaida, 1992; Frith & Snowling, 1983; Snowling et al., 1986) an even larger number of studies employing reading-level controls have not (Baddeley, Logie, & Ellis, 1988; Beech & Harding, 1984; Ben-Dror, Pollatsek, & Scarpati, 1991; Bruck, 1990; Holligan & Johnston, 1988; Olson et al., 1985; Stanovich et al., 1988; Treiman & Hirsh-Pasek, 1985; Watson & Brown, 1992). All of these studies have used the traditional matched-groups design. Using the regression strategy just described, we examined the performance of children on the regular and exception words used in a much-cited 1979 study by Baron. We are well aware that since the publication of Baron's (1979) paper, theories of lexical access have markedly evolved (see Stanovich, 1991b). However, for the purpose of the descriptive individual differences analysis that is our focus, it is only necessary to establish that these sets of words vary in their spelling-sound predictability, regardless of how defined (for example, whether by small-unit regularity or large-unit consistency) and that these words are comparable to those used in other investigations that have used the RL design.

Table 6 displays the results of the regression analyses. The first two analyses were conducted using performance on the regular and exception words, respectively, as the criterion variables. Not surprisingly, because the criterion variables reflect the ability to recognize words, WRAT Reading grade level accounted for most of the variance. Nevertheless, the RD versus NRD contrast did attain significance in the exception word analysis. Although the sign of the beta weight is in the expected direction (indicating superior performance by the RD children on exception words) it is very small in magnitude (accounting for only 0.5% unique variance).

The essential similarity in the performance of the RD and NRD children is bolstered by the separate regression analysis conducted on the magnitude of the regularity effect. Here, neither of the subject group contrasts is statistically significant. Overall, there is little indication in these results that disabled readers are relatively more impaired at reading regular words than exception words. Although this finding is theoretically problematic, it is consistent with the

TABLE 6

Regression results for regular and exception words.

| | Dependent variables 1. | 2. | 3. |
|---|---|---|---|
| | *multiple R* | | |
| WRAT grade level | .849** | .854** | .157 |
| Quadratic fit | .914** | .920** | .170 |
| Cubic fit | NS | NS | .281** |
| | *beta weight in final equation* | | |
| RD vs. NRD contrast | .021 | .070* | -.106 |
| RD-N vs. RD-D contrast | .022 | .024 | -.023 |
| | *unique variance explained* | | |
| RD vs. NRD contrast | .000 | .005 | .011 |
| RD-N vs. RD-D contrast | .000 | .001 | .001 |
| | *F ratio in final equation* | | |
| RD vs. NRD contrast | 0.35 | 4.25 | 1.56 |
| RD-N vs. RD-D contrast | 0.36 | 0.49 | 0.08 |
| | *sample size* | | |
| N | 141 | 141 | 141 |

Dependent variables:
1 = regular words
2 = exception words
3 = regularity effect

* $p < .05$
** $p < .01$
NS = not significant

results from some other studies that have used a discrete groups RL-match design (e.g. Beech & Harding, 1984; Ben-Dror et al., 1991; Olsen et al., 1985; Treiman & Hirsh-Pasek, 1985). Finally, differences in performance between RD-D and RD-N children were negligible in all three analyses.

## ANALYZING PERFORMANCE OUTSIDE OF THE PHONOLOGICAL CORE:

### WORKING AND SHORT-TERM MEMORY

The processes analyzed so far have all been subcomponents of the word recognition (and spelling) process. Differences between reading disabled children of differing IQs on these component word recognition subskills have been extremely few in number. However, the phonological-core variable difference model of reading disability (see Siegel, 1992; Stanovich, 1988a, 1988b) predicts that such differences should increase as the processes examined become more central, less modular, and further removed from the phonological core. Therefore, we examined several working and short-term memory tasks with the analytic method previously described.

The first task was a short-term memory measure modelled on the work of Shankweiler, Liberman, Mark, Fowler, and Fischer (1979) and that employed rhyming and nonrhyming letters on different trials. We also analyzed a measure of the rhyme effect in this task (the number of letters recalled on nonrhyming trials minus the number of letters recalled on rhyming trials). Additionally, we examined performance on two working memory tasks modeled on the sentence span paradigm introduced by Daneman and Carpenter (1980). One of these working memory tasks involved the retention of words, the other retention of numbers.

Table 7 displays the results of the regression analyses. On the two versions of the STM task (Rhyming and Nonrhyming) there is a tendency for the RD-D group to outperform the other two groups matched on reading level. This pattern is reflected in the regression analyses, which indicate significant negative beta weights for the RD-N versus RD-D contrast. Analyses on the magnitude of the rhyming effect yielded somewhat different outcomes. The regression analysis on the rhyming effect presented in Table 7 indicates a significant quadratic trend, a significant negative beta weight for the RD versus NRD contrast (indicating larger rhyming effects for the nondisabled subjects), and no significant contrast between RD-D and RD-N children. The performance pattern revealed in the analysis of the rhyming effect was thus similar to that obtained on the pseudo-word processing tasks: reading disabled children performed differently from nondisabled children, but no differences between RD-D and RD-N children reached statistical significance. This finding may indicate that the rhyme effect is tapping into the same phonological deficit that is the cause of the alphabetic coding problems that are associated with reading disability.

TABLE 7

Regression results for memory tasks.

| | Dependent variables | | | | |
|---|---|---|---|---|---|
| | 1. | 2. | 3. | 4. | 5. |
| | | | *multiple R* | | |
| WRAT grade level | .526** | .474** | .053 | .335** | .432** |
| Quadratic fit | NS | .482* | .088* | NS | NS |
| | | | *beta weight in final equation* | | |
| RD vs. NRD contrast | .169** | .023 | -.165** | .260** | .124 |
| RD-N vs. RD-D contrast | -.129** | -.160** | -.069 | -.263** | -.232** |
| | | | *unique variance explained* | | |
| RD vs. NRD contrast | .023 | .011 | .021 | .050 | .012 |
| RD-N vs. RD-D contrast | .016 | .025 | .005 | .065 | .053 |
| | | | *F ratio in final equation* | | |
| RD vs. NRD contrast | 21.11 | 0.35 | 13.89 | 23.08 | 2.07 |
| RD-N vs. RD-D contrast | 14.94 | 20.99 | 2.93 | 29.81 | 9.06 |
| | | | *sample size* | | |
| N | 640 | 640 | 640 | 354 | 132 |

Dependent variables:
1 = STM - rhyming
2 = STM - nonrhyming
3 = STM - rhyme effect
4 = working memory - words
5 = working memory - numbers

* $p < .05$
** $p < .01$
NS = not significant

The results from the two working memory tasks were fairly similar to those obtained from the STM task. Both regression analyses indicated positive beta weights for the RD versus NRD comparison (although only that for the Working Memory - Words task was statistically significant) and significant negative beta weights for the RD-D and RD-N comparison (indicating that RD-D children performed better than the RD-N children statistically matched on WRAT Reading level). Thus, in contrast to the situation with tasks reflecting word-level processing, in the domain of short-term and working memory, there are performance differences between reading disabled children at different IQ levels.

## ANALYZING PERFORMANCE OUTSIDE OF THE PHONOLOGICAL CORE:

### LANGUAGE TASKS

In addition to memory tasks, our battery allowed for the investigation of another domain of processing that extended outside of the phonological deficit known to be associated with reading disability. As a further test of one of the central predictions of the phonological-core variable-difference model - that processing differences associated with IQ-discrepancy should increase as the task requirements extend beyond phonological processing we examined performance on a variety of language processing tasks. The six tasks that we analyzed included the grammatical closure subtest of the Illinois Test of Psycholinguistic Abilities, two versions of an oral sentence correction task (version 2 more difficult than version 1), two versions of an oral cloze task (version 2 more difficult than version 1), and a sentence repetition task where children had to repeat back sentences containing complex syntactic structures.

Table 8 displays the results of the regression analyses. Across all six tasks, there was no strong tendency for reading disabled children to perform differently from reading-level controls. Two of the tasks (the more difficult versions of the sentence correction and oral cloze measures) displayed significant contrasts between RD-N and RD-D children. The negative sign of these two beta weights indicates that the RD-D performed better than the RD-N children. There were no differences between these two groups on the grammatical closure task, sentence repetition task, error correction 1, and oral cloze 1.

TABLE 8

Regression results for language tasks.

| Dependent variables | 1. | 2. | 3. | 4. | 5. | 6. |
|---|---|---|---|---|---|---|
| | | | *multiple R* | | | |
| WRAT grade level | .615** | .529** | .553** | .518** | .596** | .376** |
| Quadratic fit | NS | NS | .584** | .584** | .628** | NS |
| | | | *beta weight in final equation* | | | |
| RD vs. NRD contrast | .109 | .031 | .001 | .062 | -.034 | .035 |
| RD-N vs. RD-D contrast | -.096 | -.096 | -.190** | -.099 | -.236** | -.100 |
| | | | *unique variance explained* | | | |
| RD vs. NRD contrast | .010 | .001 | .000 | .004 | .000 | .001 |
| RD-N vs. RD-D contrast | .008 | .009 | .036 | .009 | .050 | .010 |
| | | | *F ratio in final equation* | | | |
| RD vs. NRD contrast | 3.84 | 0.18 | 0.01 | 0.76 | 0.56 | 0.19 |
| RD-N vs. RD-D contrast | 3.39 | 1.74 | 8.32 | 1.99 | 34.69 | 1.59 |
| | | | *sample size* | | | |
| N | 234 | 147 | 149 | 148 | 388 | 148 |

Dependent variables
1 = grammatical closure
2 = sentence correction 1
3 = sentence correction 2
4 = oral cloze task 1
5 = oral cloze task 2
6 = sentence repetition

* $p < .05$
** $p < .01$
NS = not significant

## OTHER DISCREPANCY CRITERIA

All of the analyses presented so far have been based on an absolute IQ cut-off criterion to differentiate RD-D from RD-N children. The results presented here are highly convergent with analyses conducted using other methods of determining aptitude/achievement discrepancy.

For example, analyses employing a standard-score discrepancy cut-off produced data patterns virtually identical with those shown here (see Stanovich & Siegel, 1994). Table 9 presents the results from

TABLE 9

Regression results for classification based on regression discrepancy method. Beta weights for each contrast for each variable are indicated along with proportion of variance explained (in parentheses).

| | RD vs. NRD | | RD-N vs. RD-D | |
|---|---|---|---|---|
| arithmetic grade level (WRAT) | .301** | (.073) | -.235** | (.051) |
| *Pseudoword processing tasks* | | | | |
| GFW pseudoword spelling | -.258** | (.058) | .099 | (.009) |
| GFW pseudoword reading | -.149** | (.020) | .024 | (.001) |
| Woodcock Word Attack | -.159** | (.020) | -.092** | (.007) |
| experimental pseudowords 1 | -.185** | (.027) | .014 | (.000) |
| experimental pseudowords 2 | -.240** | (.046) | .023 | (.000) |
| *Phonological coding tasks* | | | | |
| phonological choice task | -.060 | (.003) | -.084 | (.006) |
| pseudoword recognition | -.027 | (.001) | .130* | (.017) |
| *Orthographic coding tasks* | | | | |
| spelling recognition (PIAT) | .212** | (.033) | .027 | (.000) |
| experimental spelling recognition | .010 | (.000) | -.151** | (.019) |
| wordlikeness choice | .102 | (.009) | .059 | (.003) |
| *Regular and exception words* | | | | |
| regular words | .014 | (.000) | .015 | (.000) |
| exception words | .067 | (.004) | -.003 | (.000) |
| regularity effect | -.110 | (.012) | .039 | (.002) |
| *Memory tasks* | | | | |
| STM - rhyming | .197** | (.031) | -.147** | (.020) |
| STM- nonrhyming | .060 | (.003) | -.174** | (.028) |
| STM - rhyme effect | -.150** | (.018) | -.052 | (.003) |
| working memory - words | .297** | (.066) | -.324** | (.094) |
| working memory - numbers | .179 | (.020) | -.155 | (.018) |
| *Language tasks* | | | | |
| grammatical closure | .145* | (.017) | -.085 | (.006) |
| sentence correction 1 | .059 | (.003) | -.042 | (.002) |
| sentence correction 2 | .122 | (.009) | -.244** | (.044) |
| oral cloze task 1 | .103 | (.010) | -.133* | (.017) |
| oral cloze task 2 | .010 | (.000) | -.273** | (.063) |
| sentence repetition | .059 | (.003) | -.007 | (.000) |

* $p < .05$, ** $p < .01$

the use of a discrepancy criterion that is generally preferred to the standardscore discrepancy method - a regression discrepancy criterion (see Fletcher et al., 1992; Reynolds, 1985).

The results presented in Table 9 were based on the following procedure for classifying the RD-D and RD-N children. The WRAT Reading percentile score was regressed on the IQ scores of all children in our sample who were between ages 7 and 16. As before, we selected all children who were reading at grade levels 1 through 5 on the Reading subtest of the Wide Range Achievement Test, and all children with percentile scores on the WRAT $\geq$ 30 were classified as not reading disabled (NRD). All children with percentile scores $\leq$25 on the WRAT were considered reading disabled. These children were split into RD-D and RD-N groups based on the standardized residual scores that resulted from applying the regression equation from the entire 7 - 16 year-old sample. Children were classified as RD-D if their standardized residual scores were less than -1.0 and RD-N if their standardized residual scores were greater than or equal to -1.0.

The results of regression analyses conducted on all of the criterion variables using the regression-discrepancy classification method are displayed in Table 9. Visual inspection immediately reveals that the outcomes of these analyses parallel closely those conducted using the absolute IQ cut-off criterion. Reading disabled children as a group perform worse than nondisabled children statistically equated on WRAT reading level on all five pseudoword processing tasks. They display performance commensurate with their reading levels on the two phonological coding tasks. They display superiority on two of the three orthographic coding tasks and show spelling-sound regularity effects that are commensurate with their reading levels. More importantly, the results across these word-level processing tasks for the RD-D vs. RD-N contrast paralleled the results using the other discrepancy criteria in that few differences were revealed. No beta weight exceeded .151 in absolute value, and on no word-level variable did the variance explained by the RD-N versus RD-D contrast exceed 1.7%.

As in all previous analyses, differences between these subject groups were revealed on the WRAT Arithmetic subtest, both short-term memory conditions, and on both working memory tasks. The two groups did not differ significantly in the magnitude of the rhyme effect in short-term memory - again, probably because this measure reflected the phonological processing deficit that they share. The results of the analyses conducted on the language processing tasks paralleled the results obtained using the discrepancy criteria.

## CONCLUSIONS

In summary, cognitive differences between children with reading disabilities who do or do not have aptitude/achievement discrepancy all seem to reside outside of the word-recognition module. With regard to word recognition processes themselves, RD-D and RD-N show performance patterns that are remarkably similar. Both show pseudoword reading performance below that expected on the basis of their WRAT Reading levels. Both show performance on phonological coding tasks not involving production of a spelling or pronunciation (phonological choice task and pseudoword recognition) that is commensurate with their reading levels but inferior to chronological age controls. Both show indications of relative strength in orthographic processing skill: performance on some orthographic tasks is underpredicted by their WRAT Reading levels. Both demonstrate spelling-sound regularity effects that are commensurate with their reading levels.

Not surprisingly, there are cognitive differences between RD-D and RD-N children outside of the word recognition module. Some of these cognitive differences may be related to comprehension processes. Thus, there may well be reading comprehension differences between RD-D and RD-N readers who are equated on word recognition ability. These differences might well relate to certain educational issues such as the reading level to be expected of a student subsequent to remediation of their primary word recognition problem. However, it is important to note that any such differences are not indicators of the core processing problem that caused the word recognition deficit that triggered the diagnosis of reading disability in the first place - that is, phonological coding difficulties probably resulting from deficient phonological awareness. Thus, such differences outside of the word recognition module provide no rationale for a definition of reading disability based on IQ-discrepancy. Such definitions would only give the mistaken impression that children with IQ-discrepancy have distinctive genetic/neurological aetiology.

One potential caveat to the conclusions drawn here is that the discrepancy criteria that we employed were not as extreme as those employed in other studies, for example, by Rutter and Yule (1975).

We have examined some more extreme criteria for defining discrepancy in this same database and have found the results to be robust, however. Although it is always possible that the use of ever more extreme criteria for defining discrepancy would eventually alter the pattern of results, we have not found this in our sample.

Thus, IQ discrepancy appears to be at best weakly correlated with the primary phenotypic indicators of reading disability. This finding is problematic for the traditional concept of dyslexia which is inextricably linked with the idea of an aetiologically distinct type of reading disability associated with moderate to high IQ. Taylor and Schatschneider (1992) have reminded us that "IQ criteria were imposed primarily as a means of ruling out confounding variables and for assisting in the search for specific cognitive antecedents" (p. 630). It appears that the intuition that IQ discrepancy measurement would provide such assistance is mistaken. IQ discrepancy does not carve out a unique information processing pattern in the word recognition module that is the critical locus of reading disability. If there is a special group of reading disabled children who are behaviourially/ cognitively/genetically "different", it is becoming increasingly unlikely that they can be quickly picked out using reading-IQ discrepancy as a proxy for the genetic and neurological differences themselves.

Rather than becoming further distracted by the IQ issue, it may well be more fruitful for the field to explore the implications of conceptualizing reading disability as residing on a continuum of developmental language disorder (see Bishop & Adams, 1990; Catts, 1989, 1991, 1993; Fowler, 1991; Gathercole & Baddeley, 1987, 1990, 1993; Kamhi, 1992; Kamhi & Catts, 1989; Rubin & Dworkin, 1985; Rubin, & Liberman, 1983; Scarborough, 1990). For example, Gathercole and Baddeley (1987) argue that "it is possible that the alphabetic literacy skills required in reading may be more sensitive to the adequacy of speech analytic skills than other aspects of normal linguistic development, such that a mild deficit may only be detectable in reading performance. More severe subjects may result in the more generalized symptom complex associated with developmental language disorder.... This is also clearly consistent with the notion that the two populations may quantitatively differ rather than qualitatively" (p. 464). In the light of these attempts to conceptualize reading disability as a milder form of language disability, it is interesting to note that the question of whether a discrepancy defined disability is different from a disability defined purely in terms of chronological age occurs in analogous form in the area of developmental language disorder (Aram, Morris, & Hall, 1992; Cole, Dale, & Mills, 1990).

In summary, the search for neurological and genetic correlates of reading disability is being conducted with vigor in research laboratories around the world. Based on the results reported here, there appears to be no reason for such investigations to restrict their research samples in advance based on reading-IQ discrepancy. Indeed, our ability to map the multidimensional space of reading related cognitive skills would be impaired by such a procedure. No one disputes the logical possibility of distinct aetiologies within the population of poor readers. Obviously, if a group of children were not taught to read and not exposed to print, their reading disability would have a distinct causation different from that in the general disabled population. The point, instead, is that it has yet to be demonstrated that whatever distinct causes actually exist are correlated with the degree of reading-IQ discrepancy.

## FOOTNOTE

This research was supported by grant #OGP0001607 from the Natural Sciences and Engineering Research Council of Canada to Keith E. Stanovich and by grant #OGP0138452 from the Natural Sciences and Engineering Research Council of Canada to Linda S. Siegel.
Corres- pondence should be addressed to Keith E. Stanovich or Linda S. Siegel, Ontario Institute for Studies in Education, University of Toronto, 252 Bloor St. West, Toronto, Ontario, Canada M5S lV6.

## REFERENCES

Aram, D., Morris, R., & Hall, N. (1992). The validity of discrepancy criteria for identifying children with developmental language disorders. *Journal of Learning Disabilities, 25*, 549-554.

Backman, J. E., Mamen, M., & Ferguson, H. (1984). Reading-level design: Conceptual and methodological issues in reading research. *Psychological Bulletin, 96*, 560-568.

Baddeley, A. D., Logie, R. H., & Ellis, N. C. (1988). Characteristics of developmental dyslexia. *Cognition, 30*, 198-227.

Baron, J. (1979). Orthographic and word-specific mechanisms in children's reading of words. *Child Development, 50*, 60-72.

Barron, R. (1981). Reading skill and spelling strategies. In A. Lesgold & C. Perfetti (Eds.), *Interactive processes in reading* (pp. 299-327). Hillsdale, NJ: Erlbaum.

Barron, R. (1986). Word recognition in early reading: A review of the direct and indirect access hypothesis. *Cognition, 24*, 93-119.

Beech, J. R. & Awaida, M. (1992). Lexical and nonlexical routes: A comparison between normally achieving and poor readers. *Journal of Learning Disabilities, 25*, 196-206.

Beech, J. & Harding, L. (1984). Phonemic processing and the poor reader from a developmental lag viewpoint. *Reading Research Quarterly, 19*, 357-366.

Ben-Dror, I., Pollatsek, A., & Scarpati, S. (1991). Word identification in isolation and in context by college dyslexic students. *Brain and Language, 40*, 471-490.

Bisanz, G. L., Das, J. P., & Mancini, G. (1984). Children's memory for phonemically confusable and nonconfusable letters. *Child Development, 55*, 1845-1854.

Bishop, D. & Adams, C. (1990). A prospective study of the relationship between specific language impairment, phonological disorders and reading retardation. *Journal of Child Psychology and Psychiatry, 31*, 1027-1050.

Bowey, J. A., Cain, M. T., & Ryan, S. M. (1992). A reading-level design study of phonological skills underlying fourth-grade children's word reading difficulties. *Child Development, 63*, 999-1011.

Bradley, L. & Bryant, P. E. (1978). Difficulties in auditory organization as a possible cause of reading backwardness. *Nature, 271*, 746-747.

Bruck, M. (1990). Word-recognition skills of adults with childhood diagnoses of dyslexia. *Developmental Psychology, 26*, 439-454.

Bryant, P. E. & Goswami, U. (1986). Strengths and weaknesses of the reading level design: A comment on Backman, Mamen, and Ferguson. *Psychological Bulletin, 100*, 101-103.

Cardon, L. R., Smith, S., Fulker, D., Kimberling, W., Pennington, B., & DeFries, J. (1994). Quantitative trait locus for reading disability on chromosome 6. *Science, 266*, 276-279.

Carr, T. H. & Pollatsek, A. (1985). Recognizing printed words: A look at current models. In D. Besner, T. G. Waller, & G. E. MacKinnon (Eds.), *Reading research: Advances in theory and practice* (Vol. 5, pp. 1-82). Orlando, FL: Academic Press.

Castles, A., & Coltheart, M. (1993). Varieties of developmental dyslexia. *Cognition ,47*, 149-180.

Catts, H. W. (1989). Defining dyslexia as a developmental language disorder. *Annals of Dyslexia, 39*, 50-64.

Catts, H. W. (1991). Early identification of reading disabilities. *Topics in Language Disorders, 12* (1), 1-16.

Catts, H. W. (1993). The relationship between speech-language impairments and reading disabilities. *Journal of Speech and Hearing Research, 36*, 948-958.

Ceci, S. J. (1986). *Handbook of cognitive, social, and neuropsychological aspects of learning disabilities* (Vol. 1). Hillsdale, NJ: Erlbaum.

Cole, K. N., Dale, P. S., & Mills, P. E. (1990). Defining language delay in young children by cognitive referencing: Are we saying more than we know? *Applied Psycholinguistics, 11*, 291-302.

Coltheart, M. (1978). Lexical access in simple reading tasks. In G. Underwood (Ed.), *Strategies of information processing* (pp. 151-216). London: Academic Press.

Daneman, M., & Carpenter, P. A. (1980). Individual differences in working memory and reading. *Journal of Verbal Learning and Verbal Behaviour, 19*, 450-466.

DeFries, J. C., Fulker, D., & LaBuda, M. (1987). Evidence for a genetic aetiology in reading disability in twins. *Nature, 329*, 537-539.

Fletcher, J. M., Espy, K., Francis, D., Davidson, K., Rourke, B., & Shaywitz, S. (1989). Comparisons of cut-off and regression-based definitions of reading disabilities. *Journal of Learning Disabilities, 22*, 334-338.

Fletcher, J. M., Francis, D. J., Rourke, B. P., Shaywitz, B. A., & Shaywitz, S. E. (1992). The validity of discrepancy-based definitions of reading disabilities. *Journal of Learning Disabilities, 25*, 555-561.

Fletcher, J. M., Shaywitz, S. E., Shankweiler, D., Katz, L., Liberman, I., Stuebing, K., Francis, D. J., Fowler, A., & Shaywitz, B. A. (1994). Cognitive profiles of reading disability: Comparisons of discrepancy and low achievement definitions. *Journal of Educational Psychology, 86*, 6-23.

Fowler, A. (1991). How early phonological development might set the stage for phoneme awareness. In S. A. Brady & D. P. Shankweiler (Eds.), *Phonological processes in literacy* (pp. 97-117). Hillsdale, NJ: Erlbaum.

Frith, U. & Snowling, M. (1983). Reading for meaning and reading for sound in autistic and dyslexic children. *British Journal of Developmental Psychology, 1*, 329-342.

Galaburda, A. (1991). Anatomy of dyslexia: Argument against phrenology. In D. Duane & D. Gray (Eds.), *The reading brain: The biological basis of dyslexia* (pp. 119-131). Parkton, MD: York Press.

Galaburda, A. (1994). Developmental dyslexia and animal studies: At the interface between cognition and neurology. *Cognition, 50*, 133-149.

Galaburda, A. M., Sherman, G., Rosen, G., Aboitz, F., & Geschwind, N. (1985). Developmental dyslexia: Four consecutive patients with cortical anomalies. *Annals of Neurology, 18*, 222-233.

Gathercole, S. E. & Baddeley, A. D. (1987). The processes underlying segmental analysis. *European Bulletin of Cognitive Psychology, 7*, 462-464.

Gathercole, S. E. & Baddeley, A. D. (1990). Phonological memory deficits in language disordered children: Is there a causal connection? *Journal of Memory and Language, 29*, 336-360.

Gathercole, S. E. & Baddeley, A. D. (1993). *Working memory and language.* Hove UK: Lawrence Erlbaum Ltd.

Goswami, U. & Bryant, P. (1989). The interpretation of studies using the reading level design. *Journal of Reading Behaviour, 21*, 413-424.

Gough, P. B. & Tunmer, W. E. (1986). Decoding, reading, and reading disability. *Remedial and Special Education, 7*, 6-10.

Guthrie, J. T. (1973). Reading comprehension and syntactic response in good and poor readers. *Journal of Educational Psychology, 65*, 294-299.

Holligan, C. & Johnston, R. S. (1988). The use of phonological information by good and poor readers in memory and reading tasks. *Memory & Cognition, 16*, 522-532.

Humphreys, G. W. & Evett, L. J. (1985). Are there independent lexical and nonlexical routes in word processing? An evaluation of the dual-route theory of reading. *Behavioural and Brain Sciences, 8*, 689-740.

Hynd, G. S., Marshall, R., & Gonzalez, J. (1991). Learning disabilities and presumed central nervous system dysfunction. *Learning Disability Quarterly, 14*, 283-296.

Hynd, G. S., Marshall, R., & Semrud-Clikeman, M. (1991). Developmental dyslexia, neurolinguistic theory and deviations in brain morphology. *Reading and Writing: An Interdisciplinary Journal, 3*, 345-362.

Jackson, N. E. & Butterfield, E. C. (1989). Reading-level-match designs: Myths and realities. *Journal of Reading Behaviour, 21*, 387-412.

Jorm, A., Share, D., Maclean, R., & Matthews, R. (1986). Cognitive factors at school entry predictive of specific reading retardation and general reading backwardness: A research note. *Journal of Child Psychology and Psychiatry, 27*, 45-54.

Kamhi, A. G. (1992). Response to historical perspective: A developmental language perspective. *Journal of Learning Disabilities, 25*, 48-52.

Kamhi, A. & Catts, H. (1989). *Reading disabilities: A developmental language perspective.* Austin: PRO-ED.

Larsen, P., Hoien, T., Lundberg, I., & Odegaard, H. (1990). MRI evaluation of the size and symmetry of the planum temporale in adolescents with developmental dyslexia. *Brain and Language, 39*, 289-301.

Mamen, M., Ferguson, H., & Backman, J. E. (1986). No difference represents a significant finding. *Psychological Bulletin, 100*, 107-109.

Manis, F. R., Szeszulski, P. A., Holt, L. K., & Graves, K. (1990). Variation in component word recognition and spelling skills among dyslexic children and normal readers. In T. H. Carr & B. A. Levy (Eds.), *Reading and its development: Component skills approaches* (pp. 207-259). San Diego, CA: Academic Press.

Olson, R., Kliegl, R., Davidson, B., & Foltz, G. (1985). Individual and developmental differences in reading disability. In G. E. MacKinnon & T. Waller (Eds.), *Reading research: Advances in theory and practice* (Vol. 4, pp. 1-64). London: Academic Press.

Olson, R. K., Wise, B., Conners, F., & Rack, J. (1990). Organization, heritability, and remediation of component word recognition and language skills in disabled readers. In T. Carr & B. A. Levy (Eds.), *Reading and its development: Component skills approaches* (pp. 261-322). New York: Academic Press.

Olson, R. K., Wise, B., Conners, F., Rack, J., & Fulker, D. (1989). Specific deficits in component reading and language skills: Genetic and environmental influences. *Journal of Learning Disabilities, 22*, 339-348.

Pennington, B. F. (1990). The genetics of dyslexia. *Journal of Child Psychology and Psychiatry, 31*, 193-201.

Pennington, B. F., Gilger, J., Olson, R. K., & DeFries, J. C. (1992). The external validity of age- versus IQ-discrepancy definitions of reading disability: Lessons from a twin study. *Journal of Learning Disabilities, 25*, 562-573.

Pennington, B. F., Gilger, J., Pauls, D., Smith, S. A., Smith, S. D., & DeFries, J. (1991). Genetic and neurological influences on reading disability: An overview. *Journal of the American Medical Association, 266* (1), 1527-1534.

Pennington, B. F., McCabe, L. L., Smith, S., Lefly, D., Bookman, M., Kimberling, W., & Lubs, H. (1986). Spelling errors in adults with a form of familial dyslexia. *Child Development, 57*, 1001-1013.

Pennington, B. F., Van Orden, G., Kirson, D., & Haith, M. (1991). What is the causal relation between verbal STM problems and dyslexia? In S. A. Brady & D. P. Shankweiler (Eds.), *Phonological processes in literacy* (pp. 173-186). Hillsdale, NJ: Erlbaum.

Rack, J. (1985). Orthographic and phonetic coding in developmental dyslexia. *British Journal of Psychology, 76*, 325-340.

Rack, J. P., Snowling, M. J., & Olson, R. K. (1992). The nonword reading deficit in developmental dyslexia: A review. *Reading Research Quarterly, 27*, 28-53.

Reynolds, C. R. (1985). Measuring the aptitude-achievement discrepancy in learning disability diagnosis. *Remedial and Special Education, 6*, 37-55.

Rodgers, B. (1983). The identification and prevalence of specific reading retardation. *British Journal of Educational Psychology, 53*, 369-373.

Rubin, H. & Dworkin, P. (1985). The language-impaired student. In P. Dworkin (Ed.), *Learning and behaviour problems of school children* (pp. 98-115). Philadelphia, PA: W.B. Saunders Co.

Rubin, H. & Liberman, I. Y. (1983). Exploring the oral and written language errors made by language disabled children. *Annals of Dyslexia, 33*, 111-120.

Rutter, M. & Yule, W. (1975). The concept of specific reading retardation. *Journal of Child Psychology and Psychiatry, 16*, 181-197.

Scarborough, H. S. (1990). Very early language deficits in dyslexic children. *Child Development, 61*, 1728-1743.

Semrud-Clikeman, M., Hynd, G. S., Novey, E., & Eliopulos, D. (1991). Dyslexia and brain morphology: Relationships between neuro-anatomical variation and neurolinguistic tasks. *Learning and Individual Differences, 3*, 225-242.

Shankweiler, D., Liberman, I., Mark, L., Fowler, C., & Fischer, F. (1979). The speech code and learning to read. *Journal of Experimental Psychology: Human Learning and Memory, 5*, 531-545.

Share, D. L. & Stanovich, K. E. (1995). Cognitive processes in early reading development: Accommodating individual differences into a model of acquisition. *Issues in Education: Contributions from Educational Psychology, 1*, 1-57.

Shaywitz, S. E., Escobar, M. D., Shaywitz, B. A., Fletcher, J. M., & Makugh, R. (1992). Evidence that dyslexia may represent the lower tail of a normal distribution of reading ability. *The New England Journal of Medicine, 326*, 145-150.

Shaywitz, B. A., Fletcher, J. M., Holahan, J. M., & Shaywitz, S. E. (1992). Discrepancy compared to low achievement definitions of reading disability: Results from the Connecticut longitudinal study. *Journal of Learning Disabilities, 25*, 639-648.

Shepard, L. (1980). An evaluation of the regression discrepancy method for identifying children with learning disabilities. *The Journal of Special Education, 14*, 79-91.

Siegel, L. S. (1988). Evidence that IQ scores are irrelevant to the definition and analysis of reading disability. *Canadian Journal of Psychology, 42*, 201-215.

Siegel, L. S. (1989). IQ is irrelevant to the definition of learning disabilities. *Journal of Learning Disabilities, 22*, 469-479.

Siegel, L. S. (1992). An evaluation of the discrepancy definition of dyslexia. *Journal of Learning Disabilities, 25*, 618-629.

Siegel, L. S. (1993). The development of reading. In H. Reese (Eds.), *Advances in child development and behaviour* (pp. 63-97). San Diego, CA: Academic Press.

Siegel, L. S. & Ryan, E. B. (1988). Development of grammatical-sensitivity, phonological, and short-term memory skills in normally achieving and learning disabled children. *Developmental Psychology, 24*, 28-37.

Smith, S. D., Kimberling, W. J., & Pennington, B. F. (1991). Screening for multiple genes influencing dyslexia. *Reading and Writing: An Interdisciplinary Journal, 3*, 285-298.

Snowling, M. (1980). The development of grapheme-phoneme correspondence in normal and dyslexic readers. *Journal of Experimental Child Psychology, 29*, 294-305.

Snowling, M., Stackhouse, J., & Rack, J. (1986). Phonological dyslexia and dysgraphia: A developmental analysis. *Cognitive Neuropsychology, 3*, 309-339.

Stanovich, K. E. (1986a). Cognitive processes and the reading problems of learning disabled children: Evaluating the assumption of specificity. In J. Torgesen & B. Wong (Eds.), *Psychological and educational perspectives on learning disabilities* (pp. 87-131). New York: Academic Press.

Stanovich, K. E. (1986b). Matthew effects in reading: Some consequences of individual differences in the acquisition of literacy. *Reading Research Quarterly, 21*, 360-407.

Stanovich, K. E. (1988a). Explaining the differences between the dyslexic and the garden-variety poor reader: The phonological-core variable-difference model. *Journal of Learning Disabilities, 21*, 590-612.

Stanovich, K. E. (1988b). The right and wrong places to look for the cognitive locus of reading disability. *Annals of Dyslexia, 38*, 154-177.

Stanovich, K. E. (1991a). Discrepancy definitions of reading disability: Has intelligence led us astray? *Reading Research Quarterly, 26*, 7-29.

Stanovich, K. E. (199lb). Word recognition: Changing perspectives. In R. Barr, M. L. Kamil, P. Mosenthal, & P. D. Pearson (Eds.), *Handbook of reading research* (Vol. 2, pp. 418-452). New York: Longman.

Stanovich, K. E. (1992). Speculations on the causes and consequences of individual differences in early reading acquisition. In P. Gough, L. Ehri & R. Treiman (Eds.), *Reading acquisition* (pp. 307-342). Hillsdale, NJ: Erlbaum Associates.

Stanovich, K. E. (1993a). Does reading make you smarter? Literacy and the development of verbal intelligence. In H. Reese (Ed.), *Advances in child development and behaviour* (Vol. 24, pp. 133-180). San Diego, CA: Academic Press.

Stanovich, K. E. (1993b). Dysrationalia: A new specific learning disability. *Journal of Learning Disabilities, 26*, 501-515.

Stanovich, K. E., & Cunningham, A. E. (1991). Reading as constrained reasoning. In S. Sternberg & P. Frensch (Eds.), *Complex problem solving: Principles and mechanisms* (pp. 3-60). Hillsdale, NJ: Erlbaum.

Stanovich, K. E., Nathan, R. G., & Zolman, J. E. (1988). The developmental lag hypothesis in reading: Longitudinal and matched reading-level comparisons. *Child Development, 59*, 71-86.

Stanovich, K. E. & Siegel, L. S. (1994). The phenotypic performance profile of reading disabled children: A regression-based test of the phonological-core variable-difference model. *Journal of Educational Psychology, 86*, 24-53.

Steinmetz, H. & Galaburda, A. M. (1991). Planum temporale asymmetry: In-vivo morphometry affords a new perspective for neuro-behavioural research. *Reading and Writing: An Interdisciplinary Journal, 3*, 331-343.

Stevenson, J. (1988). Which aspects of reading ability show a "hump" in their distribution? *Applied Cognitive Psychology, 2*, 77-85.

Stevenson, J. (1992a). Genetics. In N. Singh & I. Beale (Eds.), *Learning disabilities: Nature, theory and treatment* (pp. 327-351). New York: Springer Verlag.

Stevenson, J. (1992b). Identifying sex differences in reading disability: Lessons from a twin study. *Reading and Writing: An Interdisciplinary Journal, 4*, 307--326.

Szeszulski, P. & Manis, F. R. (1987). A comparison of word recognition processes in dyslexic and normal readers at two reading-age levels. *Journal of Experimental Child Psychology, 44*, 364-376.

Taylor, H. G. & Schatschneider, C. (1992). Academic achievement following childhood brain disease: Implications for the concept of learning disabilities. *Journal of Learning Disabilities, 25*, 630-638.

Treiman, R. & Hirsh-Pasek, K. (1985). Are there qualitative differences in reading behaviour between dyslexics and normal readers? *Memory and Cognition, 13*, 357-364.

Vellutino, F. R. & Scanlon, D. M. (1987). Phonological coding, phonological awareness, and reading ability: Evidence from a longitudinal and experimental study. *Merrill- Palmer Quarterly, 33*, 321-363.

Vellutino, F. R. & Scanlon, D. M. (1989). Some prerequisites for interpreting results from reading level matched designs. *Journal of Reading Behaviour, 21*, 361-385.

Watson, F. & Brown, G. (1992). Single-word reading in college dyslexics. *Applied Cognitive Psychology, 6*, 263-272.

# SECTION 3

# LANGUAGE DISORDERS

D. V. M. BISHOP

# IS SPECIFIC LANGUAGE IMPAIRMENT A VALID DIAGNOSTIC CATEGORY?

## GENETIC AND PSYCHOLINGUISTIC EVIDENCE

SUMMARY. Specific language impairment (SLI) is diagnosed when a child fails to develop language normally for no apparent reason: hearing and intelligence are adequate and the social environment is unexceptional. Definitions of SLI typically specify that the child must have a substantial discrepancy between language ability and non-verbal IQ. However, data from a twin study question the validity of this requirement, and indicate that SLI is not genetically distinct from less specific disorders where language impairment occurs in the context of low average or borderline nonverbal ability. A second question concerns the heterogeneous language symptoms seen in SLI: do these correspond to distinct conditions, for to different phenotypic manifestations of a common underlying disorder, or are they merely random variations resulting from unreliable assessments? The last of these possibilities is ruled out by the finding that twins who are concordant for language disorder show good agreement in terms of the pattern of language impairment. However, systematic variation in the age and ability of children in different SLI subgroups suggest that these may correspond to variable manifestations of a core inherited language disorder, rather than distinct diagnostic entities.

### INTRODUCTION

It has long been recognised that some children fail to develop normal language for no apparent reason; hearing and intelligence are adequate, the home environment is unexceptional, yet ability to produce and/or comprehend language are well below age level. The terminology used to refer to such children has varied over the past few decades: "developmental aphasia" and "developmental dysphasia" have waned in popularity as it has become recognised that they imply more understanding of the neurological basis than is the case. More neutral diagnostic term with fewer medical overtones, such as "developmental language disorder" or "specific language impairment" (SLI) are now usually preferred.

Formulations of diagnostic criteria (e.g. American Psychiatric Association [APA], 1987; Stark & Tallal, 1981) stress three key features:

Reprinted with permission of the publisher from Bishop, D. (1994). Is specific language impairment a valid diagnostic category? *Philosophical Transactions of the Royal Society of London, Series B, Vol. 346*, pp. 105-111.



*J. Rispens et al. (eds.),*
*Perspectives on the Classification of Specific Developmental Disorders*, 139–153.

(i) language must be significantly below age level;
(ii) poor language functioning must be out of keeping with other aspects of development; this is normally interpreted as a substantial discrepancy between a language test score and non-verbal IQ;
(iii) possible physical causes (e.g. hearing loss, acquired brain damage or abnormal structure of the articulators) and recognised syndromes associated with language delay (e.g. autism) are excluded.

This definition embodies conventional wisdom about SLI, but few attempts have been made to validate the criteria; i.e. to establish that they do define a coherent disorder with a distinct aetiology. Two questions that merit further scrutiny are: (i) how distinct is specific language impairment from more general developmental delay affecting all cognitive functions? (ii) how many subgroups of SLI are there?

### *Is the Distinction between Specific Language Impairment and More Global Cognitive Impairment Valid?*

Conventional definitions of SLI stress the importance of differentiating specific speech and language disorders from more global developmental delays. An analogy may be drawn with cases where language is impaired for an obvious reason: children with profound congenital hearing loss tend to have poor oral language, yet normal non-verbal intelligence. In such cases, the non-verbal IQ is regarded as providing an estimate of "true" intellectual potential. In cases of SLI, we do not know the cause of the language impairment, but the existence of a large verbal/non-verbal discrepancy is taken as circumstantial evidence of a specific aetiology that interferes selectively with language.

This approach to the diagnosis of SLI has a clear parallel with the definition of "developmental dyslexia" or specific reading retardation, where the diagnostic criteria specify that the child's poor reading must be out of keeping with age and ability. However, as Stanovich (1994) has pointed out, there is remarkably little evidence for the validity of this approach. On the contrary, both types of child appear to have similar genetic risk factors, psychological profiles and associated problems with phonological processing (Pennington, Gilger, Olson, & DeFries, 1992; Fletcher, Francis, Rourke, Shaywitz, & Shaywitz, 1992). It therefore seems misguided to regard the IQ-reading discrepancy as a cornerstone of the diagnostic criteria for dyslexia.

Exactly the same issues apply in the case of SLI. Stark and Tallal (1981) and Aram, Morris, and Hall (1992) found that a high proportion of children who are thought on clinical grounds to have SLI fail to show a substantial discrepancy between language and non-verbal ability on psychometric tests. Such findings suggest that we need to examine carefully the validity of using a non-verbal/verbal discrepancy to identify a clinical group. Cole, Dale, and Mills (1992) have argued that one reason why we should be cautious of using a discrepancy criterion is that the reliability of non-verbal/verbal discrepancy may be unsatisfactory; they found that many children who met discrepancy criteria for SLI on one occasion failed to do so on another, and vice versa.

### *Are there Distinct Subgroups of SLI?*

A further issue is whether SLI is a unitary condition or a heterogeneous collection of disorders. There is no doubt that the clinical manifestations of SLI can be extremely variable. Some children have problems predominantly with production of speech sounds; others make many grammatical errors but appear to understand normally; cases have been described of children with severely restricted comprehension, and others of children who speak fluently in complex sentences but who give tangential answers to questions (Bishop & Rosenbloom, 1987).

Although most specialists recognise that there is considerable variation from child to child, attempts to devise a classification of SLI have not been conspicuously successful. Early studies applying multivariate methods such as cluster analysis to derive subgroups from language test data used samples far too small to give reliable results (Aram & Nation, 1975; Wolfus, Moscovitch, & Kinsbourne, 1980). Beitchman et al. (1989) applied cluster analysis to data from five speech-language measures from a large sample of 5-year-olds, including 301 children who failed a speech-language screening. They distinguished three subgroups; those with pure articulation disorders (N = 174), those with impairment only on an auditory comprehension test (N = 56), and those with low performance on all language measures (N = 87). The problem with this result is that it lacks face validity; in clinical experience it is most unusual to find a child with poor comprehension and normal expression, whereas the converse is relatively common. Furthermore, as Wilson and Risucci (1986) note, results of a cluster analysis depend crucially on the measures entered into the analysis. Standardized tests are not sensitive to all aspects of clinical presentation; e.g. it is difficult to identify pragmatic difficulties or dyspraxic speech except by clinical appraisal. Thus critical features may go unrecognised if one relies solely on test scores. Wilson and Risucci suggest that an approach which starts with clinically-defined categories and then attempts to validate these by quantitative analyses is more appropriate. They report modest success in validating a clinically derived five-subgroup classification against a classification derived from a cluster analysis. Agreement between the clinicians and the cluster analysis was 46% (Cohen's kappa = .32), which is above chance, but far from impressive, especially when one considers that the clinicians and the cluster analysis based their classifications on the same data. Furthermore, out of 93 children, only 78 could be categorised by the clinicians, and the remainder were excluded. Out of these 78, only 69 were assigned classifications by the cluster analysis program.

Two factors pose particular problems when attempting to devise a classification of SLI. First, when looking for patterns in language test data, great importance is attached to the profile of language test scores. However, discrepancies between a verbal and non-verbal test scores, or between two language scores are common in normal samples. We may illustrate this point with data from a representative sample of 179 English children who were assessed by Bishop and Butterworth (1979) in the course of studying the suitability of the revised version of the Wechsler Intelligence Scale for Children (WISC-R; Wechsler, 1974) for use in the UK. The average scaled score difference between the highest and lowest subtest was 7.6 (s.d. = 2.23), i.e. 2.5 standard deviations. The average scaled score difference between the lowest subtest and the mean of the remaining 9 subtests was 4.5 (s.d. = 1.65), i.e. 1.5 standard deviations. A flat subtest profile is very unusual; peaks and troughs in performance are commonplace and cannot be assumed to have clinical significance. The causes of such variation in normal samples is not well understood, but at least some of the unevenness in scores reflects error of measurement. Single subtests are less reliable than composites derived by summing several subtests, and differences between two subtests will be less reliable than the individual tests on which they are based. As well as error of measurement, there may be systematic differences in cognitive strengths and weaknesses of individuals that reflect specific experiences and preferences. For instance, the child who is fascinated by animals may do particularly well on a naming test that includes several animals. Factors such as these can produce peaks and troughs in test profiles that may be reliable without being very meaningful. The problem, then, is to identify systematic patterns of language impairment from a data set that is bound to contain a great deal of meaningless variation.

Second, where one does find evidence of distinct patterns, it does not necessarily follow that these correspond to different conditions. Lewis (1992) found that relatives of children with pre-school phonological disorders were affected by a wide range of speech, language and literacy problems, and she concluded that these different disorders may be variable manifestations of a broad verbal trait deficit. There may also be systematic variability in the pattern of test scores with age. For instance, Bishop and Edmundson (1987) found that a generalised expressive disorder involving speech and language often resolved into a pure phonological disorder as the child grew older. The message from these studies is clear: we should beware of assuming that different linguistic profiles correspond to aetiologically distinct disorders; the possibility remains that a single disorder might show very variable manifestation.

## TWIN DATA AS A MEANS OF VALIDATING DEFINITIONS

The twin study method is typically used in the context of behaviour genetics to address questions about aetiology. Where both twins have a disorder, they are said to be concordant, whereas when only one twin is affected, the pair is discordant. By comparing concordance rates for monozygotic (MZ) twins, who are genetically identical, and dizygotic (DZ) twins, who share only half their genes on average, one can deduce whether genes are important in causing the disorder (see Plomin, DeFries, & McClearn, 1989). However, the twin study can also help us arrive at a clearer definition of a disorder. One way of tackling questions of diagnosis and classification is to compare different characterisations of the phenotype when attempting to fit a genetic model. Rutter, Simonoff, and Silberg (1993) suggest an iterative approach where one starts with an hypothesised definition of disorder and uses genetic findings to refine the concept of the phenotype, then validating this in subsequent studies. In addition, concordant twins provide a natural form of replication study and enable one to study the question of whether different patterns of disorder simply reflect random error of measurement. If so, twins who are concordant for presence of disorder may be discordant for language profile.

In this paper, data from a twin study will be used to consider the questions outlined above. Preliminary data from this study were reported by Bishop (1992) and indicated that there was evidence of a genetic component to the aetiology. A full account is reported by Bishop, North, and Donlan (1995) and only brief details of sampling and methodology will be given here. Bishop et al. (1995) recruited 90 same-sex twin pairs where one or both twins had a specific speech or language impairment, using stringent diagnostic criteria based on definitions in the Diagnostic and Statistical Manual of the American Psychiatric Association DSM-III-R (APA, 1987). The majority of twins (90%) were aged between 7 and 10 years; the remainder were teenagers or young adults. The diagnosis of SLI was made on the basis of significantly impaired performance (scaled score of 80 or below) on any one of four language tests, with a substantial discrepancy (20 points) from non-verbal IQ, as measured by Raven's Matrices (Raven, Court, & Raven, 1986). The tests were selected to be well standardized and sensitive to different domains of language function. They included two tests of receptive language Test for Reception of Grammar (TROG) (Bishop, 1983) and WISC-R Comprehension (Wechsler, 1974), a test of sentence repetition (Semel, Wiig, & Secord, 1980), and a word finding test formed by combining items from a children's and adult's picture-naming scales (Renfrew, 1980; McKenna & Warrington, 1983). The proportion of pairs concordant for having any DSM-III-R diagnosis (i.e. speech and/or language disorder) was 54% in MZ twins (34 out of 63 pairs) and 30% in DZ twins (8 out of 27 pairs).

### *Specific and Nonspecific Language Impairment*

Although concordance was significantly higher for MZ than for DZ twins, it was well below 100 per cent. However, when Bishop et al. (1995) considered the discordant "unaffected" MZ twins, it was clear that few of them could be regarded as having normal language development. As can be seen from Figure 1, "unaffected" MZ twins frequently obtained low scores on language tests and failed to be included as affected cases simply because the discrepancy between verbal and non-verbal ability was not large enough to meet stringent criteria for SLI. The "unaffected" MZ twins did not differ significantly from their affected co-twins on two of the four language measures (TROG and Word Finding), but they did differ in terms of the Matrices non-verbal IQ, obtaining significantly lower scores than the affected twins. Figure 1 also shows the comparable data for discordant DZ twins, where the pattern was far more in line with what one would expect if the unaffected co-twins were linguistically and cognitively normal; language scores for unaffected individuals were much closer to the population mean and significantly different from affected co-twins for all four language measures, whereas non-verbal IQ was slightly above average and did not differ from that of affected individuals.

If we adopt a laxer diagnostic criterion for language disorder that includes all children who obtain any language test score below 81, and who are not mentally handicapped (i.e. IQ of 70 or above), then the concordance for MZ twins rises to 70% (with DZ concordance of 41%). Furthermore, the majority of the remaining ''unaffected'' MZ co-twins had received speech therapy for a period of 2 years or more after the age of 4 years. Including these cases as "affected" brings the MZ concordance up to 89%, compared with DZ concordance of 48%. These results lead one to draw a conclusion very similar to that stated by Stanovich (1994) regarding the dyslexia literature - namely, that there is no fundamental difference between children with language impairments who have a large discrepancy between IQ and verbal functioning, and those who do not.

FIGURE 1

Mean non-verbal and language test scores for MZ and DZ twins discordant for SLI

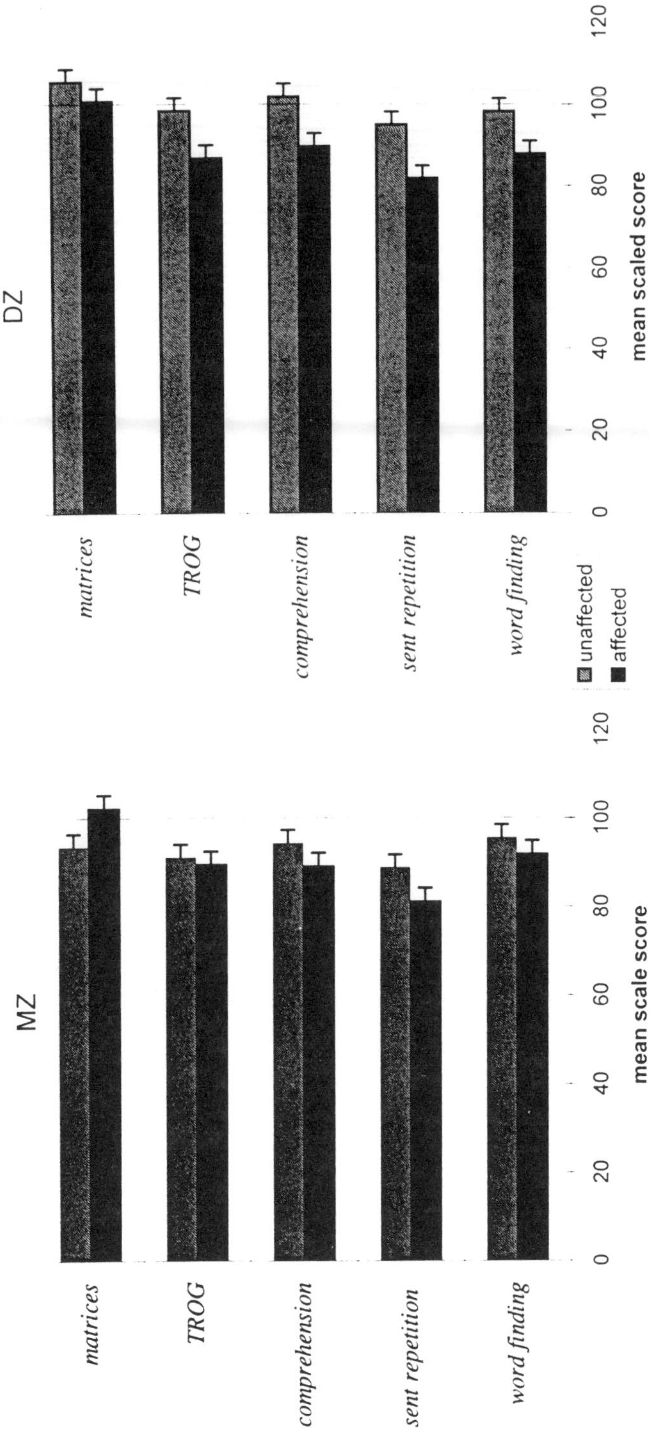

The concern is that if we were to relax discrepancy criteria we may end up with an over-inclusive definition that will select all children with borderline intelligence that has no known cause. Only empirical studies can determine how serious a problem this is. We know far less about the causes of borderline intelligence than we do about mental handicap: it could be that the majority of cases are aetiologically similar to children with SLI, or it could be that there is a host of different causal factors that can lead to the final common path of low verbal ability. If the latter is the case, then by abandoning the IQ-language discrepancy criterion we will identify a much higher proportion of cases of genetically-based developmental language disorder but only at the cost of including a great many false positive cases who have other aetiologies. It may prove to be the case that we need qualitative indicators of communicative function, rather than language test scores, in order to discriminate aetiologically distinct groups of children with low verbal abilities.

Clearly, there are no simple answers to the question of definition. In our current state of knowledge, research studies may be best advised to continue to use discrepancy criteria, simply to avoid the possibility of selecting a heterogeneous mix of children with diverse aetiologies. However, it must be recognised that in doing so, they are drawing an artificial distinction; many children with the same aetiology have equally severe language difficulties without a large IQ-language discrepancy. A diagnostic term which does not include the word "specific", such as "developmental language disorder" seems preferable to describe the condition. In terms of practical policy, there seems little justification in continuing to place heavy reliance on IQ-language discrepancies in determining who should receive extra help at school. Such decisions should be based more on whether or not the child has communicative difficulties that impair daily life and educational progress, rather than on whether they have a large difference between two test scores (Fletcher, 1992).

### *Concordance for Subgroup of Language Impairment*

When one turns to look at specific aspects of language difficulty, one is greeted by a bewildering array of symptoms. Some children are poor on all verbal tests; others have much more specific impairments with particular aspects of expression or comprehension. Concordant twins provide a useful means of testing whether patterns of language impairment reflect stable individual characteristics, or whether they are largely the result of error of measurement. The crucial question is how far there is consistency between concordant twins in terms of the pattern of impairment shown on language tests.

This analysis considered data only from 54 twin pairs who were concordant for language disorder; these included those meeting strict criteria for SLI or developmental articulation disorder, and those who have a less specific developmental language disorder, with at least one language scaled score of 80 or below, and non-verbal IQ above 70. MZ and DZ twins are treated together for this analysis; the question here is not whether genetic similarity is related to phenotypic similarity, but rather whether the pattern of disorder reflects a stable behavioural profile or whether it merely arises through random variation.

A previous analysis of this kind had been conducted by Bishop et al. (1995) to look at the stability of diagnostic category across twin pairs using the diagnostic groupings of DSM-III-R (expressive language disorder, receptive language disorder and articulation disorder). However, it was clear that these groupings did not correspond to any natural categories; many children met criteria for two or three of the subgroups and there were many instances where both twins were affected but one met criteria for receptive language disorder and the co-twin did not. However, if one ignored the child's receptive status, there was excellent agreement between twins in terms of whether or not an expressive language disorder was accompanied by an articulation disorder.

The tests used in the twin study had been selected with the aim of differentiating between different types of receptive and expressive problems, so it seemed worthwhile extending the study of twin similarity by looking at a more detailed classification system that had evolved through clinical experience. Wilson and Risucci's (1986) diagnostic framework was taken as the starting point. These authors related clinically derived categories to test scores covering nine major domains of neuropsychological functioning. Their test protocol follows a branching procedure, whereby an initial test in a given domain screens for general problems in that area, allowing further follow-up tests if the child appears to have difficulties. Thus information is potentially available on a very wide range of measures. Depending on the pattern of performance, Wilson and Risucci assigned children to one of 11 language disorder subgroups; however, because there were very small numbers in some subgroups, these were collapsed to five subgroups in their validation study.

Data from our twin study were available for only four language measures, but three of these corresponded fairly closely to measures used by Wilson and Risucci (1986). Thus, in relation to their model, WISC-R Comprehension can be regarded as an index of Auditory Cognition (equivalent to their measure AC3), Word Finding can be regarded as an index of Retrieval (RET), and Repeating Sentences as an index of Auditory Memory (equivalent to their AM1). Their battery contained no measure analogous to TROG, which is a multiple choice test specifically designed to evaluate comprehension of grammatically complex sentences when vocabulary is kept simple. This type of test, which is known to reveal grammatical difficulties in children with predominantly expressive problems (Bishop, 1979), is very different from the semantic comprehension measures used by Wilson and Risucci. They also used a range of tests designed to test visual aspects of cognitive processing. We had no tests directly analogous to their battery, but we had included the Immediate Visual Memory subtest from the British Ability Scales (Elliot, Murray, & Pearson, 1979). The test is not a pure measure of visual memory; the child is shown a card with 20 pictured items which are named by the tester, and is asked for verbal recall when the card is removed. However, there is some overlap with the Visual Memory construct of Wilson and Risucci, and this test was used here as a proxy for their VM3 test.

TABLE 1

Operational criteria for assigning individuals with SLI to diagnostic subgroups.

| construct | - | AC3 | AM1 | RS | VM3 |
|---|---|---|---|---|---|
| test | TROG | Comp | Repetition | Word Find | Vis Mem |
| **subgroup** | | | | | |
| W: global | - | - | - | - | - |
| W' | - | - | - | - | + |
| C: receptive 1 | + | - | . | . | + |
| HB: receptive 2-3 | + | - | . | . | - |
| P: receptive 4 | - | - | - | + | - |
| F: aud mem/retrieval | + | + | - | + | + |
| F': | + | + | - | - | - |
| A: expressive I | | - | - | + | + |
| S: expressive 2 | + | + | + | - | . |
| G: short-term memory | + | + | - | + | . |
| G' | - | + | - | + | . |
| N: no deficits on test* | + | + | + | + | + |

code: + scaled score of 85 or above
- scaled score below 85
. indeterminate (score can take any value)

* in this sample, the only children in this group would be those with pure articulation disorder.

On the basis of the descriptions and criteria for categories given by Wilson and Risucci, operational definitions for each subgroup were specified, as shown in Table 1. Cases were assigned a code for each measure as impaired or unimpaired simply on the basis of whether their score fell above or below 85. The pattern of codes was directly translated into categories according to the operational definitions in Table 1. Because the Wilson and Risucci classification depends on a much more complex database than was available here, it was not possible to derive criteria for every subgroup, and some categorical assignments had to be made on the basis of information that was considerably more limited than that specified by Wilson and Risucci. Subgroup H was not discriminable from subgroup B on the basis of available data, and no tests were available for diagnosing auditory processing disorders. Wilson and Risucci usually had several indices of each area of functioning and so could specify that a child showed an impairment if two out of three indices were low. Because only one index per area was available for this study, it was necessary to specify impairment on the basis of that particular test. Where one category was a logical subset of another (e.g. subgroups C and A), the more under-specified category was assigned only if the more specified category did not apply. Where a pattern was common enough in the data set to merit a category of its own, but did not exactly correspond to one of the Wilson and Risucci subgroups, a related subgroup was created, i.e. W', G' and F'. The number of possible patterns on five tests is 32; ten of these do not correspond to any subgroup in the Wilson and Risucci scheme, and twins showing these patterns were assigned no code.

Table 2 shows the conjoint classification of language disorder subgroups for each pair of twins. Numbers on the diagonal indicate concordant twin pairs where there is perfect agreement in terms of subgroup classification. The extent of agreement between twins, while far from perfect, is substantially above chance levels. In terms of specific subgroups, 20 out of 54 pairs share the same diagnosis, whereas 4.39 would be expected by chance ($Chi^2 = 262.6$, d.f. = 144; $p < .001$). If we group W with W', G with G' and F with F' agreement is even stronger, rising to 52%.

What can we conclude from this analyses? At least some of the subgroups identified by Wilson and Risucci (1986) were relatively frequent in this sample and yielded agreement between twins that was well above chance levels, demonstrating that these patterns of language score are reasonably stable phenomena and not merely reflective of error of measurement. Some subgroups, notably the receptive categories and category A (expressive 1) did not seem very coherent, though it must be recognised that assignment of cases to subgroups was based on considerably less detailed information than had been used by Wilson and Risucci.

TABLE 2

Agreement in Wilson-Risucci subgroup between 54 pairs of twins concordant for developmental language disorder.

| twin B category | twin A category W | W' | C | HB | P | F | F' | A | S | G | G' | N | none |
|---|---|---|---|---|---|---|---|---|---|---|---|---|---|
| W | 4 | 3 | . | . | . | 1 | 1 | . | . | . | . | . | 1 |
| W' | | . | 2 | . | 1 | . | . | . | . | . | . | . | . |
| C | | | . | . | 1 | . | . | 2 | . | 1 | . | 1 | 1 |
| HB | | | | 1 | . | . | . | . | . | . | . | . | . |
| P | | | | | . | . | 1 | 1 | . | 1 | 2 | . | 1 |
| F | | | | | | 4 | 2 | 2 | . | 1 | . | . | . |
| F' | | | | | | | . | . | . | . | . | . | 2 |
| A | | | | | | | | . | . | . | 1 | . | . |
| S | | | | | | | | | 1 | . | . | . | . |
| G | | | | | | | | | | 5 | 2 | . | . |
| G' | | | | | | | | | | | 3 | 2 | . |
| N* | | | | | | | | | | | | 1 | 1 |
| none | | | | | | | | | | | | | 1 |

However, good agreement between twins for subgroup of disorder does not necessarily mean that the subgroups correspond to different conditions with different causes. It could be that the same underlying disorder leads to different linguistic profiles depending on other factors such as age and cognitive abilities. Table 3 shows data compatible with that interpretation from twin pairs who are concordant for the three most common subgroups. Subgroups W (global) and G (repetition deficit) do not differ in age, but do differ in non-verbal IQ. Those in subgroup F (poor repetition and word finding, with normal comprehension) are significantly older than twins in the other two subgroups. These systematic differences between subgroups in terms of age and IQ suggest that it would be premature to
dismiss the null hypothesis of a single core inherited language deficit whose manifestation depends on level of other cognitive abilities and on stage of development.

However, we must remember that a classification is only as good as the data from which it is derived. Clinically based classifications (e.g. Bishop & Rosenbloom, 1987; Rapin & Allen, 1983) rely on language features that would not be detected with standardized language tests - e.g. key features of "semantic pragmatic disorder" are verbosity, tangential answers to questions, and problems in understanding discourse.

TABLE 3

Mean non-verbal IQ and age for twins according to language disorder subgroup.

| | W + W' global | F + F repetition + word finding | G + G' repetition only | significance* |
|---|---|---|---|---|
| | N = 20 | N = 20 | N = 28 | |
| age | 7.88<br>(1.01) | 11.49<br>(5.38) | 8.11<br>(1.48) | F (2, 65) = 8.9<br>p < .01<br>(W=G) < F |
| Matrices IQ | 90.2<br>(11.03) | 98.3<br>(12.54) | 101.1<br>(12.25) | F (2, 65) = 5.0<br>p < .01<br>W < G |

* one way analysis of variance; Scheffé test for specific contrasts.

The twin data demonstrate that some patterns of language impairment are reliable. The challenge for the future is to discover how far these patterns correspond to different disorders. Two research strategies are required. We need longitudinal studies to evaluate how language phenotypes change as the child develops, and we need to develop new assessment procedures that provide valid and reliable measures of those behaviours that appear, on clinical grounds, to characterise distinct subgroups of language disorder.

## REFERENCES

American Psychiatric Association. (1987). *Diagnostic and statistical manual of mental disorders* (3rd ed., Rev.). Washington DC: APA.

Aram, D. M., Morris, R., & Hall, N. E. (1992). The validity of discrepancy criteria for identifying children with developmental language disorders. *Journal of Learning Disabilities, 25*, 549-554.

Aram, D. M. & Nation, J. E. (1975). Patterns of language behaviour in children with developmental language disorders. *Journal of Speech and Hearing Disorders, 18*, 229-241.

Beitchman, J. H., Hood, J., Rochon, J., Peterson, M., Mantini, T., & Majumdar, S. (1989). Empirical classification of speech/language impairment in children: I. Identification of speech/language categories. *Journal of the American Academy of Child and Adolescent Psychiatry, 28*, 112-117.

Bishop, D. V. M. (1979). Comprehension in developmental language disorders. *Developmental Medicine and Child Neurology, 21*, 225-238.

Bishop, D. V. M. (1983). *The Test for Reception of Grammar*. (Available from Age and Cognitive Performance Research Centre, Department of Psychology, University of Manchester, M 13 9PL, Manchester, U.K.).

Bishop, D. V. M. (1992). The biological basis of specific language impairment. In P. Fletcher & D. Hall (Eds.), *Specific speech and language disorders in children* (pp. 2-17). London: Whurr.

Bishop, D. V. M & Butterworth, G. E. (1979). A longitudinal study using the WPPSI and WISC-R with an English sample. *British Journal of Educational Psychology, 49*, 156-168.

Bishop, D. V. M. & Edmundson, A. (1987). Language-impaired four-year-olds: Distinguishing transient from persistent impairment. *Journal of Speech and Hearing Disorders, 52*, 156-173.

Bishop, D. V. M., North, T., & Donlan, C. (1995). Genetic basis of specific language impairment: Evidence from a twin study. *Developmental Medicine and Child Neurology, 37,* 56-71.

Bishop, D. V. M. & Rosenbloom, L. (1987). Classification of childhood language disorders. In W. Yule & M. Rutter (Eds), *Clinics in Developmental Medicine: Vol. 101/102. Language development and disorders* (pp. 16-41). London: MacKeith Press.

Cole, K. N., Dale, P. S., & Mills, P. E. (1992). Stability of the intelligence quotient - language quotient relation: Is discrepancy modelling based on a myth? *American Journal on Mental Retardation, 97*, 131-143.

Elliot, C. D., Murray, D. J., & Pearson, L. S. (1979). *British Ability Scales*. Windsor: NFER-Nelson.

Fletcher, J. M. (1992). The validity of distinguishing children with language and learning disabilities according to discrepancies with IQ. *Journal of Learning Disabilities, 25*, 546-548.

Fletcher, J. M., Francis, D. J., Rourke, B. P., Shaywitz, S. E., & Shaywitz, B. A. (1992). The validity of discrepancy-based definitions of reading disabilities. *Journal of Learning Disabilities, 25*, 555-561.

Lewis, B. A. (1992). Pedigree analysis of children with phonology disorders. *Journal of Learning Disabilities, 25*, 586-597.

McKenna, P. & Warrington, E. K. (1983). *Graded Naming Test (GNT)*. Windsor: NFER-Nelson.

Pennington, B. F., Gilger, J. W., Olson, R. K., & DeFries, J. C. (1992). The external validity of age- versus IQ-discrepancy definitions of reading disability: Lessons from a twin study. *Journal of Learning Disabilities, 25*, 562-573.

Plomin, R., DeFries, J. C., & McClearn, G. E. (1989). *Behavioural genetics: A primer* (2nd ed.). New York: W. H. Freeman.

Rapin, I. & Allen, D. (1983). Developmental language disorders: Nosologic considerations. In U. Kirk (Ed.), *Neuropsychology of language, reading and spelling* (pp. 155- 184). New York: Academic Press.

Raven, J. C., Court, J. H., & Raven, J. (1986). *Raven's Progressive Matrices and Raven's Coloured Matrices*. London: H.K. Lewis.

Renfrew, C. (1980). *Word-finding vocabulary scale*. Oxford: C. E. Renfrew.

Rutter, M., Simonoff, E., & Silberg, J. (1993). How informative are twin studies of child psychopathology? In T. J. Bouchard & P. Propping (Eds.), *Twins as tools of behavioural genetics* (pp. 179-194). Chichester: Wiley.

Semel, E. M., Wiig, E. H., & Secord, W. (1980). *Clinical evaluation of language fundamentals* (Rev.). San Antonio, TX: Psychological Corporation.
Stanovich, K. E. (1994). Annotation: Does dyslexia exist? *Journal of Child Psychology and Psychiatry, 35*, 579-595.
Stark, R. E. & Tallal, P. (1981). Selection of children with specific language deficits. *Journal of Speech and Hearing Disorders, 46*, 114-122.
Wechsler, D. (1974). *Wechsler Intelligence Scale for Children* (Rev.). New York: Psychological Corporation.
Wilson, B. C. & Risucci, D. A. (1986). A model for clinical-quantitative classification generation 1: Application to language disordered preschool children. *Brain and Language, 27*, 281-310.
Wolfus, B., Moscovitch, M., & Kinsbourne, M. (1980). Subgroups of developmental language impairment. *Brain and Language, 10*, 152-171.

HEDWIG AMOROSA

# THE CLASSIFICATION OF SPEECH AND LANGUAGE DISORDERS

## INTRODUCTION

Speech and language disorders in children interfere with other aspects of development and daily life. Different professions are usually involved in the diagnosis and management of these disorders. In this paper an attempt is made to describe how speech and language disorders are seen in current classifications of various professional backgrounds. Similarities, differences and problems in classification will be discussed and a descriptive system will be proposed. Necessary research will be recommended that would allow a classification based on facts rather than on concepts.

## CLASSIFICATIONS OF SPEECH AND LANGUAGE DISORDERS

Speech and language disorders have always been considered as symptoms of neurological and psychiatric syndromes. Categories of developmental disorders were therefore included in the first psychiatric classifications in the 1950s (Rispens & Van Yperen, this volume). During the past twenty years, linguists have increasingly shown an interest in these disorders and have proposed their own classifications. In addition, neuropsychologists adapted concepts from disorders in adults to classify developmental disorders. These different classifications and proposed modifications will be considered first, before new proposals will be discussed.

### *Psychiatric Classifications*

There are two official psychiatric classifications, chapter V of the International Classification of Diseases (ICD) of the World Health Organization and the Diagnostic and Statistical Manual of Mental Disorders (DSM) of the American Psychiatric Association. Both classifications have had several revisions. The 10th revision of ICD has been published and will be the official classification system in



*J. Rispens et al. (eds.),*
*Perspectives on the Classification of Sp[illegible]ific Developme[illegible]al Disorders,* 155–180.

1996 in most European countries. In the USA, DSM-IV was published in 1994 (American Psychiatric Association [APA], 1994), but DSM-III-R is still in use.

### *ICD-10*

ICD-10 was published in 1992. The WHO developed two sets of criteria in ICD-10, one for clinical use and one for research (World Health Organization [WHO], 1992, 1993). In both classification-systems it is stressed that they are descriptive and not aetiological. Nevertheless, they describe the specific developmental disorders as strongly related to biological maturation of the central nervous system, thereby introducing aetiological factors.

*Clinical Criteria*. For ICD-10 a multi-axial form has been published (Remschmidt & Schmidt, 1994). This scheme has six axes:

I. Clinical Psychiatric Syndrome
II. Specific Developmental Disorders
III. Intellectual Level
IV. Medical Conditions
V. Associated Abnormal Psychosocial Situations
VI. Global Assessment of Psychosocial Disability.

Abnormalities in speech and language development are not only placed on the axis for specific developmental disorders, but also on other axes, in different categories (Table 1). Infantile Autism with its specific abnormalities of speech, language, and communication such as echolalia, pronominal reversal, abnormal intonation, is placed under the heading of Pervasive Developmental Disorders together with Rett's Disorder (F84.2) and Disintegrative Psychosis (F84.3), both syndromes with speech and language loss, on Axis I. Stuttering (F98.5) and Cluttering (F98.6) are individual categories within the chapter Behaviour and Emotional Disorders with Onset Specific to Childhood and Adolescence (F9). Also Elective Mutism is coded in this chapter (F94.0).

The Specific Developmental Disorders of Speech and Language (F80) are grouped together with Specific Developmental Disorders of Scholastic Skills (F81), and Specific Developmental Disorder of Motor Function (F82) on a separate axis. Specific developmental speech and language disorders are diagnosed when there is a speech and/or language disorder from the early stages of development that cannot be explained sufficiently by a backward general cognitive development, sensory deficits, neurological disease, or deprivation.

TABLE 1

Comparison of categories in current classifications of ICD-10 and DSM-IV which include speech or language symptoms as an important part of the diagnosis.

| ICD-10 | DSM-IV |
|---|---|
| **F84 Pervasive Developmental Disorders (Axis I)** | **Pervasive Developmental Disorder (Axis I)** |
| 84.0 Childhood Autism | Autistic Disorder |
| 84.1 Atypical Autism | Pervasive Developmental Disorder NOS |
| 84.2 Rett's Syndrome | Rett's Disorder |
| 84.3 Other Childhood Disintegrative Disorders | Childhood Disintegrative Disorder |
| 84.5 Asperger's Syndrome | Asperger's Disorder |
| **F94 Disorders of Social Functioning with Onset Specific to Childhood and Adolescence (Axis I)** | **Other Disorders of Infancy, Childhood, or Adolescence (Axis I)** |
| 94.0 Elective Mutism | Selective Mutism |
| **F98 Other Behaviour and Emotional Disorders with Onset Usually Occurring in Childhood or Adolescence (Axis I)** | **Communication Disorders (Axis I)** |
| 98.5 Stuttering | Stuttering |
| 98.6 Cluttering | |
| **F80 Specific Developmental Disorders of Speech and Language (Axis II)** | **Communication Disorders (Axis I)** |
| 80.0 Specific Speech Articulation Disorder | Phonological Disorder |
| 80.1 Expressive Language Disorder | Expressive Language Disorder |
| 80.2 Receptive Language Disorder | Mixed Receptive Expressive Language Disorder |
| 80.3 Acquired Aphasia with Epilepsy | |
| 80.8 Other Developmental Disorders of Speech and Language (Lisp) | Communication Disorder Not Otherwise Specified |
| **F81 Specific Developmental Disorders of Scholastic Skills (Axis II)** | **Learning Disorders (Axis I)** |
| F81.8 Other Developmental Disorders of Scholastic Skills | Disorder of Written Expression |
| **F70 Mental Retardation (Axis III)** | **Mental Retardation (Axis II)** |
| **R47 Speech- and Language Disorders not otherwise Classified (Axis IV)** | **Communication Disorders (Axis I)** |
| Dysphasia and Aphasia | Expressive Language Disorder |
| Dysarthria, Anarthria | Speech motor Deficit (Axis III) |
| **R48.2** Apraxia | |
| **R49** Voice Disorders | |

In ICD-10, there is a subdivision into five categories, namely Articulation Disorder, Expressive Disorder, Receptive Disorder, Acquired Aphasia with Epilepsy and Other Developmental Disorders of Speech and Language. In this last category, Lisp should be coded. Speech and language problems that are part of mental retardation are coded on Axis III. It is stated that in these children a great variation in their ability in different areas is common, especially language development can be particularly low. No diagnosis on Axis II is coded when a severe mental retardation is diagnosed. Acquired Aphasia (R 47.0) is listed on Axis IV.

*Research Criteria.* Research criteria of ICD-10 are closely related to clinical diagnostic criteria, but they have been operationalized and quantified to a greater degree. The research criteria for specific developmental disorders of speech and language are specified as a performance of at least two standard deviations below age-expected level as measured on an articulation or language test. Also, the performance must be at least one standard deviation below the nonverbal IQ. Furthermore, an IQ below 70 is an exclusion criterion, although it is not standardized which dimension of the IQ test has to be considered here.

Basically ICD-10 uses a categorical system for classification. Several speech and language disorders are included in psychiatric disorders such as pervasive developmental disorders or mental retardation. Others are coded as psychiatric disorders on their own such as Stuttering or Elective mutism. A third group is considered as a specific developmental disorder and closely linked to the concept of a maturational lag of the central nervous system. The Acquired aphasia with epilepsy is a curiosity, since it is an acquired neurological disorder that one could expect to be coded on Axis IV. It was included on Axis II, however, because of the close correlation in age of onset with developmental disorders and the often severe behavioural problems.

### *DSM-IV*

DSM-IV is a multi-axial system with five axes. The problem areas are distributed differently from those in the multi-axial system of the ICD.

I. Clinical Disorders
II. Personality disorders, Mental retardation
III. General medical conditions
IV. Psycho-social and environmental problems
V. Global assessment of functioning.

Speech and language problems are coded on the Axes I to III (see also Table 1). Pervasive Developmental Disorders with their speech and language abnormalities such as echolalia, pronominal reversal, abnormal intonation in Autistic Disorder or language loss in Rett's Disorder or Childhood Disintegrative Disorder are coded on Axis I. Disorders Usually First Diagnosed in Childhood or Adolescence are coded on Axis I. Elective Mutism (313.23) is coded here. The category Communication Disorders includes: Expressive Language Disorder (315.31), Mixed Receptive-Expressive Disorder (315.31), Phonological Disorder (315.39), Stuttering (307.0), and Communication Disorders Not Otherwise Specified.

The Expressive Language Disorder and the Mixed Receptive-Expressive Disorder refer to developmental and acquired disorders as well as to oral and written language. In mental retardation these classifications can be used if the impairment is in excess of the level usually associated with a low IQ. These specific disorders are not coded if a diagnosis of Pervasive Developmental Disorder is given.

Under the heading of Learning Disorders there is a category Disorders of Written Expression (315.2). It is defined as 'a combination of difficulties in the individual's ability to compose written text, evidenced by grammatical or punctuation errors within sentences, poor paragraph organization, multiple spelling errors and excessively poor handwriting' (APA, 1994, p. 52). A problem in spelling alone is not sufficient to warrant this diagnosis. Important is the impairment in written expression. Learning disorders such as a reading disorder can be diagnosed together with a pervasive developmental disorder, but the communication disorders cannot.

Mental retardation, coded on Axis II, is defined as "significantly subaverage general intellectual functioning that is accompanied by significant limitations in adaptive functioning in at least two of the following skill areas: communication, self-care, home living, social/ interpersonal skills, use of community resources, self-direction, functional academic skills, work, leisure, health, and safety" (APA, 1994, p. 39). The condition is usually accompanied by speech and language disorders.

DSM-IV uses a multi-axial format as it comes to the classification of speech and language disorders. Disorders of fluency such as stuttering are now considered Communication Disorders. Communication disorders can be coded together with mental retardation if they are in excess of the delay that can be expected on the basis of the IQ. These disorders can also be coded if they are part of an acquired disorder, but not if they are part of a pervasive developmental disorder. DSM-IV states why communication disorders are included into a psychiatric classification: "They are included to familiarize clinicians with the ways in which Communication Disorders present and to facilitate their differential diagnosis" (APA, 1994, p. 55).

### *Proposed Changes*

Van Yperen and Rispens (1990) and Van Yperen, Van Berckelaer-Onnes, and Rispens (1992) proposed a revision of the section on specific developmental disorders in psychiatric classification-systems. These authors objected to the operationalization of the discrepancy criterion between language and intelligence. Also, they pointed out that information is lost if an existing language problem cannot be coded when mental retardation or an environmental factor is assumed to be the main cause of the language disorder. In their classification, the speech or language disorder is coded whenever it occurs, independent of possible causes. With additional digits the type of disorder, e.g. expressive or receptive language disorder, as well as the assumed nature, e.g. specific, environmental or others can be coded. In a study on the reliability of these diagnoses, the authors showed that the categorical classification of ICD-10 is not very reliable. However, reliable diagnoses can be made when only the existence of an expressive or receptive language disorder has to be stated. Their proposed new classification includes speech and language disorders in mental retardation, the specific developmental disorders, stuttering, and cluttering, but it is not stated whether it also includes the speech and language disorders in pervasive developmental disorders or the acquired disorders.

## *Other Classifications*

Table 2 shows a number of classifications that were proposed by various researchers. Neurolinguistic models were used by Wilson and Risucci (1986) and Beitchman et al. (1989). The authors included very different information as a basis for their classification and came to different results. Wilson and Risucci originally derived 9 subgroups which they condensed into 5. It is not quite clear how the best number of subgroups is determined in this or other studies. Rapin and Allen (1983) proposed a medical classification with several subgroups in which they tried to relate neurological, psychiatric, and psycholinguistic information. They were interested in classifying all types of speech and language disorders in children. Linguists and neuropsychologists were mainly interested in subdividing the group of children with specific disorders.

TABLE 2

Comparison of several classifications of speech and language disorders in children.

| **Wilson & Risucci** (1986) | **Rapin & Allen** (1983) | **Aram & Nation** (1975) | **Bishop & Rosenbloom** (1987) | **Beitchman et al.** (1989) |
|---|---|---|---|---|
| Expressive Disorder (A,S)* | Phonologic Syntactic Syndrome<br>Severe Expressive Group with Good Comprehension | Formulation- Repetition Deficit | Specific Problems with Syntax and Phonology | ---- |
| Receptive Disorder (B,C,H,P)* | Syntactic Pragmatic Disorder | Repetition Strength Pattern<br>Nonspecific Formulation Repetition<br>Comprehension Deficit | Poor Understanding and Limited Verbal Expression | Poor Comprehension |
| Auditory Memory and Retrieval (F)* | ---- | Syntactic and Speech Programming Disorder | ---- | ---- |
| Global Deficit (W)* | Verbal Auditory Agnosia | Generalized Low Pattern | Generalized Delay | Low Overall |
| No Deficit (N)* | ---- | ---- | ---- | High Overall |
| ---- | Phonologic Production and Speech Planning | Phonologic Deficit | Speech Limited in Quality and/or Quantity but Other Language Skills Normal | Poor Articulation |
| ---- | Semantic Pragmatic S. without Autism<br>Autistic S. with Echolalia | ---- | Specific Problems with Pragmatics and Semantics | ---- |
| ---- | Mute Autistic Syndrome | ---- | Severe Impairment of Nonverbal and verbal Communication | ---- |

* The letters stand for several subgroups that were combined by Wilson and Risucci. (Adapted from Wilson & Risucci, 1986)

Aram and Nation (1975) used results of various language tests chosen to represent the different aspects of linguistics in order to divide a group of 19 children into subgroups by cluster analysis. Bishop and Rosenbloom (1987), in contrast, used the linguistic model and divided each area (e.g. phonology, semantics, etc.) into an expressive and a receptive mode and each subdivision into 'delayed' and 'deviant' development. This theoretical model included sixteen subgroups. The authors tried to fit known clinical cases into this system. They also related some of these subgroups to known medical causes of speech and language disorders. Most of the specific disorders fell into the group 'Aetiology unclear'. Bloom and Lahey (1978) differentiated between disorders of language form (mainly grammar), language content (mainly semantics) and language use (mainly pragmatics). In some children one area was mainly impaired, while in other children combinations of impairment were found. Fletcher (1992) saw the linguistic approach towards classifying children's disorders as too narrow and therefore proposed a 'speech and language production model' as the basis for subdividing the group. His use of language data to verify these subgroups was partly successful.

The classification of children with speech and language disorders by different approaches and by different theoretical models led to three subgroups, which are found in most studies. The first and largest group is formed by children who have an expressive disorder which usually includes problems with correct word order, morphology, and a limited vocabulary. A second smaller group includes children with problems in language comprehension. A third group comprises children with a global disorder, a combined disorder in phonology, semantics and grammar. Additional subgroups differ from study to study. It is impossible to decide from the descriptions whether the children in similar subgroups are similar to each other, or whether they would have been put into a different subgroup in another study. It is also unclear which theoretical model is most appropriate and how to decide on criteria for the number of subgroups.

## DISCUSSION OF THE CLASSIFICATIONS

### *Similarities and Differences*

The psychiatric classifications ICD-10 and DSM-IV are categorical classifications. The categories are defined by a number of typical symptoms, of which some are obligatory, while other are optional.

Usually a typical case or prototype is described. The cut-offs are more or less well defined. The goal for clinical classification is to leave as few cases as possible undiagnosed. Both classifications code speech and language abnormalities on several axes (Table 1): stuttering and cluttering are often coded with clinical psychiatric syndromes. Other speech and language disorders are only coded as part of another diagnosis such as autism or mental retardation. Both systems have a category for specific developmental disorders, where the speech and language impairment is related to the cognitive development of the child.

In ICD-10 and DSM-IV changes have been made to increase the compatibility of the two systems but differences still remain. ICD-10 gives more consideration to aetiological information and the course of diseases than DSM-IV. Therefore, ICD-10 lists the Landau-Kleffner-Syndrome (acquired aphasia and epilepsy) as a separate category, while DSM-IV does not. In DSM-IV, however, this disorder would be categorized as a Mixed Receptive-Expressive Language Disorder in the section Communication Disorder on Axis I and as a neurological disease on Axis III. This example shows that DSM-IV has gone towards the direction of coding speech and language impairments in a more dimensional way if they interfere with age-appropriate communication. Also problems both with oral and written language and developmental and acquired disorders can be coded as expressive disorders. But DSM-IV has not used this approach consistently. If a mixed expressive-receptive language disorder exists in a child with autism besides the other typical features of autism, then this symptom is not classified under the heading of Communication Disorder.

Another difference between the two classifications concerns the Disorder of Written Expression in DSM-IV and the Specific Spelling Disorder in ICD-10. The disorder of written expression excludes pure spelling disorders and there is no category for pure spelling disorders in DSM-IV. The problems of written expression are obvious in some children, but usually these children have similar problems of forming correct sentences and organizing a story in oral language. Therefore, these problems would be coded as Expresssive Language Disorders in ICD-10. If the deficit is not seen in the oral language, ICD-10 proposes to classify the Disorder of Written Expression under Other Developmental Disorders of - Scholastic Skills (F81. 8). The other classifications distinguish the same main subgroups as ICD-10 and DSM-IV, but each study describes additional subgroups.

## *Reliability*

Reliability has been studied mainly for psychiatric classifications. In DSM-III-R, overall kappas for interrater agreement for specific developmental disorders ranged from .51 to .77. For the multi-axial version of ICD-9 agreement varies from 70 to 80 % (Remschmidt, Schmidt, & Göbel, 1983; Skovgaard, Isager, & Jorgensen, 1988). Some of these classifications were done from summary reports on the children written by the attending clinician. Van Yperen et al. (1992; see also Rispens & Van Yperen, this volume) did a more thorough study on the classification of speech and language disorders with ICD-10. They studied the classification done on 97 preschool children consecutively admitted to a preschool treatment centre. The diagnoses by different raters were compared. The agreement was satisfactory for the existence of an impairment, like receptive or expressive language disorder (Kappa .77 and .66 respectively). The reliability for an articulation disorder was very low, namely Kappa .30. When specification of the category was required, such as specific disorder, environmental deprivation or other, reliability fell to a Kappa below .60, and was mainly below .40.

The differences in the results of the studies may be explained by the type of information provided to the raters. In a final report, the information has been selected with diagnostic criteria in mind and usually only information that is clear is included. Information in files usually contains all the available data, unsorted, so that each rater has to formulate his own report, include and exclude information. Another difference between these studies pertains to the age of the child. Preschoolers, especially those with behaviour problems and language delays, are much more difficult to assess than older children. The reliability between raters depends not only on the information supplied to the rater, but also on the age and the behavioural problems of the child and to the speech and language impairment.

There are not enough studies to allow a final conclusion about the reliability of the diagnostic categories of ICD-10 and DSM-IV. More research is certainly needed.

## *Operationalization and Measurement*

In the studies on reliability, the operationalization and measurement of speech and language disorders and cognitive abilities varied from subject to subject. In some children both language skills and IQ were measured by standardized tests, but often clinical judgement was used to evaluate either or both. Measurements of both the language skills and cognitive abilities are required as research criteria and recommended as part of the clinical criteria for psychiatric classification. The ICD-10 or DSM-IV definitions of specific developmental disorders of speech and language state that there is a discrepancy between speech and language development and mental age. Therefore, normal development in these areas has to be defined and decisions have to be made as to what constitutes a significant delay or impairment. According to the definition, delay must be sufficiently severe to fall outside the limit of two standard deviations. This implies, as the research criteria state explicitly, that language tests have to be used.

### *Measures of Language*

The relevant areas covered by a language test depend on the linguistic or psycholinguistic model that is used to construct the test. Few tests include pragmatics. Grammatical features are tested with real words or 'non-words', to determine whether the child can use the underlying rule to generate the correct form. Language comprehension is tested mainly as comprehension of words or sentences, seldom as comprehension of paragraphs or longer text.

Language tests give an overall account of the language abilities and are constructed to differentiate between children within the normal range. The tasks in the test are selected to give a normal distribution in the overall test result, with 2.3% of the population falling beyond two standard deviations. The guidelines for exclusion from or inclusion into the standardization group will determine the number of children with speech and/or language delay that will be included. This will influence the decision whether a child is considered to have a speech or language disorder.

Several authors investigated the agreement between the clinical judgement of a speech and language disorder and performance below one or two standard deviations in a language test. Howlin and Kendall (1991) found that different language tests administered to the same children showed high intercorrelation. However, if age equivalents as stated by the test authors were used, differences up to two years were found between tests done with the same child.

Von Suchodoletz and Höfler (1996) report that children who had been judged as normal in their speech and language development in a clinical examination showed subnormal scores in the language test (Heidelberger Sprachentwicklungstest). Aram, Morris, and Hall

(1992) report similar results for a group of American children, who were investigated as a control group within a longitudinal study. In this group of over 300 eight year old children the authors found that 47% were language impaired if a difference of one SD between a language test (PPVT-R; Tokentest for Children, Rapid Automatized Naming, Sentence Subtest of the Clinical Evaluation of Language Functions) and IQ was used. With a criterion of two SD's still 18% of the children had to be considered language impaired.

The opposite has also been found, namely that children who have a speech and/or language impairment according to clinical evaluation often do not perform below one or two SD in language tests (Amorosa, Kleinhans-Lintner, & Fisser, 1980). Aram et al. (1992) found, in children between 3 and 5;11 years of age referred by professionals for developmental disorders of speech and language, that only 51% could be diagnosed as language impaired if a discrepancy between chronological age and language test (TELD) of one SD was required, and 23% if a discrepancy of two SD was required. This observation was true not only when a composite score of tests was used, but also when only relevant subtests were considered (Von Suchodoletz & Höfler, 1996). Plante and Vance (1995) suggested individual empirically based cut-off scores for two language tests for preschool children. On these two tests, the children considered language impaired by clinicians scored at least one standard deviation below the mean in only 40% or 75% of the cases (depending on the tests used).

These results raise the question whether we can use language tests designed to measure overall language performance or differentiate among 'normal' children for the diagnosis of a language impairment. This obviously has to be doubted seriously (Howlin & Kendall, 1991). Children with scores in the lower range of these tests are not necessarily children with a language disorder. Moreover, the validity of most language tests has not been examined sufficiently (McCauley & Swisher, 1984).

Problems also arise when individual subtests of language tests are used to define a sample of language impaired children (McCauley & Demetras, 1990). Esser (1991) used the subtest 'association of sounds' from the ITPA in their Mannheim longitudinal study to define a group of children they labelled 'receptive language disorder'. Although the operationalization is well done, the validity of what is measured remains unanswered.

A similar problem has been discussed with regard to behaviour disorders, when questionnaires are used. In a study by Remschmidt and Walter (1990) on the CBCL the authors used overall scores to determine the psychiatric disorder, but they also used critical items. A higher score on these critical items would in itself be considered sufficient to warrant intervention, independent of the total scores. A similar rule may be used with language disorders. Specific abnormalities (e.g. grammatical errors such as positioning the verb consistently at the end of an utterance in German) suffice to warrant a diagnosis of a disorder in certain age-groups, independent of a total test score.

Analysis of spontaneous speech, as preferred by clinical linguists cannot solve the problem since the evaluation usually gives a profile of the stages of development related only vaguely to age. Moreover only language production is analyzed, not language comprehension.

If tests are used to measure the degree of speech and language impairment, these tests must be validated by clinical ratings of the degree of impairment in relevant speech and language areas.

### *Measures of Intelligence*

In the Multi-axial Classification (Remschmidt & Schmidt, 1994) it is stated that a nonverbal test of reasoning should be used to determine the intelligence of the children with specific developmental disorders of speech and language. The research criteria state that the IQ has to be more than 70, but do not mention whether a full scale IQ, a verbal IQ or a performance IQ is required. Language and cognitive abilities are highly interactive. According to Howlin and Rutter (1987), there is a 'constructive interaction' between the two. The form of this interaction changes, depending on the experience and maturation of the child. Tests of general intelligence correlate highly with language tests in the order of .60 or more, indicating that similar abilities are required. The correlation between language skills is lower with the performance IQ. Also there are children with good formal language skills despite of a low IQ.

Which tests are most appropriate to determine the cognitive abilities of children with specific developmental speech and language disorders is still a question. Sometimes a full scale IQ is used. Because of the high correlation between verbal IQ and the language tests, a child would have to obtain a very high performance IQ to be considered specifically language impaired. Another possibility is to use nonverbal intelligence tests or the performance IQ. These tests vary according to which functions are included. For example, the Snijders-Oomen test (1977) has no subtest that assesses memory functions, while the nonverbal scale of the Kaufman Assessment Battery includes three subtests out of six that assess memory functions. Yule (1987) asks whether the results of normal children may be generalized to children with handicaps. Especially when profiles of the scores on the subtests deviate considerably, it might be in-appropriate to use a summed score such as the performance IQ to describe the cognitive abilities of the child.

Often, one-dimensional tests, such as the Raven Matrices or the Columbia Mental Maturity Scale, or individual subtests from performance scales are used. The results of these tests are less reliable than when multi-dimensional tests are used. The use of individual subtests creates a problem, because the standard test procedure cannot be used, so that it is difficult to interpret the results (Yule, 1987).

In sum, it may be difficult to obtain a reliable measurement of the nonverbal intelligence of children with speech and language disorders.

### *Discrepancy Between Language and IQ*

In both the clinical and the research classification, a discrepancy between language performance and age must be established for the diagnosis of a specific developmental disorder. In addition a discrepancy between language and nonverbal IQ is required. In the research criteria, in the former the discrepancy must be two SD's, in the latter one SD. An IQ below 70 is an exclusion criterion. In clinical classification the criterion is not clearly specified: "... below the appropriate level for his or her mental age..." for articulation disorder and the receptive language disorder, and "... markedly below the appropriate level for his or her mental age..." for the expressive language disorder (WHO, 1992, pp. 236-238).

Considering the problems identified in the above discussion of language tests and the measurement of intelligence in language impaired children, a discrepancy definition is clearly based on highly questionable procedures. Aram et al. (1992) addressed the question of discrepancy definitions in a study and found that the number of children referred by experienced clinicians with the diagnosis of a specific disorder of speech and language who were actually given this diagnosis, depended on the criteria applied. Only 40-60% of the children were classified as 'specific disorder' when the discrepancy criteria were used. The discrepancy definition of specific developmental disorders is closely related to the concept of a maturational lag and has to be discussed in relation to the different concepts underlying classifications.

## CONCEPTS

Different attempts to classifying children with speech and language disorders and especially those with the „specific“ disorders are related to the underlying models of language learning and speech production. There are linguistic and neuropsychological models. The theoretical background of classification in ICD-10 which leads to categorical classification is the concept of language disorders caused by a maturational lag. DSM-IV leans instead towards a model in which speech and language is considered as an important factor in many areas of child development which should be looked at in a multi dimensional way.

### *Linguistic and Neuropsychological Concepts*

Linguists consider a model that includes the different components of language, phonology, grammar, semantics and pragmatics, as the most appropriate way to describe language disorders in children. Often, this model includes the idea of language function as an independent module in brain functioning with an innate language acquisition device. The assumption is that if this module is not working properly, the person is unable to generate the appropriate rules of grammar. Fletcher (1992) has criticised this approach as too narrow and prefers a psycholinguistic model of the speech production process as the basis for the description of subtypes of children with speech and language disorders.

There are other problems with linguistic models. Most methods and systems developed in linguistics are developed to describe the competence of a mature speaker, but they are then used to analyze production data of children having problems learning a first language. The systematic descriptions are used as if they show the production process of an individual speaker who is producing an individual utterance. Many linguists seem to imply that language learning and language production are independent of other abilities such as memory, auditory perception, attention or others.

Neuropsychological models, in contrast, consider many different functions that are seen as important for language learning in their analysis. The functions included are partly derived from adult models of language functioning. Often each of these functions is included with equal weight and at all stages of development. However, it has been shown that certain functions might be important at one stage but not at another. For example, as studies from blind persons have shown (Fraiberg, 1977), visual information seems to be important in early but not in later development.

*Categorical Concept*

The concept for the specific developmental disorders is categorical, which means that these disorders are entities which are different from speech and language disorders in, for example, Autism or in Mental Retardation. The category is closely related to the concept of a maturational lag in brain development that specifically delays speech and language development in otherwise normal children. ICD-10 refers to "impairment or delay of functions closely related to biological maturation of the central nervous system" (Cooper, 1991, p. 262). The categorical concept of a specific disorder can have three meanings: 1. The disorder is temporary (the child will catch up in time); 2. The disorder is isolated (the child is otherwise normal); 3. The symptoms are different from those in children with 'nonspecific' disorders of speech and language.

*Temporary Impairment*

This concept of temporary impairment has been challenged. Longitudinal studies have shown that many children do not outgrow their problems. Bishop and Edmundson (1987) assessed children at the age of 4, 5;6 and 8 years, and found that 44 % of the children originally diagnosed with a clinically significant delay in speech or language no longer fulfilled the criteria for severe language impairment. However, while the group had improved, the language performance was still below the language level of the control group at the age of 8 years. Similar findings are reported by Fundudis, Kolvin, and Garside (1979). They reexamined children at the age of 7-8 years, who did not join three words into a meaningful utterance at the age of 3 years. The children who met the criteria for a specific speech and language disorder were still having speech and language problems at follow-up.

In a longitudinal study, Schakib-Ekbatan and Schöler (1994) followed children with specific developmental disorders of speech and language between the ages of 6 and 17. They showed that short term memory in the auditory modality and the performance in specific language tasks remained at a very low level without significant increases over the last few assessments. Rutter and Mawhood (1991) reported a follow-up study of children originally seen at the age of 7;6 years. These children had a severe receptive language disorder, but a nonverbal IQ above 70. At the age of 24 they had gained conversational language, but the expressive language was considered adequate in only one third of the group. Twenty-one percent had a receptive language level equivalent to children aged below 10 years of age or less.

These studies show that most children with specific developmental disorders do not outgrow their difficulties but continue to have problems into adolescence or adult life, in contrast to what would be expected from a delay in maturation of brain structures.

### *Isolated Disorder*

The children with specific developmental disorders are supposed to develop normally in all other respects. Their cognitive abilities have to be within the normal range, as well as their hearing. The criterion that there is no neurological or psychiatric abnormality and that there is a normal psychosocial environment, are required as part of the definition. Cromer (1988) and Johnston (1992), however, describe cognitive deficits in these children in spite of an average IQ. Several complex mental activities have been found to be impaired in groups of language disordered children, such as hierarchical planning (Cromer, 1988), symbolic functioning (Morehead, 1972) or more basic mechanisms such as short term memory (Amorosa, in press; Gathercole & Baddeley, 1993; Kirchner & Klatzky, 1985). Each one of these mental activities does not explain the language disorder in itself (Johnston, 1992), but the studies show that cognitive dysfunctions of different types are observed in these children. Besides the cognitive deficits, examinations found an increase in fine and gross motor impairments and neurological abnormalities (Amorosa, 1989; Noterdaeme, Amorosa, Ploog, & Scheimann, 1988).

Moreover, children with specific developmental speech and language disorders are much more likely to have a psychiatric diagnosis than children with normal speech and language development. However, no specific diagnosis combines with developmental disorders (Amorosa, Von Benda, & Wagner, 1986;

Cantwell & Baker, 1985; Esser, Lehmkuhl, & Schmidt, 1983). Some psychiatric problems seem to be caused mainly by the language disorder, but often the two disorders coexist from the beginning or the psychiatric disorder clearly precedes the language disorder.

### *Differences with Nonspecific Disorders of Speech and Language*

The concept of a specific disorder implies that children with specific developmental speech and language disorders show abnormalities that are not usually seen in children, neither in younger normal children, nor in children with nonspecific speech and language disorders. There have been intensive discussions about deviance or delay of language development (Rutter, Mawhood, & Howlin, 1992). The problem has not been resolved, but it seems clear that children with a specific speech and language disorder do not show abnormalities that cannot be found at a certain stage in normal language development.

In the formal aspects of grammar, the language of autistic children does not differ from the language of children with specific developmental disorders (e.g. Von Benda, 1984) or children with Down's Syndrome (Tager-Flusberg et al., 1990). The children do differ in the way they use language for communication. Also, they often learn the language at different rates, but usually in the same sequence as normal children do.

Mentally retarded children differ considerably in degree of speech and language impairment. The group studied most frequently are children with Down's Syndrome. In these children a discrepancy between language development and nonverbal IQ has been found. However, no difference was observed in many aspects of language, when the children were parallelled for stage of language development (Fowler, 1986). Fundudis et al. (1979), in their longitudinal study, divided a group of children with residual speech and language disorders into three subgroups with different IQ levels. No difference was found in the profiles of the language tests except that all scores of the subtests were higher in the group with the higher IQ.

These studies show that there are no qualitative differences - neither in the sequence in which different aspects of language are acquired, nor in the types of discrepancies with adult language that children use - between children with specific developmental disorders of speech and language, normal children, children with mental retardation, or autistic children. The differences are quantitative. This questions the specificity of the 'specific' developmental disorders, but it does not say anything about the fact whether or not the different groups of children learn language in the same way as normal children do.

The difference between a specific language disorder and a language disorder in a child with a low IQ was also questioned in a study by Cole and Dale (1986). They found that therapy with language impaired children did not differ significantly between children with a 'specific disorder' and those with a 'nonspecific' disorder linked to an IQ below 70.

The concept of a maturational lag as underlying specific developmental disorders is difficult to prove or disprove (Bishop & Edmundson, 1987). Specific developmental disorders as a category in the classification are not specific in the sense that they are isolated or qualitatively different from the disorders in normal younger children or children with other psychiatric disorders. They are also not temporary delays that are easily improved by therapy.

### *The Multi-Dimensional Framework*

During the last few years there has been some discussion whether the categorical classification of psychiatric disorders is the best way of subdividing children with problems. The multi-axial classification was introduced because important aspects of a case could not be coded sufficiently with just one diagnosis. In this way, IQ was introduced in a dimensional description. In the multi-axial form of the ICD-10 the IQ is coded independent of other aspects of the case and independent of other diagnoses given. There are several reasons for considering the area of speech, language and communication as equal in importance as IQ, especially in children.

1. Speech and language disorders interfere with communication that is appropriate in complexity for the overall development of the child. Disorders of speech sound production or fluency make it difficult to understand the child. The person interacting with the speech impaired child is often unsure of what the child wants to communicate and will often be reluctant to engage in verbal interaction or will structure or dominate the interaction to avoid misunderstandings. Since the child often does not get the appropriate feedback to what it said, the language development will not be supported as much as in children with normal speech. Also the relationship with the caregivers will be less stable and supportive. The same is true for the expressive language disorders.

The child's ability to express itself is often far less complex as would be necessary for the child's developmental status. In children with a receptive disorder, communication often breaks down unnoticed by the person interacting with the child. Also, the child often does not understand the feedback given verbally. Misunderstandings are common, but are often attributed to inattention or disobedience of the child.

2. Communicative breakdowns influence the socio-emotional development of the child. Kammerer (1988), in a study of deaf children, showed that the degree of perceived communicative ability in children and parents was highly related to psychiatric disorder. The lower the ability to communicate with the family and important others, the higher the risk for social and emotional problems. Rutter and Mawhood (1991) also showed that children with specific developmental disorders have a raised frequency of socio-emotional disorders.

3. Speech and language disorders also interfere with cognitive development. Sometimes it is stated that concepts have to be formed first and then they are labelled. However, if the same object is named reliably with the same sounds that can be remembered, it is easier to form a concept of the object. Concepts that have a name can be talked about, elaborated, changed, adjusted and used in daily life. Howlin and Rutter (1987) state that the development of language and cognition should be seen as 'constructive interaction'. The impairment of one will affect the development of the other.

4. Problems in speech and language development are important for school achievement. Verbal IQ is an important predictor of school achievement in the normal population. Most teaching and interacting in school is done by oral language, supplemented increasingly by written language in all types of schools. Children with speech and language problems, especially those with receptive disorders, will have major problems in school unless great care is taken to compensate for their handicap.

DSM-IV has taken the importance of speech, language, and communication problems into account and has moved towards a more comprehensive approach, by including disorders in sign language, acquired disorders and fluency disorders into the category of communication disorders. However, DSM has not gone all the way. The speech and language disorders of autism and mental retardation are still excluded.

A comprehensive approach takes into account that speech and language are the most important means for a differentiated communication and that impairment interferes with socio-emotional and cognitive development and school achievement. All of these are important risk factors for psychiatric disorders. This approach takes in consideration that speech and language development is not so highly correlated with IQ that including the IQ in the classification sufficiently describes speech and language function in the child.

## PROPOSAL FOR A CLASSIFICATION AND SUGGESTIONS FOR FURTHER RESEARCH

The classification of speech and language disorders in ICD-10 and DSM-IV is not satisfactory. Speech and language disorders can be found on several axes. Some are grouped with the psychiatric disorders or included in them, even though they are not necessarily a symptom of the disorder. Sometimes they are part of a developmental disorder, a neurological disease or mental retardation. The operationalization of the categories for the specific disorders of speech and language is questionable, due to problems of validity and reliability of measurement. Furthermore, it is unclear whether the differentiation between, for example, the specific disorders and mental retardation is adequate. It is also questionable whether the differentiation within the categories of Communication Disorder (DSM-IV) or Developmental Disorders of Speech and Language (ICD-10) is adequate.

Speech and language are two independent areas, but also language in itself is not a uni-dimensional concept. For the description in a medical or psychiatric classification, it is at the moment questionable whether linguistic differentiation into phonological, semantic and grammatical impairment will be the best system. ICD and DSM settled for a subdivision based on knowledge derived from adult neurology including three broad categories: Articulation Disorder (in ICD-10) and Phonological Disorder (in DSM-IV), Expressive, and Receptive Language Disorder. These are also the most stable categories in the other classifications described. The reliability for these categories was sufficient according to the study by Van Yperen et al. (1992), except for the articulation disorder. Clinically it is important to differentiate between children who have problems expressing themselves but who understand well and those who have problems comprehending age-appropriate language directed at them. Besides these three categories, the fluency disorders (stuttering and cluttering), should be included as well as elective mutism, since both interfere with communication through language. In my view five types of speech and language deficits should be coded with the additional possibility to code absence of speech or language:

80. 0 No speech or language;
80. 1 Disorders of speech sound production;
80. 2 Fluency disorder (Stuttering, Cluttering);
80. 3 Expressive language disorder;
80. 4 Receptive language disorder;
80. 5 Use of speech and language in communication.

These areas are judged independent of each other and independent of other classifications (e.g. those on Axis I of the multi-axial ICD-scheme). In this way, the mute autistic child has the diagnosis 'Early infantile autism' on Axis I and 'no speech or language' on Axis II, whereas the IQ is coded on Axis III.

In this system all other types now coded under the heading F80 in ICD-10 can be coded according to the type of speech or language disorder on Axis II and according to the cause on Axis IV. For example, the Landau-Kleffner Syndrome would be classified with its behavioural abnormalities, if they are present, on Axis I, its language comprehension problems on Axis II and the epilepsy or as Landau-Kleffner Syndrome on Axis IV; the language deficit in severe deprivation is coded on Axis II and the lack of stimulation is coded on Axis V. The only category that is not sufficiently coded this way is the category for the specific developmental disorders, since the full scale IQ is the basis of coding on Axis III and not the nonverbal IQ as required for the diagnosis of a specific disorder of speech and language. In ICD-10 the second digit after the decimal point could be used to code the severity of the deficit or the degree of interference with age-appropriate communication.

To operationalize the diagnoses it will be necessary to do further research. Speech and language tests to assess normal variation of language development are not sufficient. Their validity for the assessment of clinically relevant abnormalities in speech and language development has to be established. Critical symptoms related to specific ages might be more important signs of disorder than a low overall test score. The critical items will be different not only for different ages but also for different languages. Studies of reliability of judgement and importance of these factors for management, therapy and course of the behavioural disorder are necessary to decide which information would be most useful.

The present subdivision of speech and language disorders is clinically oriented, based on classifications derived from adult aphasia. Further research should be done to investigate whether other factors might be more important for the course and treatment of these disorders. These factors could be:

- the ability to analyze an acoustical signal on-line, i.e. fast enough to follow speech;
- the ability to keep enough auditorily presented information in short term memory;
- the ability to form sufficiently differentiated concepts and to keep them stored in memory together with their names;
- the ability to set up a well-structured lexicon that makes fast retrieval possible;
- the ability to use feedback consistently in a parallel processing system to develop correct grammar.

These factors might be important for learning a language. Deficits in one or several factors might be responsible for the language problems we see in the children. If we study these factors we might come to a different subdivision of the speech and language disorders, which may be related more closely to brain functioning, to therapeutic requirements, or outcome prediction than the present system.

## REFERENCES

American Psychiatric Association. (1994). *Diagnostic and statistical manual of mental disorders* (4th ed.). Washington, DC: American Psychiatric Association.

Amorosa, H. (1989). *Die Untersuchung kindlicher Sprechbewegungsstörungen mit Hilfe der akustischen Analyze*. Habilitationsschrift, Ludwig-Maximilian Universität, München.

Amorosa, H. (in press). Störungen des Kurzzeitgedächtnisses bei Sprachentwicklungsstörungen. *Fundamenta psychiatrica.*

Amorosa, H., Kleinhans-Lintner, J., & Fisser, U. (1980). Eine Untersuchung mit dem Tokentest an sprachentwicklungsverzögerten und teilleistungsgestörten Kindern. *Zeitschrift für Kinder-und Jugendpsychiatrie, 8*, 288-299.

Amorosa, H., Von Benda, U., & Wagner, E. (1986). Die Häufigkeit psychiatrischer Auffälligkeiten bei 4-8 jährigen mit unverständlicher Spontansprache. *Zeitschrift für Kinder- und Jugendpsychiatrie, 14*, 289-295.

Aram, D.M., Morris, R., & Hall, N.E. (1992). The validity of discrepancy criteria for identifying children with developmental language disorders. *Journal of Learning Disability, 25*, 549-554.

Aram, D.M. & Nation, J.E. (1975). Patterns of language behaviour in children with developmental language disorders. *Journal of Speech and Hearing Research, 18*, 229-241.

Beitchman, J.H., Hood, J., Rochon, J., Peterson, M., Mantini, T., & Majumdar, S. (1989). Empirical classification of speech/language impairment in children I.

identification of speech/language categories. *Journal of the American Academy of Child and Adolescent Psychiatry, 28*, 112-117.

Bishop, D. & Edmundson, A. (1987). Specific language impairment as a maturational lag: Evidence from longitudinal data on language and motor development. *Developmental Medicine and Child Neurology, 29*, 442-459.

Bishop, D. & Rosenbloom, L. (1987). Childhood language disorders: Classification and overview. In W. Yule & M. Rutter (Eds.), *Clinics in developmental medicine: Vol. 101/102. Language development and disorders* (pp. 16-41). London: MacKeith Press.

Bloom, L. & Lahey, M. (1978). *Language development and language disorder.* New York: Wiley.

Burgemeister, B. B., Hollander Blum, L., & Lorge, I. (1959). *Columbia Mental Maturity Scale.* New York: World Book Company.

Cantwell, D. P. & Baker, L. (1985). Psychiatric and learning disorders in children with speech and language disorders: A descriptive analysis. *Advances in Learning and Behavioural Disabilities, 4*, 29-47.

Cole, K. N. & Dale, P. S. (1986). Direct language instruction and interactive language instruction with language delayed preschool children: A comparison study. *Journal of Speech and Hearing Research, 29*, 193-205.

Cooper, J. E. (1991). *Pocket guide to the ICD-10 classification of mental and behavioural disorders.* World Health Organization, Geneva, Churchill Livingstone, Edinburgh.

Cromer, R. F. (1988). The cognition hypothesis revisited. In R. Kessel (Ed.), *The development of language and language researchers: Essays in honour of Roger Brown* (pp. 223-248). Hillsdale: Erlbaum.

Esser, G. (1991). *Was wird aus Kindern mit Teilleistungsschwächen? Der langfristige Verlauf umschriebener Entwicklungsstörungen.* Stuttgart: Enke Verlag.

Esser, G., Lehmkuhl, G., & Schmidt, M. (1983). Die Beziehung von Sprechstörungen und sprachlichen Entwicklungsrückständen zur zerebralen Dysfunktion und psychiatrischen Auffälligkeiten bei 8 jährigen. *Sprache, Stimme, Gehör, 2*, 59-62.

Fletcher, P. (1992). Sub-groups in school-age language-impaired children. In P. Fletcher & D. Hall (Eds.), *Specific speech and language disorders in children.* London: Whurr Publishers.

Fowler, A. E. (1986). The development of language structure in children with Down Syndrome. *Haskins Laboratories Status Report on Speech Research, 88*, 221-262.

Fraiberg, S. (1977). *Insights from the blind.* New York: Merridian.

Fundudis, T., Kolvin, J., & Garside, R. F. (1979). *Speech retarded and deaf children: Their psychological development.* London: Academic Press.

Gathercole, S. E. & Baddeley, A. D. (1993). *Working memory and language.* Hove: Lawrence Erlbaum.

Howlin, P. & Kendall, L. (1991). Assessing children with language tests - which test to use? *British Journal of Disorders of Communication, 26*, 355-367.

Howlin, P. & Rutter, M. (1987). The consequences of language delay for other aspects of development. In W. Yule & M. Rutter (Eds.), *Clinics in developmental medicine: Vol. 101/102. Language development and disorders* (pp. 271-294). London: MacKeith Press.

Johnston, J. R. (1992). Cognitive abilities of language impaired children. In P. Fletcher & D. Hall (Eds.), *Specific speech and language disorders in children* (pp. 105-116). London: Whurr Publishers.

Kammerer, E. (1988). *Kinderpsychiatrische Aspekte der schweren Hörschädigung.* Stuttgart: Enke Copythek.

Kaufman, A. S. & Kaufman, N. L. (1983). *Kaufman Assessment Battery for Children (K-ABC).* Circle Pines, MN: American Guidance Service Inc.

Kirchner, D. & Klatzky, R. (1985). Verbal rehearsal and memory in language disordered children. *Journal of Speech and Hearing Research, 28*, 556-564.

McCauley, R. J. & Demetras, M. J. (1990). The identification of language impairment in the selection of specifically language-impaired subjects. *Journal of Speech and Hearing Disorder, 55*, 468-475.

McCauley, R. J. & Swisher, L. (1984). Psychometric view of language and articulation tests for preschool children. *Journal of Speech and Hearing Disorders, 49*, 34-42.

Morehead, D. (1972). Early grammatical and semantic relations: Some implications for a general representational deficit in linguistically deviant children. *Papers and Reports in Child Language Development, 4*, 1-12.

Noterdaeme, M., Amorosa, H., Ploog, M., & Scheimann, G. (1988). Quantitative and qualitative aspects of associated movements in children with specific developmental speech and language disorders and in normal preschool children. *Journal of Human Movement Studies, 15*, 151-169.

Plante, E. & Vance, R. (1995). Diagnostic accuracy of two tests of preschool language. *American Journal of Speech-Language Pathology, 4*, 70-76.

Rapin, I. & Allen, D. A. (1983). Developmental language disorder: Nosologic considerations. In U. Kirk (Ed), *Neuropsychology of language, reading, and spelling* (pp. 155-185). New York: Academic Press.

Raven, J. (1981). *Coloured Progressive Matrices.* London: Lewis.

Raven, J. (1987). *Standard Progressive Matrices.* London: Lewis.

Remschmidt, H. & Schmidt, M. (Hrsg.) (1994). *Multi-axiales Klassifikationsschema für psychische Störungen des Kindes- und Jugendalters nach ICD-10 der WHO.* Bern: Huber.

Remschmidt, H., Schmidt, M., & Göbel, D. (1983). Erprobungs- und Reliabilitätsstudie zum multi-axialen Klassifikationsschema für psychiatrische Erkrankungen im Kindes- und Jugendalter. In H. Remschmidt & M. Schmidt (Hrsg.) *Multi-axiale Diagnostik in der Kinder- und Jugendpsychiatrie*, (pp. 43-75). Bern: Huber.

Remschmidt, H. & Walter, R. (1990). *Psychische Auffälligkeiten bei Schulkindern.* Zürich: Hofgrefe.

Rutter, M. & Mawhood, L. (1991). The long-term psychological sequelae of specific developmental disorders of speech and language. In M. Rutter & P. Casaer (Eds.), *Biological risk factors in childhood psychopathology* (pp. 233-259). Cambridge: Cambridge University Press.

Rutter, M., Mawhood, L., & Howlin, P. (1992). Language delay and social development. In P. Fletcher & D. Hall (Eds.), *Specific speech and language disorders in children* (pp.63-78). London: Whurr Publishers.

Schakib-Ekbatan K. & Schöler, H. (1994). Zur Persistenz von Sprachentwicklungsstörungen: Ein 10jähriger Längsschnitt neun spezifisch sprachentwicklungsgestörter Kinder. *Arbeitsberichte aus dem Forschungsprojekt "Dysgrammatismus", 22*, Pädagogische Hochschule Heidelberg.

Skovgaard, A. M., Isager, T., & Jorgensen, O. S. (1988). The reliability of Child psychiatric diagnosis: A comparison among Danish child psychiatrists of traditional diagnosis and a multi-axial diagnostic system. *Acta Psychiatrica Scandinavica, 77*, 469-476.

Snijders, J. T. & Snijders-Oomen, N. (1977). *Snijders-Oomen nonverbale Intelligenztestreihe*. Wolters-Noordhoff, Groningen.

Tager-Flusberg, H., Calkins, S., Nolin, T., Baumberger, T., Anderson, M., & Chadwick-Dias, A. (1990). A longitudinal study of language acquisition in autistic and Down syndrome children. *Journal of Autism and Developmental Disorders, 20*, 1-21.

Van Yperen, T. A. & Rispens, J. (1990). The classification of specific developmental disorders: An alternative to DSM and ICD. In P. J. Drenth, J. A. Sergeant, & R. J. Takens (Eds.), *European Perspectives in Psychology, Vol 1.* (pp. 219-234). Chichester: Wiley.

Van Yperen, T. A., Van Berckelaer-Onnes, I. A., & Rispens, J. (1992). Classification of specific developmental disorders: Moving away from the hierarchical model of DSM and ICD. *European Journal of Psychiatry, 6*, 223-235.

Von Benda, U. (1984). Untersuchungen zur Intonation autistischer, sprachentwicklungsgestörter und sprachunauffälliger Kinder. *Forschungsberichte des Instituts für Phonetik und sprachliche Kommunikation, 20*, 1-232.

Von Suchodoletz, W. & Höfler, C. (1996). Stellenwert des Heidelberger Sprachentwicklungstests (HSET) in der Diagnostik von Kindern mit Sprachentwicklungsstörungen. *Zeitschrift für Kinder- und Jugendpsychiatrie, 24*, 4-11.

Wilson, B. C. & Risucci, D. A. (1986). A model for clinical quantitative classification, Generation I: Application to language-disordered preschool children. *Brain and Language, 27*, 281-309.

World Health Organization. (1992). *ICD-10: International classification of diseases and related health problems (10th rev.)*. Geneva: World Health Organization.

World Health Organization. (1993). *Tenth Revision of the International Classification of Diseases, Chapter V (F): Mental and Behavioural Disorders. Diagnostic Criteria for Research.* Geneva: World Health Organization.

Yule, W. (1987). Psychological assessment. In W. Yule & M. Rutter (Eds.), *Clinics in developmental medicine: Vol. 101/102. Language development and disorders* (pp. 312-323). London: MacKeith Press.

TOM A. VAN YPEREN

# SPECIFIC LANGUAGE AND SPEECH DISORDER: PURIFYING THE CONCEPT

## INTRODUCTION

Children with language or speech impairments are often easily recognized in clinical practice. Cases that show these impairments, but have no mental retardation, pervasive developmental disorder, a physical handicap or a depriving environment, almost intuitively give the idea that some specific disorder exists. From this perspective, the concept of Specific Developmental Disorders of Language and Speech (SDD-LS) is appealing (see also Rispens & Van Yperen, this volume). From a scientific point of view, however, the evidence for the validity of a category must be based on more than intuition. The category must be analyzed theoretically and empirically in detail, purifying it from invalid connotations and illogical elements. The preceding chapters by Amorosa and Bishop showed that the validity of the ICD and DSM categories for SDD-LS are, at least, questionable. Amorosa argued that there are no qualitative differences between children with the specific developmental disorder of language or speech, normal children, children with mental retardation, or autistic children. The differences appear to be quantitative only. Bishop argued that the distinction between Specific Language Impairment (SLI) and global cognitive impairment is invalid. She found that there are no fundamental differences between SLI discrepants and non-discrepants.

The purpose of this paper is to offer a more detailed conceptual analysis of the SDD-LS categories in ICD and the corresponding categories in DSM. It is important to discuss the distinction between the various categories in classification systems such as ICD and DSM in the context of the general, structural characteristics of these classification schemes. The approach taken in this chapter differs from the preceding two chapters, in that it will focus on the taxonomic aspects of the classification of SDD-LS. From this perspective we will take a look at the way the categories are defined and how the boundaries with other categories are marked. I will focus on three (related) issues:



*J. Rispens et al. (eds.),*
*Perspectives on the Classification of Specific Developmental Disorders*, 181–206.

- The first is in what kind of a conceptual network the categories are defined. We will take a closer look at the classification model in which the SDD-LS category of ICD and DSM is placed. Furthermore, I will discuss the concepts that mark the boundaries and the core of the category.
- The second issue is what the psychometric aspects are of the differentiation that is made between the SDD-LS category and various other categories. From this perspective, the consequences for the empirical validation of the concept are discussed.
- The third issue is whether ICD and DSM offer the best taxonomic solution in the classification of this disorder, given the current state of knowledge. Several alternatives will be presented.

This chapter will conclude with a discussion on how SDD-LS should be classified in schemes such as DSM and ICD, in view of the difficulties with the SDD-LS category described in this and the preceding two chapters.

## THE CONCEPTUAL NETWORK

The categories for the specific developmental disorders in ICD-10 and DSM-IV constitute a part of a complex conceptual framework. This framework is based on three principles.

Amorosa (this volume) already mentioned one principle: the ICD-10 and DSM-IV are categorical classifications, in which typical cases or prototypes are described. In this section, I will argue that the SDD-LS concept, however, does not represent a simple category, but forms part of a hierarchical disease model, in which disorders are defined as higher-order or lower-order prototypes. The logical consequence is that the same patterns of language and speech impairment can belong to different disorders, just as different patterns can also belong to one and the same disorder.

A second principle in the conceptual framework is that the SDD-LS category is largely defined by exclusionary criteria. In this section I will discuss the possible concepts behind the exclusionary criteria of mental retardation, physical abnormality, severe environmental deprivation, and pervasive developmental disorder, used to mark the boundaries with SDD-LS.

A third principle is that the disorder that falls within the boundaries of the SDD-LS category is attributed a specific nature (the 'core' of the category). I will look at the explanations and examples that are offered by ICD and DSM to describe this core.

### *The SDD-LS Category: a Prototype within a Hierarchy*

The categorical model in ICD-10 and DSM-IV is characterized by a hierarchical as well as a prototypical definition of syndromes. In a hierarchical model, symptoms and syndromes are ordered in hierarchies, according to their diagnostic priority. Diagnostic priorities developed in psychiatry are usually placed in the following hierarchy:

| | |
|---|---|
| highest position: | organic disorders |
| ↑ | functional disorders |
| ↓ | neuroses |
| lowest position: | reactive disorders and other symptoms |

Normally, disorders that have an organic cause or nature are placed in a higher position than functional disorders (i.e. disorders without a clear organic cause or nature). Functional psychoses prevail over neuroses. Reactive disorders, that are caused by stressful events and are usually only of a short duration, are placed at the bottom of the hierarchy, together with other symptoms (Foulds, 1976; Morey, 1987; Silberman, 1971). If a symptom, for example anxiety, has a clear organic cause, it is seen as a part of this organic syndrome. Only if there is no clear organic cause, the symptom can be considered as part of a lower order syndrome. Before anxiety can be classed as a reactive disorder, it should be excluded that this symptom is part of a functional psychosis or a neurosis.

A similar hierarchy is used in the classification of language and speech impairments. The model here is:

| | |
|---|---|
| higher position: | intellectual retardation, physical handicaps, pervasive developmental disorders or environmental deprivation; |
| lowest position: | SDD-LS (i.e. language and speech impairments not due to any of the above mentioned conditions). |

In this model, if language and speech symptoms can be attributed to conditions like intellectual retardation, physical handicaps, pervasive developmental disorders or environmental deprivation, these other conditions are considered as superordinate syndromes that include the language or speech symptoms. SDD-LS can only be diagnosed if these higher order syndromes can be excluded. A particular language or speech symptom (like difficulty in word finding, limited speech, difficulty acquiring new words, or misarticulations) as such does not determine the category that is to be classified. If this symptom can be attributed to a higher order syndrome, this higher order syndrome is classified. Only if the symptom cannot be attributed to any of these conditions, the SDD-LS category may be adequate.

The hierarchical classification model is complicated by the conceptualization of each of the categories as prototypes. A prototype is the theoretical ideal of the manifestation of a disorder. It represents a complete picture of the disorder, covering all the individual variations in manifestation. It is a theoretical standard that is approached in different degrees in reality. The more a disorder matches this theoretical standard, the more it typifies the theoretical ideal (Horowitz, Wright, Lowenstein & Parad, 1981). Many categories in DSM and ICD represent prototypes (Carson, 1991; Frances et al., 1991). The label of the category (for example Phonological Disorder) stands for the theoretical ideal, or the complete picture of the disorder. The description that follows the label often contains a list of symptoms that covers the variation of manifestations of the disorder. For example, the description of the DSM-IV Phonological Disorder reads that "The essential feature ... is failure to use developmentally expected speech sounds that are appropriate for the individual's age and dialect (...). This may involve errors in sound production, use, representation, or categorization such as, but not limited to, substitutions of one sound for another (use of /t/ for target /k/ sound) or omissions of sounds (e.g., final consonants)" (American Psychiatric Association [APA], 1994, p. 61). A child need not manifest all these symptoms for a phonological disorder to be diagnosed. Sometimes one or a few are enough.

The prototypical classification model results in categories that each contain a heterogenic collection of syndromes. This is one of the reasons why the SDD-LS categories are not homogeneous: *by definition* the category covers a range of individual variations. But also the higher order syndromes are heterogeneous. Language or speech impairments may be present in these syndromes, but they are no necessary symptoms. The result is that language and speech disorders can be classified in different categories. The categories that are used in these classifications, however, not always imply a language or a speech disorder. Consider, for example, four different cases:

Anne is a six-year-old girl that shows the symptoms of a language and speech disorder; there are no signs of mental retardation, pervasive developmental disorder, physical handicap or environmental deprivation. The diagnosis is SDD-LS.

Bert is a twelve-year-old boy with a mild mental retardation, and a minor language/speech disturbance. The diagnosis is Mild Mental Retardation. Because the language/speech disturbance is only minor, and not in excess of the intellectual level, there is no diagnosis of SDD-LS.

Chris is a five-year-old boy with a mild mental retardation and a severe language/speech impairment that is, however, not in excess of the intellectual level. The diagnosis is Mild Mental Retardation. Since the language/speech disturbance - although severe - is not in excess of the intellectual level, there is no diagnosis of SDD-LS.

David is a seven-year-old boy with a mild mental retardation and a profound language and speech disturbance. He is diagnosed as having a Mild Mental Retardation and SDD-LS; the latter applies because the language and speech impairment is in excess of the intellectual level.

Following the classification criteria in ICD and DSM, both Anne and David are diagnosed with SDD-LS, with David also receiving the additional diagnosis of Mental Retardation. From a clinical point of view, the symptoms of the language impairment of David may differ considerably from those of Anne. However, the prototypical model in ICD and DSM implies that these differences are often contained within the boundaries of the same category (i.e. SDD-LS). The same applies to the higher-order classification for mental retardation in the case of Bert and Chris. Both children have the diagnosis Mental Retardation. This classification, however, implies no language or speech disorder. In the case of Chris, a language/speech disturbance was present, whereas in the case of Bert it was not.

Note that, in the hierarchical model, also an identical constellation of signs in language or speech performance can be considered as a language or speech syndrome in one case, but not in another. For example, Anne and Chris may have quite the same pattern of language and speech behaviour. However, since Chris' language and speech performance falls within the same level as his general intelligence, his language and speech impairment is considered as a part of the superordinate syndrome of mental retardation.

In sum, ICD and DSM each represent a conceptual network in which syndromes are defined as prototypes within a hierarchy. Hence, the ICD/DSM concept of SDD-LS can only be understood and evaluated in the context of this comprehensive network. It may explain the lack of qualitative differences between language and IQ discrepants and non-discrepants, as reported by Amorosa (this volume) and Bishop (this volume). It may well be the result of this very complex conceptual network, that makes it possible that the same language and speech patterns are assigned to different categories, that are each in their turn very heterogenic.

### *The Meaning of the Exclusionary Criteria*

Exclusionary criteria are crucial in the definition of SDD-LS. For example, in DSM-IV, criteria C and D for the Expressive Language Disorder are that "Criteria are not met for ... a Pervasive Developmental Disorder. If Mental Retardation, a speech motor or sensory deficit, or environmental deprivation is present, the language difficulties are in excess of those usually associated with these problems" (APA, 1994, p. 58; see also Amorosa, this volume).

It is important to understand the meaning of these exclusions for the concept of SDD-LS. In the hierarchical disease model, the language or speech impairments that belong to the conditions that are excluded are of a higher order than the SDD-LS syndrome. These conditions may be different from SDD-LS because

- they may have a known pathogenesis (e.g. language disturbances due to a neurological trauma);
- they may have a course, familial pattern or differential treatment that is clearly distinct from SDD-LS (e.g. language impairment due to severe environmental deprivation).

But an exclusionary criterion may also have nothing to do with the hierarchical disease model. For example, Yule and Maughaum (this volume) argued that the use of IQ is merely because IQ is a convenient predictor of the specific skill. In their opinion, the use of IQ here is purely empirical. Yule and Maughaum's approach shows that an exclusionary criterion may not have to be related in a direct or a meaningful way to the condition that is to be identified (cf. Morey & McNamara, 1987). This can be further illustrated by a simple example. Suppose you live in a street where Mr. Smith is always at home when the man next door, Mr. Jones, is not. This pattern of absence and presence happens to exist due to the different jobs Mr. Smith and Mr. Jones each have. One day, you want to pay a visit to Mr. Jones. However, when you look outside your window you see that Mr. Smith is at home. You decide to visit Mr. Jones another time, because now you know he won't be home. Similarly, mental retardation may exclude the diagnosis of SDD-LS, not because of a 'deeper' underlying hierarchical disease model, but simply because the presence or absence of mental retardation is a convenient identifier. The rule than is: if a mental retardation is present, the specific developmental disorder is not (unless the language or speech difficulties exceed the level of intellectual functioning). This rule does not necessarily imply that mental retardation and SDD-LS are negatively related in a meaningful way. The mental retardation may serve as a negative identifier for a SDD-LS, because the presence of mental retardation may happen to coexist with an absence of SDD-LS.

Now, why are the exclusionary criteria used to define SDD-LS? Are they really just convenient identifiers, or do they imply a hierarchical disease model? In the following sections, the relationship of the exclusionary criteria with language and speech is discussed in more detail in order to shed light on why these criteria are used.

### *Intelligence Level*

The taxonomic model used to differentiate between SDD-LS and a general intellectual impairment, known as the discrepancy model, is rather complex. This complexity is clarified by the figure presented by Yule and Maughaum (this volume). Figure 1 shows an elaboration of this figure for the concept of SDD-LS. The model is based on the fact that, at a group level, language performance correlates with intelligence, but that the relationship is not perfect. Statistically, the conceptual model implies that the variance in language performance can be partitioned into unique variance, variance shared with intelligence, and error. On the basis of the shared variance, language performance can be predicted from IQ. Figure 1 shows a regression line that represents the best estimate of language performance associated with different IQ-levels, assuming that the correlation between language and IQ is .50. The Figure shows several areas that refer to different groups:

A The area between the two cut-off lines parallel to the regression line represents the normal variation in language based on the IQ-level of children that are not mentally

retarded. Cases in this field are excluded from the diagnosis of SDD-LS.
(Note that this field contains a small shaded area that represents children that have a language impairment that is severe - two standard deviations below the mean - but still within the normal range given the child's IQ).

SDD The second area is defined by language performance that is below the normal variation given the child's age and IQ. This area contains cases of SDD-LS, such as Anne, who was described above.

MR A third area in Figure 1 represents the cases of mental retardation. This area contains three subgroups: cases of mental retardation without a severe language impairment (MR-X; e.g. Bert), cases with a non-specific language impairment (MR-A; e.g. Chris), and cases in which SDD-LS is a comorbid disorder (SDD-MR; e.g. David).

The issue here is why the IQ is used as an identifier to exclude disorders that do not belong to the SDD-LS area. It is important to note that ICD and DSM differ somewhat in their definition of the discrepancy. In DSM the definition is based explicitly on nonverbal intelligence. In ICD, the manual (World Health Organization [WHO], 1992) refers only to 'mental age' and 'general level of cognitive functioning'. The same applies for speech disorders as defined by ICD, except that the ICD manual not only states that the articulation disorder should be beyond the normal variation given the child's mental age, but also that nonverbal IQ should be within normal limits. DSM uses another approach towards the Phonological Disorder, where intelligence is only involved in that, if Mental Retardation is present the speech difficulties should be in excess of those usually associated with this condition. Clearly, ICD and DSM do not apply the same principles for using intelligence as an exclusionary factor. The lack of consensus on this matter results in a rather confusing and puzzling difference between the two systems.

But what is even more puzzling is that DSM explicitly states that *nonverbal* IQ should be used as an exclusionary criterion. In the definition of mental retardation limitations in communication or verbal and speech abilities are mentioned as possible features. In

FIGURE 1

Schematic representation of the relationship between language and IQ in the concept of the specific developmental language disorder.

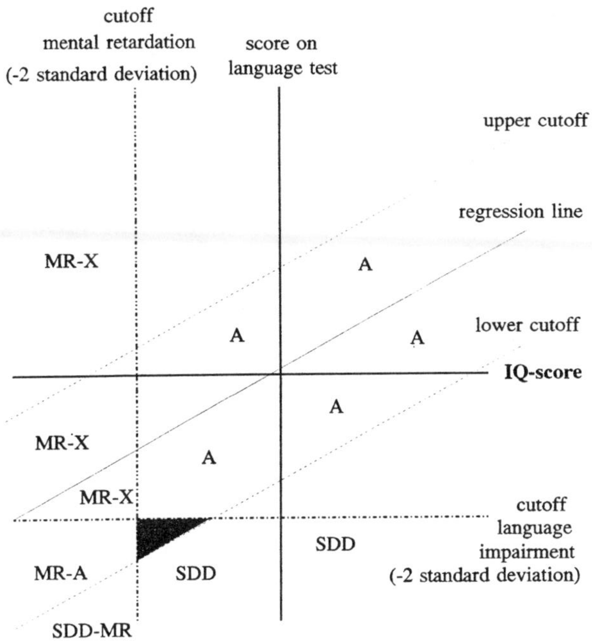


Legend:

| | | |
|---|---|---|
| — | = | regression line predicting language (y) from IQ (x) in a space defined by actual language and IQ scores (z-standardized) ($r_{xy}$=.50; see e.g. Stevenson & Richman, 1976) |
| - - - | = | lower and upper cut-off defined by: Observed - Predicted language score = $\pm 1.65 \cdot \sqrt{(1-r^2_{xy})}$ (see e.g. Willson & Reynolds, 1984) |

Notes:

1) in drawing the area for MR and SDD, no difference was made between non-verbal and total IQ;

2) a lower cut-off can also be defined using an expression like

$$70 = \frac{\text{language age}}{\text{mental age}} \times 100.$$

(e.g. Cohen, Paul, & Volkmar, 1987). The principle is very similar to the regression based formula (see also Burns, 1982), provided that the correlation between language and mental age is known, and Figure 1 is extended with a third dimension to account for chronological age.

a hierarchical classification model, a language/speech deficit may be considered a symptom of the higher-order prototype of mental retardation. This diagnostic hierarchy may reflect the widely accepted notion that verbal ability contributes to general intelligence. By using the nonverbal IQ, however, the hierarchical classification model fits less well, because there is no clear hierarchical relation between verbal ability and nonverbal intelligence (not as clear as in verbal ability and general intelligence). Then why should the nonverbal IQ be used? One could argue that nonverbal intelligence, and the way this is operationalized in most tests, is conceptually related to language abilities. Language tests and verbal- and nonverbal IQ-test may tap certain shared cognitive abilities and achievements, such as analytic skills that support the production and understanding of language, or vocabulary that serves to solve spatial problems. Therefore, nonverbal intelligence may be used as an exclusionary criterion in the definition of the specific developmental language disorder because of the common factor connecting language and nonverbal intelligence. In the literature (Bishop, 1994; Paul, 1992; Stevenson, 1984; Whitehurst & Fishel, 1994), nonverbal IQ is mentioned as a strong predictor in the development of children with a language disorder. Children with a language as well as a nonverbal intellectual deficit generally show less developmental progress in language compared to children with a language deficit and a normal nonverbal IQ. This means that there may be some causal mechanism that connects language and nonverbal intelligence. Therefore, the use of nonverbal IQ as an exclusionary criterion in the diagnosis of SDD could serve to differentiate between language problems that may have different causes. DSM and ICD do not shed any light on the causal mechanisms that may be involved. This is in line with the 'a-theoretical' or 'theoretically unenterprising' orientation of these schemes (Sartorius, 1988). However, the question is: can there be reasons other than causality for using nonverbal IQ as an exclusionary factor? As discussed earlier, Amorosa (this volume) and Bishop (this volume) argued that there are no qualitative differences between language impaired children with and without a discrepant non-verbal IQ. Another possibility is, then, that nonverbal IQ indeed serves merely as a convenient identifier, in the sense that the co-occurrence of a low language level and a relatively low non-verbal IQ just happens to indicate the absence of SDD-LS. But then, the only way to know whether or not the non-verbal IQ is an accurate identifier is to know what we are looking for. At the moment, however, we seem to be more sure on what the specific developmental disorder in language is not, instead of what it is (see also below). If non-verbal IQ would really be just an identifier, it would only be a means to make a good guess. Another reason for using the nonverbal IQ could be that the exclusion of areas A and MR-A in Figure 1 is simply for reasons of efficiency. Because intelligence and language are associated (conceptually and/or empirically), low intelligence and language impairment will be frequent comorbid conditions. The discrepancy-rule, then, would avoid redundancy in the classification of disorders. But this explanation is also unsatisfactory, because it is unclear why in that case nonverbal IQ should be used as a predictor, instead of, for example, verbal IQ. Hence, the conclusion can only be that it is obscure why intelligence, or a particular intelligence factor, is involved as an exclusionary criterion in the diagnosis of the specific developmental language disorder.

With regard to the speech disorders, DSM-IV sheds some light on the matter. The manual states: "Although there may be an association with clear causal factors such as ... cognitive impairments (e.g., Mental Retardation) ..., at least 2.5% of preschool children present with Phonological Disorders of unknown or suspect origin, which are often referred to as functional or developmental." (APA, 1994, p. 62). Note that cognitive impairment is presented here as a causal factor. This indicates that in the identification of the DSM phonological disorder, intelligence is not involved just because it is a convenient identifier or only to avoid redundancy in classification.

The purpose of this section was to find out why IQ, and in particular the non-verbal IQ, is used as an exclusionary criterion. My conclusion is that, on logical grounds, it is unclear why intelligence is involved in the diagnostic criteria. Although for the DSM phonological disorder this involvement is more or less explained in terms of causality, a similar clarifying statement can neither be found for the DSM language disorders, nor that of the ICD. There seem to be no qualitative differences between language impaired children with and without a discrepant non-verbal IQ. It is possible that the IQ is used solely as a convenient identifier or to prevent redundancy in classification. However, this explanation is not satisfying, since it is not clear what type of IQ (general or non-verbal) should be used for this purpose.

### *Hearing Deficits and Other Physical Abnormalities*

It seems safe to say that ICD and DSM exclude impairments due to physical factors, because there is a causal relationship between language/speech and these factors. It is known that even mild hearing loss may cause language or speech disturbances, especially in young children and in chronic or recurrent cases (Freeman & Blockberger, 1987; Goorhuis-Brouwer, 1988; Whitehurst & Fishel, 1994). Other known causal factors in language or speech disturbances due to physical abnormalities are neurological trauma, as in aphasia, and deformations of the speech apparatus.

However, ICD and DSM do not by definition exclude the classification of a specific developmental disorder if a physical deficit is present. In ICD, the hearing deficit or other physical abnormality should constitute a sufficient explanation for the language or speech impairment. In all other cases, for example when the physical abnormality is a complicating factor but not a sufficient direct cause, the language or speech disorder should be included in the category for the specific developmental disorder. Since "a hard and fast distinction will be impossible to make" (WHO, 1992, p. 235), in effect, the exclusionary criterion in ICD-10 will only apply to the cases in which the hearing defect or physical abnormality is a clear cause of the language or speech impairment. In DSM-IV, a SDD-LS should be diagnosed if the language or speech disturbance is in excess of the level usually associated with the physical deficit (APA, 1994, p. 55). This conceptualization implies the same type of discrepancy model as in Figure 1, but now in terms of the association of the language skills with physical deficits. A difference with the model involving IQ is that the area of association could be interpreted more in terms of a causal relation. The text in DSM-IV, however, offers no clear explanation in this matter.

### *Severe Environmental Deprivation*

ICD and DSM also refer to environmental deprivation as an exclusionary factor. In the literature, the differentiation between the specific developmental and environmentally determined language disorders is well accepted (e.g. Bishop & Rosenbloom, 1987; Cantwell & Baker, 1985). Reviews of cases with extreme environmental deprivation (e.g. Skuse, 1984) show convincingly that social isolation causes a severe language delay. Also in less extreme cases clinicians diagnose language impairments that, in their opinion, can be attributed to circumstances like physical, sexual or emotional abuse or severe parental neglect (Van Yperen, 1990; Van Yperen & Rispens, 1996). The assumption that environmental factors may cause language delay is validated by the observation that language abilities often improve rapidly when the child is placed in a better environment (Ingram, 1972; Rutter & Lord, 1987; Skuse, 1984).

However, research on the effect of environmental factors on language disorders more in general has been limited. Factors like family size, social class, and quality of family interaction often correlate with the child's language skills (Beitchman et al., 1989; Beitchman, Hood & Inglis, 1992; Puckering & Rutter, 1987; Von Castell et al., 1985), but the causal mechanisms involved are not clearly understood. It seems that milder forms of abuse and neglect are seldomly the primary cause of language disorder (Paul, 1992). In other words, with the exception of extreme cases, the relationships between environment and language that are known from research are mostly correlational.

The text in ICD-10 is clearly formulated in terms of causality. In the main category for Specific developmental disorders of speech and language (F80), we read: "The conditions are not directly *attributable* to (...) environmental factors" (WHO, 1992, p. 234, emphasis added). Under the category for Expressive language disorder (F80.1) the manual states that "Inadequate involvement in conversational interchanges, or more general environmental deprivation, may play a major or contributory role in the impaired development of expressive language. Where this is the case, the *causal* factor should be noted by means of the appropriate Z code from chapter XXI of ICD-10" (WHO, 1992, p. 238, emphasis added). These statements seem to imply that the exclusionary criterion pertains to cases in which the environment can be considered as the direct cause of the language impairment, and not to those in which the level of performance is only correlated with the environmental conditions.

In DSM-IV, the exclusionary criterion again resembles the IQ-discrepancy rule. The criterion here is that if environmental deprivation is present, the language difficulties should be in excess of those usually associated with this problem. Although the text is put less clearly in terms of causality, and more in terms of general association, also in DSM-IV the intention may be to refer only to extreme cases of environmental deprivation in which there is a clear causal relation. Again, however, the manual is not clear at this point.

In sum, the exclusion of environmental deprivation may refer to the hierarchical disease model for only those cases in which the deprivation has been extreme, so that the language deficit clearly has a different pathogenesis and a different prognosis, as compared to SDD-LS. It may not refer to the more general correlation between environmental conditions on the one hand, and language performance on the other. This is, however, more clearly the case for ICD than for DSM.

*Pervasive Developmental Disorder*

Diagnostic criteria in ICD and DSM state that for the diagnosis of a specific language disorder, criteria for pervasive developmental disorder should not be met. The model applied here is not the same as with the factors discussed above. There is no discrepancy-concept involved. The criterion is simple: if a pervasive developmental disorder is diagnosed, the specific developmental language disorder is excluded. In the case of autism, this exclusionary rule fits the hierarchical disease model in which the 'lower' symptom of the language impairment belongs to the higher-order syndrome (autism), if other symptoms of this syndrome are also present. Autism is considered here as a disorder in which the language or speech impairment is part of a broader communicative disturbance that is essentially different from SDD-LS with respect to pathogenesis, course, prognosis, and/or treatment (see also Bishop & Roosenbloom, 1987; Rutter & Lord, 1987).

In some cases of Pervasive Developmental Disorder Not Otherwise Specified (PDD-NOS), however, the language disorder is not hierarchically, but arbitrarily excluded from SDD-LS. The DSM-IV criteria for the PDD-NOS category allow the inclusion of cases with only "a severe and pervasive impairment in the development of ... verbal and nonverbal communication skills ..." (APA, 1994, p. 77). This creates an overlap with the concept of SDD-LS, considering that in the case of a receptive language disorder conversational skills may also be very poor (see APA, 1994, p.59). The question is what is implied by the concepts 'pervasive' versus 'specific' developmental, and to what extent nonverbal communication should be affected. The problem is that there are no clear answers in this matter (Happé & Frith, 1991). ICD-10 avoids this problem by narrowing the criterion that applies to the category for receptive language disorder: here, only cases with autism are to be excluded, not the PDD-NOS also.

In all, the exclusionary criterion may be intended to exclude language and speech impairments that are essentially different from SDD-LS. In that case, the exclusion fits the hierarchical model. In DSM-IV, however, this exclusion is far too drastic. By using the entire PDD category as an exclusionary criterion (instead of just the subcategory for autism) a conceptual overlap is created that in some cases leads to an arbitrary attribution of a language impairment to either PDD-NOS or SDD-LS.

### *Conclusions*

The aim of this section was to shed light on the issue why a number of exclusionary criteria are used to identify SDD-LS. As regards to hearing impairment, neurological trauma or environmental deprivation, there are good reasons for assuming that, at least in severe cases and for ICD more clearly than for DSM, they serve as identifiers for language or speech disorders with different pathogenesis. In this respect, these exclusionary criteria fit the hierarchical disease model. Mental retardation and autism include language and speech impairments as behavioural features of superordinate syndromes. In the hierarchical disease model this implies that the language and speech impairments can be symptoms of disorders that are considered different from SDD-LS in course, prognosis or treatment.

However, the taxonomic model that defines SDD-LS is not only based on a hierarchical disease model. ICD and DSM also use another type of exclusion. Language and speech should also be discrepant with what can be expected on the basis of the child's IQ. In addition, in DSM this discrepancy model is also applied to somatic and environmental conditions. This implies that there is a general association between the degree of deprivation in the environment, the degree of physical impairment, and the level of intellectual functioning on the one hand, and language and speech performance on the other. The nature of this association is, however, unclear. It is obscure whether it is used to mark a boundary between disorders with a distinctive pathogenesis, course, prognosis or treatment, or to serve as an identifier that just happens to be negatively associated with SDD-LS. Therefore, it remains unclear why a number of exclusionary criteria are involved in the definition of SDD-LS.

### *The Core of the Concept*

Up to this point, I discussed two elements in the conceptual network that defines SDD-LS: the hierarchy of prototypes in which the category is defined, and the meaning of the exclusionary criteria. A third element to discuss is the description of the core of the SDD-LS concept in terms of what is typical for this disorder.

Almost all information in the manuals of ICD-10 and DSM-IV pertains to the exclusionary criteria and the behavioural features of the disorders. Descriptions pertaining to the underlying nature of SDD-LS are almost completely absent. In ICD we find a few bits of information on the pathogenesis of the disorder: there may be an impairment or a delay of functions strongly related to biological maturation of the central nervous system, and there are indications that genetic factors may be involved in many cases (WHO, 1992, p. 233). However, this information is provided in the description of the overall category of the psychological disorders that includes both the pervasive and the specific developmental disorders. In other words, these attributes are not described as being characteristic for SDD-LS only.

The scarcity of information in ICD and DSM on the nature is in contrast with the literature, that offers many hypotheses. However, there is still no conclusive evidence of what the disorder actually is. Bishop (1992, pp. 52-53) even speaks of a chaos in which "Every investigator has a different explanation, and each advances evidence that seems to support their viewpoint." Despite all these explanations, the pathogenesis of SDD-LS is still unknown.

As regards to the behavioural features, in the literature specific developmental language disorder is described as a 'catch all' category (Cantwell & Baker, 1987), that should at least be subdivided into an expressive and a receptive language disorder. The relevance of this expressive-receptive distinction was demonstrated in epidemiology (e.g. Silva, Williams, & McGee, 1987), as well as in clinical studies (e.g. Goorhuis-Brouwer, 1988; Love & Thompson, 1988). The descriptions in ICD and DSM, however, show that the categories for expressive and receptive language disorders still contain a heterogeneous set of disorders. Therefore, in other classifications (e.g. Bloom & Lahey, 1978; Bishop & Rosenbloom, 1987), a further differentiation on the basis of linguistic-behavioural aspects of language has been suggested in order to account for subgroups that go beyond the expressive/receptive dichotomy. The relevance of these subgroups may be questioned. Differences with respect to behavioural features do not necessarily imply differences in the underlying condition (Bishop, this volume). I explained earlier that this is a normal phenomenon in a prototypical classification model. The consequence of this model is that, although the study of behavioural features may help to find subgroups with a different core, these groups will only become meaningful 'sub-syndromes' if it is hypothesized that these subgroups are essentially different in other respects than merely the symptoms.

A complication in testing hypotheses on meaningful sub-syndromes, is that the SDD-LS is actually a residual category. Because the category is mainly defined by exclusionary criteria, it can only become a meaningful entity if this residue is further explained. However, since ICD and DSM offer no hypothesis on what constitutes the core of SDD-LS, the category does not clearly exceeds the status of a diagnostic residue.

In conclusion, there is no well established core of the SDD-LS concept. Therefore, we depend highly on exclusionary criteria (see also Paul, 1992). The consequence is that the SDD-LS category refers to a diagnostic residue that contains a very heterogeneous cocktail of conditions, waiting to be further disentangled. The hypothesis in ICD and DSM is that this residue contains the core of the SDD-LS disorder. But ICD and DSM offer no more detailed hypothesis on the nature of this core. Therefore, another plausible explanation is that this residue contains only error variance. Yet another alternative is that the residue is nothing but a container of other superordinate syndromes that are yet to be discovered and to be excluded, just like the language and speech impairments that are excluded because they are attributable to mental retardation, physical impairments, pervasive developmental disorder or environmental circumstances. If we continue to discover these superordinate syndromes, and go on to exclude the related language and speech symptoms from the SDD-LS category, we may end up with a category that contains nothing more than some residual error, or even a category that is empty (see also Robinson, 1991).

## PSYCHOMETRIC ISSUES

In search of the core of the SDD-LS category, the concept has to be defined in operational terms. The diagnostic criteria in ICD and DSM give only general directions in this respect. The criteria have to be operationalized in more detail. As Amorosa (this volume) discussed, this not an easy task. Operationalization of the exclusion involving IQ can serve as a good example of the problems involved. As in the field of learning disabilities, different formulae have been suggested in order to operationalize this exclusion (see e.g. Aram, Morris, & Hall, 1992; Cantwell & Baker, 1985, 1987; Cohen, Paul, & Volkmar, 1987; Stevenson & Richman, 1976). Figure 2 illustrates important variations that are possible with the category for language disorder. It shows that the criteria for 'language impairment' (1) and 'mental retardation' (2) may vary, depending of the cut-offs used. The 'severe discrepancy cut-off' canbe selected in various ways. The angle of this line with the horizontal axis can be increased by selecting a language and intelligence test that show higher correlation, and decreased by choosing tests with lower correlation (3). Furthermore, one could choose either a more stringent or a tolerant criterion for the 'severity' of the discrepancy (4), and adjust this severity-criterion to the different IQ-levels at which it is applied (5). The number of cases in different diagnostic groups (language impaired and not language impaired, secondary or specific language disorder) can be adjusted by selecting the appropriate operationalization. Note that children in the shaded area in Figure 2 may receive very different diagnoses (e.g. no language impairment, only language impairment, specific developmental language disorder, mental retardation, borderline intelligence), depending on the operationalization used. It will be clear that in a meta-analyses of studies in which different operationalizations are used, this category of chameleons may obscure general trends in the results.

Figure 2 pertains only to the operationalization of the discrepancy with IQ. The range of possibilities is further increased by the different options in the operationalization of the other exclusionary criteria. For example, since DSM states that in cases of hearing loss or environmental deprivation, the level of functioning should be in excess of that usually associated with these factors, this implies the introduction of more discrepancy formulae than just the one that involves IQ. All in combination, the number of possible variations is so large, that determining the impact of the operationalization on the results becomes a necessary object for study itself.

The conclusion is that the search for the core of the SDD-LS category should take the operationalization fully into account. Since we have no standard to test the accuracy of this operationalization, the quest for the core also comes to experimenting with formulae, tests, and cut-offs.

FIGURE 2

Five ways to adjust the number of cases with specific developmental language disorder.

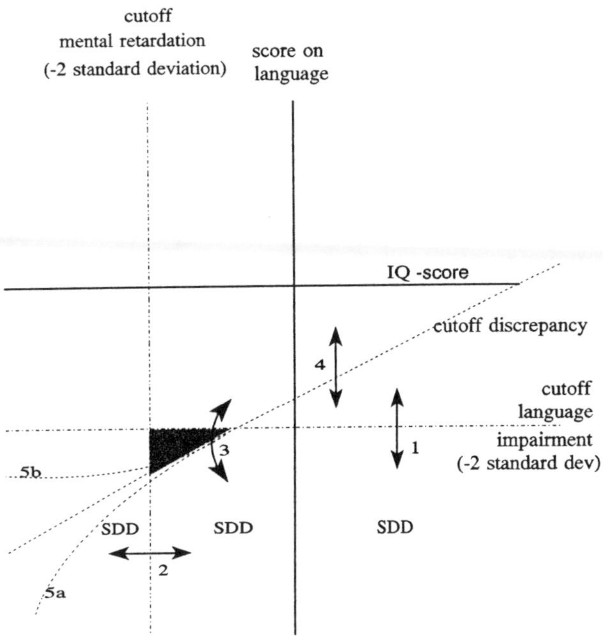


Legend:

1 = lower or raise the language cut-off
2 = lower or raise the IQ cut-off
3 = select tests to adjust the regression coefficient
4 = lower or raise the discrepancy cut-off
5 = account for an increase (a) or decrease (b) of language variance at the ends of the IQ-continuum

## HOW SHOULD LANGUAGE/SPEECH DISORDERS BE CLASSIFIED?

For a taxonomist, the classification of the SDD-LS will be a cause of concern. In the first place, the definition of the category is predominantly in terms of exclusionary criteria. Secondly, the residue is attributed a specific, but unknown nature. Thirdly, the identification of SDD-LS is difficult, since it involves not only an estimation of the seriousness of the impairment, but also inferences on causal factors and on the significance of the discrepancy with expected functioning given other disorders of the child. Fourthly, whereas the ICD and DSM offer no detailed classification criteria, and also the literature does not offer a well-accepted operationalization, in the identification of the disorders the clinicians often have to rely on their own inferences.

It is the task of a taxonomist to find out how SDD-LS should be defined in a comprehensive classification scheme. A main drawback of the categories in ICD and DSM is that, since the clinicians have to rely strongly on their inferences, the identification of SDD-LS becomes highly susceptible to interrater disagreement (Van Yperen, Van Berckelaer-Onnes, & Rispens, 1992; see also Rispens & Van Yperen, this volume). Moreover, for the purpose of determining the need for language/speech therapy, classification of the presence or absence and the severity of the language/speech impairment seems more important than the distinction between SDD-LS versus non-SDD-LS (Amorosa, this volume). In DSM and ICD, however, most language/speech impairments are only coded when not due or when in excess of other disorders (i.e. when the impairment can be characterized as an SDD-LS). Otherwise, these impairments are often hierarchically included in superordinate, prototypical defined categories (mental retardation, environmental deprivation, pervasive developmental disorder) that are not sufficiently indicative for the presence of a language/speech impairment. In other words, with the classification of one of these superordinate syndromes, the important information that a language or a speech impairment is present, is lost. In view of all the conceptual and taxonomic uncertainties involved in the classification of the different types of language and speech impairments, it seems highly desirable to prevent this loss of information. Instead of (or in addition to) the current hierarchical model, it is important that classification schemes provide for categories in which the presence of language and speech impairments can be classified, irrespective their nature.

There are several taxonomic alternatives to adapt the classification schemes in the desired way. One option is to add to the scheme a comprehensive, internationally standardized symptom list that documents the symptoms of the syndromes that are categorized. This method was used in the scheme of the Group for the Advancement of Psychiatry [GAP] (1966). In addition to, for example, a diagnosis of mental retardation, the clinician could indicate on a symptom list whether the language was severely disturbed or not. Another option is that ICD and DSM abandon the categories for specific developmental disorders, and adopt the rule that disorders of language or speech should always be coded in 'symptom'- categories like Expressive Language Disorder Not Otherwise Specified. In multi-axial schemes like DSM and MAS (Rutter, Shaffer, & Sturge, 1979; Remschmidt & Schmidt, 1994), these categories could be placed on one axis, together with other impairments in psychological functioning, while conditions that are related to these impairments could be placed on other axes. For example, this would lead to a scheme with

- an axis for psychopathological disorders, including e.g. pervasive developmental disorder and elective mutism;
- an axis for impairments in psychological functioning, including impairments in language, speech, motor coordination and scholastic skills, irrespective the nature;
- an axis for the classification of the general intellectual level, including mental retardation;
- an axis for physical conditions, including hearing deficit and neurological trauma;
- an axis for adverse environmental conditions, including social, emotional and intellectual deprivation.

(See also Amorosa, this volume).

Although this ensures the classification of *all* language and speech impairments, a drawback is that diagnostic information is documented 'cross-sectionally' (Helmchen, 1980, 1983). If a clinician attributes a language impairment to a low intelligence, the information concerning the language impairment and the intelligence level is recorded on separate axes. The fact that the clinician attributed this language impairment to the intelligence level (and thereby excluding an SDD diagnosis) is not recorded explicitly.

To overcome these problems, the categories for the impairments in psychological functioning could contain subcategories that differentiate after the 'nature' of the disorder, as inferred by the diagnostician. This type of axis was proposed by Van Yperen et al. (1992), and covered impairments in scholastic skills, language, speech and motor coordination. Figure 3 offers an example of the categories for language impairments in this scheme. The scheme can be used on different levels. If one prefers a clinical oriented scheme, level III can be used (if necessary, with more subcategories that those displayed in the figure). At this level, the impairment is coded for the presumed 'nature', as differentiations are determined by causal attributions and other clinical inferences. The level includes the SDD-LS categories. Classifications at level III can always be recoded into level II or I, where information on the impairments is summarized in categories that refer, more or less, to linguistic/ behavioural attributes only.

FIGURE 3

Example exhaustive scheme for language disorders.

| Level I | Level II | Level III |
|---|---|---|
| 2x.xx Language Disorder | 21.xx Expressive type | 21.1x Specific developmental |
| | | 21.2x Due to understimulation |
| | | 21.8x Other (e.g. related to intellectual or physical impairment) |
| | | 21.9x Unspecified |
| | 22.xx Receptive type | 22.1x Specific developmental |
| | | 22.2x Due to understimulation |
| | | 22.8x Other (e.g. related to intellectual or physical impairment) |
| | | 22.9x Unspecified |
| | 23.9x Other language disorder | |
| | 24.9x Unspecified language disorder | |

Code at last position:
2 = certainty: a disorder; 1 = uncertainty: borderline disorder/ normal variation.

An advantage of this scheme is that classifications on the presence or absence of language/speech impairment are always available on level II or I, whereas clinical information pertaining to the 'nature' is coded on level III. An important drawback of this scheme is that in some populations of, for example, mentally retarded children, classifications on different axes are often redundant (Van Yperen, 1990; Van Dijk & Meijel, 1994). Whatever model is preferred, it is clear that there are several alternative options for the classification of language or speech impairments. In my view, pending the debate on the scientific status of the SDD-LS categories, ICD and DSM should adopt one of the alternative models presented here, in order to 'intercept' the disadvantages of the current coding scheme.

## SUMMARY AND CONCLUSIONS

The purpose of this paper was to offer a detailed analysis of the SDD-LS concept and the way this disorder is classified in ICD and DSM. In these schemes the categories for SDD-LS are conceptualized in a hierarchical model with categories representing prototypes, and defined as impairments of language and speech not due or in excess of a number of other conditions. This model has two consequences: 1. Language and speech impairments excluded from these categories are considered as symptoms of superordinate conditions (mental retardation, environmental deprivation, physical impairment, pervasive developmental disorder). 2. The SDD-LS categories comprise a heterogenic diagnostic residue.

In discussing the nature the exclusionary criteria, it was concluded that some of these are used to distinguish language and speech impairment that are presumed to have a different pathogenesis, course, prognosis or treatment. Other seem to serve merely as convenient identifiers. However, the logic behind these exclusions is not always clear. Especially the rule that language/speech functioning should be discrepant with what can be expected on the basis of the child's IQ, somatic condition, and environment needs further clarification. The nature of the association of language or speech functioning with environmental and somatic factors and IQ *in general* is not explained. It is obscure whether ICD and DSM use this discrepancy rule in order to exclude an impairment with, for example, a distinctive pathogenesis, or simply because it happens to contribute to the identification of SDD-LS.

In the search for the core of SDD-LS, a problem is that the exclusionary criteria identify a diagnostic residue that will contain a cocktail of attributes. Because ICD and DSM offer no clear hypothesis on the core of the SDD-LS category, this residue remains meaningless. In research aimed at finding the core, the SDD-LS concept can be operationalized in many ways. Because there is no standard to test the accuracy of an operationalization, this research also comes to finding the best formulae, tests, and cut-offs.

In all, the SDD-LS concept is, despite its long history, still immature. It is time to purify the concept from everything what it is not and consider it for what it is. Although the clinical pictures of children like Anne, Bert, Chris and David are undoubtly realistic, we cannot say that the SDD-LS concept is a meaningful and valid category to typify some of these cases. We have to keep in mind that the specific nature of SDD-LS is far from being established as a fact. The concept still refers to a diagnostic residue of which it is hypothesized that it represents a specific language or speech disorder. Research has not resulted in firm evidence that supports this hypothesis.

This residual and hypothetical status of the SDD-LS concept is no problem, as long as taxonomic precautions are taken to overcome the disadvantages of the inferences involved in the classification of the disorder, and to compensate for the adverse consequences of the hierarchical and prototypical scheme in which the category is defined. In my view, one of the best precautions is that ICD and DSM create main categories for language and speech impairments (primarily based on behavioural features), offering a further differentiation in primary and secondary disorders only within these categories.

## REFERENCES

American Psychiatric Association. (1994). *Diagnostic and statistical manual of mental disorders* (4th ed.) Washington, DC: American Psychiatric Association.

Aram, D. M., Morris, R., & Hall, N. E. (1992). The validity of discrepancy criteria for identifying children with developmental language disorders. *Journal of Learning Disabilities, 28*, 549-554.

Beitchman, J. H., Hood, J., Rochon, J., Peterson, M., Mantini, T., & Majumdar, S. (1989). Empirical classification of speech/language impairment in children, I. Identification of speech/language categories. *Journal of the American Academy of Child and Adolescent Psychiatry, 28*, 112-117.

Beitchman, J. H., Hood, J., & Inglis, A. (1992). Familial transmission of speech and language impairment: A preliminary investigation. *Canadian Journal of Psychiatry, 37*, 151-156.

Bishop, D. V. M. (1992). The underlying nature of specific language impairment. *Journal of Child Psychology and Psychiatry, 33*, 3-66.

Bishop, D. V. M. (1994). Developmental disorders of speech and language. In M. Rutter, E. Taylor, & L. Hersov (Eds.), *Child and adolescent psychiatry: Modern approaches* (pp. 546-568). Oxford: Blackwell.

Bishop, D. & Rosenbloom, L. (1987). Childhood language disorders: Classification and overview. In W. Yule & M. Rutter (Eds.), *Clinics in developmental medicine, Vol 101/102: Language development and disorders* (pp. 16-41). London: Mac Keith Press.

Bloom, L. & Lahey, M. (1978). *Language development and language disorders*. New York: Wiley.

Burns, E. (1982). Linear regression and simplified reading expectancy formulas. *Reading Research Quarterly, 4*, 359-371.

Cantwell, D. P. & Baker, L. (1985). Speech and language: Development and disorders. In M. Rutter & L. Hersov (Eds.), *Child and adolescent psychiatry: Modern approaches* (2nd ed.) (pp. 526-544). Oxford: Blackwell.

Cantwell, D. P. & Baker, L. (1987). *Developmental speech and language disorders*. New York: The Guilford Press.

Carson, R. C. (1991). Dilemmas in the pathway of the DSM-IV. *Journal of Abnormal Psychology, 100*, 302-307.

Cohen, D. J., Paul, R., & Volkmar, F.R. (1987). Issues in the classification of pervasive developmental disorders and associated conditions. In D. J. Cohen, A. M. Donnellan, & R. Paul (Eds.), *Handbook of autism and pervasive developmental disorders*. New York: Wiley.

Foulds, G. A. (1976). *The hierarchical nature of personal illness*. London, Academic Press.

Frances, A. J., First, M. B., Widiger, T. A., Miele, G. M., Tilly, S. M., Davis, W. W., & Pincus, H. A. (1991). An A to Z guide to DSM-IV conundrums. *Journal of Abnormal Psychology, 100*, 407-412.

Freeman, R. & Blockberger, S. (1987). Language development and sensory disorder: Visual and hearing impairments. In W. Yule & M. Rutter (Eds.), *Clinics in developmental medicine, Vol. 101/102: Language development and disorders* (pp. 234-247). London: Mac Keith Press.

Goorhuis-Brouwer, S. M. (1988). *Gesprekspartners? Taalontwikkelingsstoornissen als pedagogisch probleem, een verkenning*. Dissertatie, Rijksuniversiteit Groningen. Leuven: Acco.

Group for the Advancement of Psychiatry (1966). *Psychopathological disorders in childhood: Theoretical considerations and a proposed classification* (Rep. No. 62). New York: Group for the Advancement of Psychiatry.

Happé, F. & Frith, U. (1991). How useful is the "PDD" label? *Journal of Child Psychology and Psychiatry, 32*, 1167-1168.

Helmchen, H. (1980). Multi-axial systems of classification. Types of axes. *Acta Psychiatrica Scandinavica, 61*, 43-55.

Helmchen, H. (1983). Multi-axial classification in psychiatry. *Comprehensive Psychiatry, 24*, 20-24.

Horowitz, L. M., Wright, J. C., Lowenstein E., & Parad, H. W. (1981). The prototype as a construct in abnormal psychology, 1: A method for deriving prototypes. *Journal of Abnormal Psychology, 90*, 568-574.

Ingram, T. T. S. (1972). The classification of speech and language disorders in young children. In M. Rutter & J. A. M. Martin (Eds.), *The child with delayed speech*. (pp. 13-32). London: Heinemann.

Love, A. J. & Thompson, M. G. G. (1988). Language disorders and attention deficit disorders in young children referred for psychiatric services: Analysis of prevalence and a conceptual synthesis. *American Journal of Orthopsychiatry, 58*, 52-64.

Morey, L. C. (1987). The foulds hierarchy of personal illness: A review of recent research. *Comprehensive Psychiatry, 28*, 159-168.

Morey, L. C. & McNamara, T. P. (1987). On definitions, diagnosis, and DSM-III. *Journal of Abnormal Psychology, 96*, 283-285.

Paul, R. (1992). Language and speech disorders. In S. R. Hooper, G. W. Hynd, & R. E. Mattison (Eds.), *Developmental disorders: Diagnostic criteria and clinical assessment* (pp. 209-237). Hillsdale, NJ: Lawrence Erlbaum.

Puckering, C. & Rutter, M. (1987). Environmental influences on language development. In W. Yule & M. Rutter (Eds.), *Clinics in developmental medicine, Vol. 101/102: Language development and disorders* (pp. 103-128). London: Mac Keith Press.

Remschmidt, H. & Schmidt, M.H. (Hrsg.) (1994). *Multi-axiales Klassifikationsschema für psychische Störungen des Kindes- und Jugendalters nach ICD-10 der WHO*. Bern: Verlag Hans Huber.

Robinson, R. J. (1991). Causes and associations of severe and persistent specific speech and language disorders in children. *Developmental Medicine and Child Neurology, 33*, 943-962.

Rutter, M. & Lord, C. (1987). Language disorders associated with psychiatric disturbance. In W. Yule & M. Rutter (Eds.), *Clinics in developmental medicine, Vol. 101/102: Language development and disorders* (pp. 206-233). London: Mac Keith Press.

Rutter, M., Shaffer, D., & Sturge, C. (1979). *A guide to a multi-axial classification scheme for psychiatric disorders in childhood and adolescence* (3rd ed.). London: Department of Child and Adolescent Psychiatry, Institute of Psychiatry.

Sartorius, N. (1988). International perspectives of psychiatric classification. *British Journal of Psychiatry, 152*(Suppl. 1), 9-14.

Silberman, R. M. (1971). CHAM. *A classification of psychiatric states.* Dissertation. Gemeentelijke Universiteit Amsterdam, Amsterdam, the Netherlands.

Silva, P. A., Williams, S., & McGee, R. (1987). A longitudinal study of children with developmental language delay at age three: Later intelligence, reading and behaviour problems. *Developmental Medicine and Child Neurology, 29,* 630-640.

Skuse, D. (1984). Extreme deprivation in early childhood: Theoretical issues and a comparative review. *Journal of Child Psychology and Psychiatry, 25,* 543-572.

Stevenson, J. (1984). Predictive value of speech and language screening. *Developmental Medicine and Child Neurology, 26,* 528-538.

Stevenson, J. & Richman, N. (1976). The prevelance of language delay in a population of three-year-old children and its association with general retardation. *Developmental Medicine and Child Neurology, 18,* 431-441.

Van Dijk, A. & Meijel, A. (1994). *Classificatie en zwakzinnigenzorg.* Research thesis. Department of Educational Sciences, University of Utrecht, Utrecht.

Van Yperen, T. A. (1990). *Multi-axiale classificatie van specifieke ontwikkelingsstoornissen: Een studie over as II van het MAC.* Unpublished dissertation, University of Leiden, Leiden, the Netherlands.

Van Yperen, T. A., Van Berckelaer-Onnes, I. A., & Rispens, J. (1992). The classification of specific developmental disorders: moving away from the hierarchical model in DSM and ICD. *The European Journal of Psychiatry, 6,* 223-235.

Van Yperen, T. A. & Rispens, J. (1996). Classification of the Environmentally Determined Language Disorder in ICD and DSM. *The European Journal of Psychiatry, 10,* 45-58.

Von Castell, R., Meier, R., Biener, A., Artner, K., Dilling, H., & Weyerer, S (1985). Sprach- und Intelligenzleistungen gegenüber sozialer Schicht und Familiensituation. *Praxis der Kinderpsychologie und Kinderpsychiatrie, 34,* 120-123.

Whitehurst, G. J. & Fishel, J. E. (1994). Practioner review: Early developmental language delay: What, if anything, should the clinician do about it? *Journal of Child Psychology and Psychiatry, 35,* 613-618.

Willson, V.L. & Reynolds, C.R. (1984). Another look at evaluating aptitude-achievement discrepancies in the diagnosis of learning disabilities. *Journal of Special Education, 18,* 477-487.

World Health Organization. (1992). *The ICD-10 classification of mental and behavioural disorders. Clinical descriptions and diagnostic guidelines.* Geneva: World Health Organization.

# SECTION 4

# DEVELOPMENTAL MOTOR DISORDERS

SHEILA E. HENDERSON AND ANNA L. BARNETT

# DEVELOPMENTAL MOVEMENT PROBLEMS

## INTRODUCTION

Since the turn of the century, case histories of children who appear physically and intellectually normal yet lack the motor competence necessary to cope with the demands of everyday living have appeared in the literature (e.g. Brenner & Gillman, 1966; Dupre as cited in Ford, 1966; Gubbay, 1975; Henderson & Hall, 1982; Orton, 1937; Walton, Ellis, & Court, 1962). Recent longitudinal studies of such children have allowed us to make progress in understanding the natural history of this "condition", demonstrating that its manifestations are not simply transitional difficulties, devoid of personal, social and educational consequences (Geuze & Borger, 1993; Losse et al., 1991). Observations such as these have encouraged the postulation of a separable disorder of movement skill acquisition, requiring aetiological, diagnostic, and remedial attention, in its own right. This stance has, in turn, been taken up and endorsed in recent editions of the influential diagnostic manuals published by the World Health Organization [WHO] (1992) and the American Psychiatric Association [APA] (1994), respectively the *International Classification of Diseases* 10 (ICD-10) and the *Diagnostic and Statistical Manual of Mental Disorders* IV (DSM-IV). The relevant entries are headed "Specific developmental disorder of motor function" (ICD-10) and "Developmental coordination disorder," (DSM-IV). (For a historical overview of the broader context in which these entries occur see Rispens & Van Yperen, this volume).

While recognition by these bodies has helped to raise the profile of specific movement disorders among professionals in medicine and education, the problem of the reliability and validity of the classification schemes they propose have not yet been properly addressed empirically. In the absence of such studies, we thought it most useful at this juncture to subject the formulation of the entries in the most recent manuals to a critical examination, setting them in the context of developments in this field and providing an indication of the problems that seem likely to arise in the application of these taxonomies.

Our paper begins with a consideration of the labels given to the disorder in ICD-10 and DSM-IV, then proceeds to an analysis of the



*J. Rispens et al. (eds.),*
*Perspectives on the Classification of Specific Developmental Disorders*, 209–230.

diagnostic criteria proposed. The two manuals differ in the way they specify diagnostic criteria for each developmental condition. For ease of reference, we have elected to use the DSM-IV headings in the following discussion.

## TERMINOLOGY: WHAT'S IN A NAME?

Many different terms have been applied to the childhood disorder of concern here (see Table 1). Some, such as "physical awkwardness" are purely subjective but have the advantage of drawing attention to a common feature of such children's movement. Others venture beyond description, implying the existence of a distinct clinical entity with a standard set of signs which lead to differential diagnosis, e.g. "clumsy child syndrome". Yet others carry with them some general assumptions about the underlying nature of the dysfunction e.g. "dyspraxia", "sensory-integrative dysfunction".

Some authors use such terms interchangeably. Others have taken the view that they actually describe slightly different groups of children (see Missiuna & Polatajko, 1995 for a review). Not surprisingly, this situation has led to confusion both in research and clinical practice. In the research field, the loose employment of overlapping terms with ill-defined boundaries has often been combined with underspecified methods of sample selection, with the inevitable consequence that different studies cannot be compared and a cumulative body of systematic knowledge established. In clinical practice, Missiuna and Polatajko have pointed out that there is a high correlation between the particular terms used to describe this condition, the assessment instrument favoured and the form of therapy ultimately selected. For example, a child diagnosed as suffering from *sensory-integrative dysfunction* will usually turn out to have been assessed on a test battery stemming from Ayres' (1972) work, and is likely to be treated by means of Ayres' therapeutic methods. This form of assessment and treatment is totally different from that favoured, for example, by Laszlo et al. (1988). The latter use the term *kinaesthetically blind* to describe their "clients" and offer a form of treatment directed exclusively towards the improvement of the child's kinaesthetic sensitivity.

In selecting the key terms to be used in their manuals, the authors of ICD-10 and DSM-IV seem to have ignored or deliberately departed from common parlance. Neither the term "Specific Developmental Disorder of Motor Function" (SDD-MF) nor the term "Developmental Coordination Disorder" (DCD) had any precedent in existing literature. Presumably any argument for continuity of terminology was

TABLE 1

Some of the terms commonly used to denote movement difficulties in children.

| Term | Author(s) |
|---|---|
| Clumsy,<br>Developmental Clumsiness | British Medical Journal (1962)<br>Dare & Gordon (1970)<br>Gordon (1969)<br>Gubbay (1975)<br>Gubbay, Ellis, Walton, & Court (1965)<br>Henderson & Hall (1982)<br>Hulme, Biggerstaff, Moran, & McKinlay (1982)<br>Hulme & Lord (1986)<br>Keogh, Sugden, Reynard, & Calkins (1979)<br>Knuckey & Gubbay (1983)<br>McKinlay (1978)<br>Van Dellen & Geuze (1988)<br>Walton, Ellis, & Court (1962) |
| Apraxia,<br>Developmental Apraxia,<br>Developmental Dyspraxia,<br>Dyspraxia-Dysgnosia | Cermak (1985)<br>Denckla (1984)<br>Gubbay (1978)<br>Lesny (1980)<br>Orton (1937)<br>Walton, Ellis, & Court (1962) |
| Physically Awkward | Wall (1982)<br>Wall, Reid, & Paton (1990) |
| Poorly Coordinated | Johnston, Short, & Crawford (1987) |
| Motor Infantilism | Annell (1949) |
| Delayed Motor Development | Illingworth (1968) |
| Children with Movement Difficulties | Henderson, May, & Umney (1989)<br>Sugden & Keogh (1990) |
| Minimal Brain Damage | Forsström & Von Hofsten (1982) |
| Minor Neurological Dysfunction | Schellekens, Scholten, & Kalverboer (1983)<br>Touwen (1993) |
| Perceptuo-Motor Dysfunction | Laszlo, Bairstow, Bartrip, & Rolfe (1988) |

overridden by the desire to impose a standard form of words, such as *developmental xxx disorder,* throughout the developmental domain. This consideration seems to have weighed most heavily in the formulation of DSM-IV.

A quite different reason for starting afresh is the desirability of adopting a standard set of descriptive terms that are as free as possible from particular theoretical commitments. Not only are many of the terms in current usage confusing and imprecise, some have become so larded with theoretical presuppositions that they are no longer able to serve as neutral designations. For instance, ICD- 10 explicitly rejects the term "minimal brain dysfunction" (MBD) because of its "many different and contradictory meanings". Such a term is at its most dangerous when it masquerades as an ostensive definition of a class of individuals who exhibit common, observable features. As a label for clumsiness, MBD has an extraordinary number of unwanted properties. Nothing in the phrase itself refers explicitly to difficulties in acquiring movement skills. Clumsiness is visible, even if its ultimate explanation has to be cast in more abstract terms. In contrast, MBD is, almost by definition, invisible and not directly measurable. It has to be inferred from signs, which usually have no obvious connection with the child's difficulties, which are sometimes not in themselves motor and which are often reliant on a subjective clinical judgement. Thus, no clear boundary is discernable between (i) the purportedly uncommitted employment of the label MBD as an alternative to clumsiness, and (ii) its usage to denote a presumptive patho-physiological substrate which supposedly "accounts for" the observable functional impairments (e.g. clumsiness).

To the practitioner in this area, the terms *motor function* (ICD-10) and *coordination* (DSM-IV) are often regarded as interchangeable. Among researchers in the field, however, they are rarely used as synonyms and there is much debate about their exact coverage. For example, many students of motor control reserve the term *function* to describe purposeful action in everyday life. *Coordination*, on the other hand, has a more limited meaning, often defined as the "behaviour of joints and muscles in relation to each other" (Schmidt, 1988). On this basis, the term *motor function* lies closer, in its semantics, to *praxis,* with its implication of purposive action, than it does to the term *coordination*. In consequencc, thc analogous pair *dysfunction* and *dyspraxia* also become more closely allied.

However, for others, the term *dyspraxia* has a much more specific meaning. For these researchers, an instructive comparison exists with established usage in the literature dealing with acquired disorders, where a clear line is drawn between deficits of movement planning or praxis and deficits of movement execution. Disorders of execution, it follows, would require to be denied admission entirely from a developmental classification rooted in the term *dyspraxia* (see e.g. Sugden & Keogh, 1990). Even more specific is the definition of dyspraxia proposed by Denckla and Roeltgen (1992) who reserve the term dyspraxia for a disorder of gesture!

## DIAGNOSTIC CRITERIA: COMING OF AGE?

Does the attainment of an entree to these manuals signify that the condition "clumsiness" has completed the hard climb from loose description to standardized diagnostic procedure? Let us examine, first, the way these two schemes set out to assess the motor core.

### *Criterion A: the Motor Core*

ICD-10 and DSM-IV provide similar descriptions of the range of difficulties that may be experienced by children with specific motor problems. Both manuals describe movement at a "functional" level, referring to everyday goal directed action and acknowledging that the pattern of motor difficulties varies with age (see Table 2). Both specify that chronological age and general intelligence be considered in the process of diagnosis, but only the ICD manual specifies a cut-off point for motor impairment in relation to age. Moreover, the two manuals differ radically in the way they deal with intellectual ability, an issue which is dealt with separately below.

There are numerous problems relating to the assessment of motor impairment in children that are yet to be solved. First, is the absence of a "gold standard," equivalent to the WISC, in the cognitive domain. Although the Movement Assessment Battery for Children (Henderson & Sugden, 1992), the Test of Motor Impairment (Stott, Moyes, & Henderson, 1984) and the Bruininks-Oseretsky Test of Motor Proficiency (Bruininks, 1978), together with Ayres' Southern California Sensory Integration Tests (1989) probably comprise the most frequently used standardised tests, none enjoys the status of the WISC, with its supportive data base accumulated from very extensive usage.

A second problem to be solved concerns the need for an agreed quantitative criterion for the degree of "impairment" required for a child's performance to be judged as abnormal and to warrant application of the syndrome label. As noted above, ICD-10 commits itself to a criterial cut-off point at two standard deviations below the age norm, on a standardised test of fine or gross motor coordination. However, the absence of large-scale studies which provide information on the distribution of motor scores across the population means that there is no sound basis for judging what cut-points are most valid.

Within the medical profession, a rule of thumb designates children falling below the 10th centile as "impaired". In contrast, psychologists and educators often opt for the higher value of 15%. In the developed world, where resources for children with mild to moderate impairments are becoming increasingly stretched, the level at which such cut-off points are set have far-reaching implications for clinical practice and education. In the United States, for example, state legislation often dictates the eligibility criteria for special education and therapy-related services.

Another issue that remains unresolved is the question of what a fully comprehensive assessment of perceptuo-motor impairment should contain. Although we lack an agreed taxonomy of motor skills, common sense and clinical experience have led to some consensus. As Table 2 shows, both manuals mention a range of everyday life skills

TABLE 2

"Motor elements" of DSM-IV and ICD-10.

| Specific Developmental Disorder of Motor Function (ICD-10, WHO, 1992, p. 250). | Developmental Coordination Disorder (DSM-IV, APA, 1994, pp. 54-55). |
|---|---|
| The child's motor coordination, on fine or gross motor tasks, should be significantly below the level expected on the basis of his or her age and general intelligence. This is best assessed on the basis of an individually administered, standardized test of fine and gross motor coordination. The difficulties in coordination should have been present since early in development (i.e. they should not constitute an acquired deficit).<br><br>(It is usual for the motor clumsiness to be associated with some degree of impaired performance on visuo-spatial cognitive tasks.) | **Criterion A**<br>Performance in daily activities that require motor coordination is substantially below that expected given the person's chronological age and measured intelligence. This may be manifested by marked delays in achieving motor milestones (e.g., walking, crawling, sitting), dropping things, 'clumsiness', poor performance in sports, or poor handwriting. |
| | **Criterion B**<br>The disturbance in Criterion A significantly interferes with academic achievement or activities of daily living. |

which may be broadly categorised as either requiring "gross motor control" (e.g. walking, running, or hopping), or "fine motor control" (e.g. bead threading or cutting with scissors). For many of these skills, performance can be fairly easily quantified and age norms are available. Other skills which clumsy children find exceptionally difficult to acquire are remarkably hard to measure. "Self-help" skills such as tying shoe laces, fastening buttons and using a knife and fork are good examples. They can be examined qualitatively with good reliability (e.g. Barnett & Henderson, 1992) but without some knowledge of the child's past experience at home and school, it may be difficult to interpret failure when it occurs. Especially among younger children, an inability to fasten buttons or put on a sweater may simply be due to the fact that the child is cared for by a minder who does everything for him/her. Similarly, a child's handwriting is difficult to evaluate unless one knows how he has been taught in school and whether he has additional literacy problems. Finally, some aspects of performance such as the control of eye movements and vocal articulation have traditionally been treated separately from other aspects of motor functioning. Despite the fact that these aspects are often impaired in clumsy children they are not included in standardised assessment instruments.

In sum, although they vary in their coverage, the assessment instruments that are commonly described as functional, share two useful characteristics. They offer (a) a reliable way of determining whether a child's performance is below that expected for his/her age and provide (b) some information on the range and severity of the child's movement difficulties. Such tests play a crucial role not only in the identification of children with difficulties but in the subsequent decision making about service provision. Whenever we move beyond this level of analysis, however, to consider treatment, the issue as to what should be assessed becomes more complex. Central to this debate is the question of whether DCD/SDD-MF comprise a unitary condition or a heterogeneous collection of disorders.

## *One Disorder or Many?*

From the beginning, clinical and educational reports of children described as "clumsy" have emphasised the variation between children both in the severity and pattern of their problems. In the research literature, however, two rather different responses to this variation can be found.

On one hand, experimental psychologists intent on finding underlying causes of "clumsiness", proceeded as if they were dealing with a unitary phenomenon, explicable in terms of a single, often highly specific, processing deficit. For instance, one theory states that an impairment of sensory integration underlies poor coordination, while another holds that poor kinaesthetic acuity is the cause. Yet another favours a deficit in visual perception. None of these theories have been properly tested. The assessment instruments which purport to measure the deficits often have inadequate reliability and the question of how one such deficit might interact with another is never addressed. As far as the diagnostic process is concerned, this leaves practitioners with little specific guidance on how to determine the therapeutic needs of the child. Indeed, as noted by Missiuna and Polatajko (1995), many children are simply exposed to the form of assessment and treatment favoured by the adult involved.

While some researchers were treating variations in performance as if they simply represented different manifestations of the same disorder, others were exploring the possibility that identifiable sub-groups of DCD/SDD-MF exist. Various sub-types have been proposed by pediatricians (Gubbay et al., 1965; Touwen, 1979). For example, Gubbay et al. proposed two sub-types, one type having an isolated developmental apraxia or agnosia, while the other purportedly displayed evidence of dysfunction in pyramidal or cerebellar pathways. No empirical support for this subgrouping has been forthcoming. David et al. (1981) proffered a rather less idiosyncratic distinction between children who have difficulties in the *planning* of their actions and children who had difficulty in the *execution* of movements. This received endorsement in the ICD-9 classification of "Specific Motor Retardation" (WHO, 1989), which used the terms "dyspraxia" and "clumsiness" to refer to planning-impaired and execution-impaired sub-types, respectively. However, in a clinical setting, it is most unusual to find a child with only one of these difficulties. Two attempts have been made to validate these sub-types statistically, without success (Ayres, Mailloux, & Wendler, 1987; Dewey & Kaplan, 1992). Such afflictions seem likely to have caused the silent demise of this popular distinction on the rough road from ICD-9 to ICD-10.

Statistical approaches to the determination of subgroups, have also been pursued by Hoare (1994), Miyahara (1994) and Henderson, Jongmans, Dubowitz, & Demetre (in preparation). All studied children of school age who were clearly identified as "clumsy" but each used rather different sets of test items. On the whole there was very little agreement amongst the clusters or sub-types proposed. However one rather interesting finding was common to all three studies. This comprised a dissociation between performance on static and dynamic balance. Indeed, Miyahara found instances of balance abilities which deviated markedly from performance on other tasks, in either direction. There were some children whose balance was good in comparison to their performance on running and catching tasks and others whose balance seemed exceptionally poor in comparison to other locomotor tasks.

These attempts to identify subtypes purely on grounds of internal cohesion and coherence call urgently for validation. External criteria that merit consideration include the use of structural or functional brain imaging techniques to identify a pathological substrate, the use of responsiveness to different types of therapy, and the use of selective interference techniques borrowed from experimental psychology.

In our own investigations we have preferred, at this early stage, to concentrate our attempts at validation on one particularly interesting subtype that emerged as one of six clusters reported in Jongmans (1993). These children appeared to have particular difficulty with form board tasks. By showing that they also differed from the remainder of our sample on a series of "constructional" tasks not included in the cluster analysis, we were able to substantiate predictively the specificity of the deficit. From this use of similar measures applied to different tasks to establish concordance, we then turned to the use of quite different measures on the original task. Using videotape records of the children's form-board performance, we were able to show that this subgroup were also set apart by qualitative differences in performance.

Although it would be churlish to claim that no progress has been made in addressing the question of whether DCD/SDD-MF comprises a single disorder or not, the message from the studies just reviewed is quite clear. We simply do not have available to us at this time even the minimal amount of empirical evidence required to support a position taken on these issues.

### *Criterion B - a Retrograde Step?*

Criterion B states: "The diagnosis is made only if this impairment significantly interferes with academic achievement or activities of daily living." (APA, 1994, p.53). As it is now formulated in DSM-IV, it includes two rather different elements. The first suggestion is that the diagnosis should only be made if the motor impairment significantly interferes with the activities of daily living. Since this part of the assessment process is likely to determine whether a child gains access to service provision or not, it would have been helpful to have guidance on how competence in the activities of daily living should be rated.

The second suggestion contained in Criterion B is that the diagnosis should only be made if the motor impairment significantly interferes with academic achievement. In our view, this phrase is not only difficult to operationalize, it actually takes us back 20 years in its implications for the diagnosis and treatment of children with movement difficulties. To evaluate this criticism, it is necessary to consider the picture of these children that has unfolded over the last two decades.

Until quite recently, it was common for pediatricians to assume that the prognosis for children identified as having movement problems in the early years was quite benign. From this comfortable stance, it was easy to slide into a relaxed position in which inaction was the considered view and parents were simply told that the child would "grow out of it". Moreover, if such children were good readers, teachers were often dismissive of parental concern about the child's "clumsiness".

In retrospect, it is easy now to enquire how a few, poorly documented, case histories in which recovery was reported could have sustained the weight of these assumptions, seeming to establish the reality of an effortless recovery process, justifying an almost universal prescription of non-intervention. However, in order to obtain a secure position on these difficult issues, longitudinal studies employing standardised, norm-referenced tests were required.

*Recent Follow-up Studies*

Using this methodology, four recent studies have called into question the view that "clumsiness" is a problem of early childhood with few implications for later development. In 1983, Knuckey and Gubbay published the first longitudinal study of children selected exclusively on the basis of motor competence. They describe an eight year follow-up of "clumsy" children and age-matched controls, first seen between the ages of eight and ten. When these children were retested as teenagers on a series of gross and fine motor tasks, the clumsy group remained consistently less proficient.

In 1991, we reported the outcome of a ten year follow-up of 17 "clumsy" children first identified between the ages of five and seven along with pair-wise matched controls (Losse et al., 1991). All the children were in mainstream schools. When these 34 children were teenagers, three different evaluations of their motor performance were obtained. They were tested on a standardised test of motor competence, the TOMI (Stott et al., 1984) and on a battery of neuro-developmental tests (Shafer et al., 1986), both administered by assessors blind to the original classification of the children. In addition, blind ratings were derived from the children's PE records over the ten years. There was good agreement between these three sources of information. Almost all of the children identified as having motor difficulties soon after they began primary school had similar problems as teenagers (see Table 3).

TABLE 3

Motor problems and physical self concept at sixteen years of age for a group of children first identified as having movement difficulties at age six.
( -- indicates unavailable data)

| Subject | OMI Score | Neuro-developmental test score | Attainment in physical education | Other motor problems | Physical Self-Concept |
|---|---|---|---|---|---|
| 1. | very poor | very poor | poor | yes | poor |
| 2. | -- | -- | poor | yes | -- |
| 3. | very poor | average | poor | no | poor |
| 4. | average | average | poor | yes | poor |
| 5. | very poor | very poor | average | no | poor |
| 6. | poor | very poor | average | yes | average |
| 7. | poor | poor | poor | yes | poor |
| 8. | average | poor | average | yes | average |
| 9. | poor | poor | poor | yes | average |
| 10. | poor | average | poor | yes | poor |
| 11. | -- | -- | average | yes | -- |
| 12. | average | poor | poor | yes | average |
| 13. | very poor | poor | average | yes | poor |
| 14. | poor | very poor | poor | yes | poor |
| 15. | average | poor | poor | yes | poor |
| 16. | poor | average | average | no | poor |
| 17. | very poor | average | poor | yes | poor |

Our objective measures revealed a distinct lack of coordination as did the many comments from their teachers. Although some "clumsy" pupils were described as trying hard in PE, none were rated as "good" on the achievement scales used by the schools. In other subjects, problems in art & crafts and difficulty with handling equipment in science were frequently noted. Untidy handwriting and poor presentation of written work were almost universal themes. We drew an even more pessimistic conclusion than Knuckey and Gubbay (1983), emphasising our failure to find support for the benign view of "clumsiness". Two subsequent investigations have obtained broadly similar findings to those we reported (Cantell, Smyth, & Ahonen, 1994; Geuze & Borger, 1993).

### *Educational consequences*

In addition to demonstrating that spontaneous recovery is far from universal in this group of children, these studies also demonstrate that withholding a diagnosis simply because there is no apparent effect on academic attainment at that stage is a dangerous business. Although inevitability is never claimed, many studies have demonstrated that being "clumsy" in the early years carries with it an increased risk of other learning difficulties later (e.g. Drillien & Drummond, 1983; Hadders-Algra, Huisjes, & Touwen, 1988; Silva & Ross, 1980). Also, three of the longitudinal studies just mentioned show that these problems do not disappear in secondary school. Indeed, for some children the restrictions imposed by their motor difficulties seem to result in school performance that is substantially below that which would have been predicted on the basis of their IQ and this seems especially true when the movement problems are accompanied by problems of attention (Gillberg & Gillberg, 1989; Gillberg, Gillberg, & Groth, 1989).

### *Social-emotional concomitants*

Fortunately, the conclusion that there is a strong association between poor motor coordination and social-emotional problems in childhood no longer has to rest on anecdotal evidence. The publication of Wall et al.'s (1990) comprehensive review was swiftly followed by several studies which extended our knowledge of the range of difficulties these children encounter. For instance, Schoemaker and Kalverboer (1994) demonstrate that even as young as six, children's lack of confidence in their physical competence invades other domains. Not only did the children with movement problems judge themselves to be less competent socially on the Harter scale but they also rated themselves as more introverted and anxious than their well coordinated peers. At the other end of the age spectrum, too, further evidence of the co-occurrence of social, emotional and coordination problems is accumulating. Two of the longitudinal studies mentioned (Cantell et al., 1994; Losse et al., 1991) showed that "clumsy" teenagers are not only very aware of their physical difficulties but in many cases this has consequences for their social and emotional well-being.

*Summary*

What this literature reveals is that the incorporation of judgemental criteria confined to the area of academic achievement into a formal classification scheme for movement difficulties is a dangerous enterprise. The narrow reference to academic achievement fails to take account of the preschool child whose social adjustment is jeopardised by the inability to play with peers, or the high achieving teenager who attempts suicide because of social isolation. Also, strict adherence to any such criterion in the early years may exclude many children who would have benefited greatly from intervention and, most importantly, the inclusion of any such criterion detracts from the importance of motor competence in its own right.

## *Criterion C: A Medical Question?*

Both the DSM-IV and ICD-10 manuals lay stress on the exclusion of children with an identifiable neurological disorder. In a relatively small number of cases, exclusion is straightforward. For example, some children in the very early stages of muscular dystrophy are referred to a paediatrician because they are observed to be "clumsy". Very soon, however, key clinical symptoms, such as muscle weakness, are identified which lead to definitive tests and a clear differential diagnosis.

At the most severe end, the diagnosis of cerebral palsy is also not a problem. Signs of neurological dysfunction, such as extreme abnormalities of reflexes, posture or tone can be detected in the neonatal period and almost immediately begin to affect the child's ability to move (e.g. Dubowitz & Dubowitz, 1981). Beyond this point, however, the process of differential diagnosis is much more complex. As Denckla and Roeltgen (1992, p. 456) point out in their exemplary discussion of the issues, "Immediately there arises the problem of drawing a clear line of demarcation between 'cerebral palsy' and lesser disabilities of motor function and control". Two relevant issues seem worth mentioning. First is the problematic use of underspecified tests as signs of neurodevelopmental impairment, without formal evidence of their reliability and validity. Second, are the problems posed by continuing advances in the technologies of brain imaging, which require constant revision of our notion of detectable pathology.

With regard to the presence/absence of these "soft" signs among children with a specific developmental disorder of motor function, the ICD-10 (WHO, 1992, p. 25) entry states :

"In most cases a careful clinical examination shows marked neurodevelopmental immaturities such as choreiform movements of unsupported limbs, or mirror movements and other associated motor features, as well as signs of poor fine and gross motor coordination (generally described as "soft" neurological signs because of their normal occurrence in younger children and their lack of localizing value). Tendon reflexes may be increased or decreased bilaterally but will not be asymmetrical".

Although no one doubts that such signs are more common among children with movement difficulties than among typically developing children (Forsström & Von Hofsten, 1982; Henderson & Hall, 1982; Losse et al., 1991; Schellekens et al., 1983), practical and theoretical problems continue to make it difficult to evaluate their significance. Some of the difficulty lies in the nature of the signs and their measurement. Denckla and Roeltgen (1992) identify two kinds of sign: (1) subtle versions of traditional neurological abnormalities such as choreiform movements, asymmetries of tone and minor degrees of ataxia and (2) the immature-for-age collection, wherein a milestone is either not met at all or is qualitatively less well accomplished than expected at the age of testing. For the first group of items, clear instructions about what degree of abnormality should be classed as "minor" or "subtle" is often lacking and data on the reliability with which these signs can be elicited is rarely available. It is, therefore, not uncommon for paediatrician to disagree about whether a particular pattern of such signs warrants the diagnosis of cerebral palsy or not. For the "immature-for-age group" of signs, it is the absence of normative data that usually makes interpretation difficult. Even more important than the practical issues, however, is the question of what these signs actually mean in terms of the integrity of particular neural structures. With only a few exceptions, our knowledge of the evolution of these signs is incomplete and we know almost nothing of the relationships between their appearance/ disappearance and neurological development. Consequently, from a diagnostic viewpoint, the significance of the difference between a "clumsy" child who does show these signs and one who does not is unclear.

Recent advances in brain imaging techniques are also making it more difficult to draw a neat distinction between "identifiable neurological conditions" and the so-called "specific" impairments of motor function. Whereas in the past, technological restrictions made it difficult to draw any conclusions about underlying pathology among children who presented with "clumsiness without accompanying intellectual deficits", recent follow-up studies of preterm, low-birthweight and other children "at risk" are yielding data which blurs the distinction between conditions such as cerebral palsy and DCD even more. For example, it is now possible to detect small lesions in the brains of children classified as DCD which would previously have gone undetected. Also, we know that a number of children who meet all behavioural criteria for DCD at school age have brain lesions at birth, which resolve and are no longer evident on later MRI scans (Jongmans, Henderson, de Vries, & Dubowitz, 1992). The questions we are then faced with are these: "In the individual case, does this exclude the child from the DCD category?" and more generally "Does the presence of a brain lesion, however small or transitory, constitute a medical condition?".

### *Criterion D - Specificity and Intellectual Ability*

Almost the entire focus of the debate on "specificity" in the context of developmental disorders has centred on the notion of an unexpected discrepancy between a child's intellectual ability and his/her attainment.

In contrast to areas of attainment such as reading, however, in the area of movement the discrepancy notion has received little attention. No one has discussed the possibility that IQ may not be the most appropriate predictive variable against which any discrepancy in motor attainment might be judged. Why not physical development, for example? No attempt has been made to find out whether the motor difficulties experienced by intelligent children differ in any way from those experienced by the less intellectually able child and the literature on subtypes within DCD/SDD- MF reviewed above offers no information on the cognitive abilities of the children involved. Consequently, there is no empirical support either for or against the specificity notion in relation to intellectual ability in the motor domain.

In spite of this, ICD-10 and DSM-IV take rather different lines on the relationship between intellectual and motor functioning. On the one hand, WHO continues to use "normal IQ" as a mandatory diagnostic criterion. As an exclusion criterion, the research version of ICD-10 (WHO, 1993, p. 147) proposed an "IQ below 70 on an individually administered standardised test" (which happens to be the criterion used in most research studies of DCD/SDD-MF in children). In the non-research version, however, the objective criterion is rejected in favour of the phrase "... not solely explicable in terms of general intellectual retardation..." (WHO, 1992, p. 250). In contrast, the DSM-IV scheme explicitly states that the "specificity" of the disorder lies in the gap between intellectual and motor ability, the gap lying anywhere along the intellectual spectrum. Thus, Criterion D states: "If Mental retardation is present, the motor difficulties are in excess of those usually associated with it" (APA, 1994, p. 55).

In spite of the differences between them, both classificatory systems face the same problem when it comes to selecting the most appropriate index of intellectual ability for this group of children. At the present time, some authors use global IQ as a criterion for diagnosing DCD/SDD-MF, others use verbal IQ alone and yet others use a discrepancy between verbal and performance IQ. Indeed high verbal and low performance IQ is used by some clinicians as the only criterion for DCD or SDD-MF. Apart from the fact that such variation is intrinsically unsatisfactory, there are two specific problems. The ICD-10 (WHO, 1992, p. 250) entry explicitly states that "It is usual for the motor clumsiness to be associated with some degree of impaired performance on visuo-spatial cognitive tasks" and there is strong support for this statement in existing literature (e.g. Henderson, Barnett, & Henderson, 1994; Hulme & Lord, 1986; Powell & Bishop, 1992). Since the visuo-spatial tasks that these children fail are precisely those employed in the performance sections of IQ tests then it seems unreasonable to penalise the children twice by calculating a full scale IQ from the sum of the verbal and performance components. The other problem concerns the use of a V-P discrepancy as a criterion. Recently, a number of studies have shown that a V-P discrepancy is not an invariant characteristic of children with low scores on tests of motor competence. In fact, it is possible to find children who have performance IQs that are considerably higher than their verbal IQs (Barnett, 1992; Jongmans, 1993). In our view, any such data needs to be recorded in a child's clinical file but for the purposes of initial classification, the best strategy would be to rely exclusively on verbal IQ as a criterion.

In addition to the general problem just mentioned, the DSM-IV classification scheme, in which intellectual retardation is no longer a criterion for exclusion from the diagnosis of DCD, presents other difficulties. In this case, it is the absolute difference between a child's score on a motor and intellectual test that matters regardless of where they lie on the IQ scale. Thus, it is theoretically possible for a child with Down's Syndrome or Fragile X syndrome to have a "developmental coordination disorder". While this approach has considerable merit on theoretical grounds, in that it encourages a new look at the nature of movement difficulties across the intellectual spectrum, in our view it is premature to attempt to incorporate it into a formal classification scheme. Normative data for the entire spectrum of movement difficulties in children is not available (in fact, there are no motor tests which have adequate sensitivity at both ends of the performance range) and the literature offers no suggestions as to how a discrepancy between intellectual and motor ability might be established.

In sum, the question of how motor ability should be considered in relation to intellectual ability is one which urgently needs attention, not only to allow us to adjudicate between the two options offered in ICD-10 and DSM-IV, but also so that we can determine whether we should be treating bright children and not-so-bright children with motor problems in the same way or not. In the next section, we now turn to the thorny issue of co-morbidity and its implications for differential diagnosis.

### *Associated Features and Overlap with Other Disorders*

As noted above, the existence of children whose lack of competence in the motor domain contrasts sharply with their academic and social success is not in doubt. Although such specificity is provocative for the theorist, the salience of such cases often leads to overestimation of their incidence. Far more common are descriptions of children whose movement problems are accompanied by at least some of the following: poor motivation and low self esteem (e.g. Shoemaker & Kalverboer, 1994), depression and social isolation (e.g. Hellgren, Gillberg, Gillberg, & Enerskog, 1993; Losse et al., 1991), hyperactivity & distractibility (Gillberg & Gillberg, 1989), and under achievement at school (all of the above). The high incidence of these problems in association with "clumsiness" raises a number of issues relevant to the design of classificatory schemes.

At a fundamental level, the frequent co-existence of motor difficulties with impairments of attention, language or reading (all of which represent defining features of other "specific" disorders) has led some to take an extreme position on the question of specificity, calling into question the very existence of separable childhood "syndromes" centred on attention, language, motor dysfunction, etc. The editors of this volume, as well as some of the contributors, might put themselves in this camp.

A related issue which concerns those who focus on the aetiology of developmental disorders, is the question of whether early brain damage can ever result in highly specific impairments, confined to one domain of development (Caron & Rutter, 1991; Henderson, et al., 1994; Powell & Bishop 1992). On the assumption that this is highly unlikely, co-occurrence should be the norm and specificity the exception.

On a more practical level, the question of how to deal with co-occurring problems often becomes one of pragmatism. Knowledge of what services are available may well override any clear priorities that are set for the child. If the occupational therapist's lists are full then help with reading may come first for the child with a combination of motor and reading problems, regardless of the assessor's judgement. Another problem stems from ignorance of the true significance of motor disorders, which when found in combination with another developmental impairment, are often viewed as less important.

## CONCLUSIONS

As noted by Rispens and Van Yperen (this volume), the use of the term "specific" in relation to the classification of childhood disorders has changed over the years without clear explication. Indeed, in some regards the development of the classification schemes seems to have proceeded without any real empirical justification. This certainly seems to have been the case in relation to "specific" movement disorders in children. We have very little data pertaining either to the elements within the classification schemes or to the broader issues that need to be addressed. In the space available to us here, we have focused on some of the more microscopic problems that need to be solved before the larger questions can be addressed.

## REFERENCES

American Psychiatric Association. (1987). *Diagnostic and statistical manual of mental disorders* (3rd ed., rev.). Washington DC: American Psychiatric Association.
American Psychiatric Association. (1994). *Diagnostic and statistical manual of mental*

*disorders* (4th ed.). Washington DC: American Psychiatric Association.

Annell, A. L. (1949). School problems in children of average or superior intelligence: A preliminary report. *Journal of Mental Science, 95*, 901-909.

Ayres, J. A. (1972). *Sensory integration and learning disorders*. Los Angeles, CA: Western Psychological Services.

Ayres, J. A. (1989). *Sensory Integration and Praxis Test*. Los Angeles, CA: Western Psychological Services.

Ayres, J. A., Mailloux, Z. K., & Wendler, C. L. W. (1987). Developmental dyspraxia: Is it a unitary function? *Occupational Therapy Journal of Research, 7,* 93-110.

Barnett, A. L. (1992). *Manual competence in clumsy children*. PhD Thesis, University of London, Institute of Education, London.

Barnett, A. L. & Henderson, S. E. (1992). Some observations on the figure drawings of clumsy children. *British Journal of Educational Psychology, 62*, 341-355.

Brenner, M. W. & Gillman, S. (1966). Visuo-motor ability in school children - A survey. *Developmental Medicine and Child Neurology, 8,* 686-703.

British Medical Journal. (1962). Clumsy children. *British Medical Journal*, 1665-1666.

Bruininks, R. H. (1978). *The Bruininks-Oseretsky Test of Motor Proficiency*. Circle Pines, MN: American Guidance Service.

Cantell, M. H., Smyth, M. M., & Ahonen, T. P. (1994). Clumsiness in adolescence: Educational, motor, and social outcomes of motor delay detected at five years. *Special Issue of Adapted Physical Activity Quarterly, 11,* 115-129.

Caron, C. & Rutter, M. (1991). Co-morbidity in child psychopathology: Concepts, issues and research strategies. *Journal of Child Psychology and Psychiatry, 32,* 1063-1080.

Cermak, S. (1985). Developmental dyspraxia. In E. A. Roy (Ed.). *Neuropsychological studies in apraxia and related disorders* (pp. 225-248). Amsterdam: Elsevier Science Publishers B.V.

David, R., Deuel, R., Ferry, P., Gascon, G., Golden, G., Rapin, I., Rosenberger, P., & Shaywitz, B. (1981). *Proposed nosology of disorders of higher cerebral function in children*. Minneapolis, MN. Child Neurology Society.

Dare, M. T. & Gordon, N. (1970). Clumsy children: A disorder of perception and motor organisation. *Developmental Medicine and Child Neurology, 12*, 178-185.

Denckla, M. B. (1984). Developmental dyspraxia. The clumsy child. In M. K. Levine & P. Satz (Eds.), *Middle childhood: Development and dysfunction*. Boston: University Park Press.

Denckla, M. B. & Roeltgen, D. P. (1992). Disorders of motor function and control. In I. Rapin & S. J. Segalowitz (Eds), *Handbook of neuropsychology, Vol. 6: Child Neuropsychology* (pp. 455-476). Amsterdam: Elsevier Science Publishers B.V.

Dewey, D. & Kaplan, B. (1992). Subtyping of developmental motor deficits. *Journal of Clinical and Experimental Neuropsychology, 14,* 50.

Drillien, C. & Drummond, M. (1983). *Clinics in developmental medicine, Vol. 86: Developmental screening and the child with special needs: A population study of 5000 children*. London: S.I.M.P. with Heinemann Medical.

Dubowitz, L. M. S. & Dubowitz, V. (1981). *The neurological assessment of the preterm and fullterm newborn infant*. London: S.I.M.P. with Heinemann.

Ford, F. R. (1966). *Diseases of the nervous system in infancy childhood and adolescence* (5th ed). Springfield: Thomas.

Forsström, A. & Von Hofsten, C. (1982). Visually directed reaching of children with motor impairments. *Developmental Medicine and Child Neurology, 24,* 653-661.

Geuze, R. & Borger, H. (1993). Children who are clumsy: Five years later. *Adapted Physical Activity Quarterly, 10,* 10-21.

Gillberg, I. C. & Gillberg, C. (1989). Children with preschool minor neurodevelopmental disorders IV: Behaviour and school achievement at age 13. *Developmental Medicine and Child Neurology, 31,* 3-13.

Gillberg, I. C., Gillberg, C., & Groth, J. (1989). Children with preschool minor neurodevelopmental disorders V: Neurodevelopmental profiles at age 13. *Developmental Medicine and Child Neurology, 31,* 14-24.

Gordon, N. S. (1969). Helping the clumsy child in school. *Special Education, 58,* 19-20.

Gubbay, S. S. (1975) *The clumsy child: A study of developmental apraxia and agnosic ataxia.* London: W.B. Saunders Co. Ltd.

Gubbay, S. S. (1978). The management of developmental apraxia. *Developmental Medicine and Child Neurology, 20,* 643-646.

Gubbay, S. S., Ellis, E., Walton, J. N., & Court, S. D. M. (1965). Clumsy children: A study of apraxic and agnosic defects in 21 children. *Brain, 88,* 295-312.

Hadders-Algra, M., Huisjes, H. J., & Touwen, B. C. L. (1988). Perinatal risk factors and minor neurological dysfunction: Significance for behaviour and school achievement at nine years. *Developmental Medicine and Child Neurology, 30,* 482-491.

Hellgren, L., Gillberg, C., Gillberg, I. C., & Enerskog, I. (1993). Children with deficits in attention, motor control and perception (DAMP) almost grown up: General health at sixteen years. *Developmental Medicine and Child Neurology, 35,* 881-893.

Henderson, S. E., Barnett, A. L., & Henderson, L. (1994). Visuospatial difficulties and clumsiness. On the interpretation of conjoined deficits. *Journal of Child Psychology and Psychiatry, 35,* 961-969.

Henderson, S. E. & Hall, D. (1982). Concomitants of clumsiness in young school children. *Developmental Medicine and Child Neurology, 24,* 448-460.

Henderson, S. E., May, D. S., & Umney, M. (1989). An exploratory study of goal-setting behaviour, self-concept and locus of control in children with movement difficulties. *European Journal of Special Needs Education, 4,* 1-15.

Henderson, S. E. & Sugden, D. A. (1992). *Movement Assessment Battery for Children.* The Psychological Corporation, Harcourt Brace Jovanovich.

Hoare, D. (1994). Subtypes of developmental coordination disorder. *Special Issue of Adapted Physical Activity Quarterly, 11,* 158-169.

Hulme, C., Biggerstaff, A., Moran, G., & McKinlay, I. (1982). Visual, kinaesthetic and cross-modal judgements of length by normal and clumsy children. *Developmental Medicine and Child Neurology, 24,* 461-471.

Hulme, C. & Lord, R. (1986). Clumsy children: A review of recent research. *Child: Care, health and development, 12,* 257-269.

Illingworth, R. S. (1968). The clumsy child. In M. Bax & R. McKeith (Eds.), *Minimal cerebral dysfunction* (pp. 26-27). London: Heinemann Medical Books.

Johnston, O., Short, H., & Crawford, J. (1987). Poorly coordinated children: A survey of 95 cases. *Child: Care, health and development, 13,* 361-367.

Jongmans, M. J. (1993). *Perceptuo-motor competence in prematurely born children at school age: Neurological and psychological aspects.* PhD Thesis, University of London, Institute of Education, London.

Jongmans, M. J., Henderson, S. E., de Vries, L. S., & Dubowitz, L. M. S. (1992). Duration of periventricular densities in preterm infants and neurological outcome at 6 years of age. *Developmental Medicine and Child Neurology, 69,* 9-13.

Keogh, J. F., Sugden, D. A., Reynard, C. L., & Calkins, J. A. (1979). Identification of clumsy children: Comparisons and comments. *Journal of Human Movement Studies, 5,* 32-41.

Knuckey, N. W. & Gubbay, S. S. (1983). Clumsy children: A prognostic study. *Australian Pediatric Journal, 19,* 9-13.

Laszlo, J. I., Bairstow, P. J., Bartrip, J., & Rolfe, U. T. (1988). Clumsiness or perceptuo-motor dysfunction? In A. M. Colley & J. R. Beech (Eds.), *Cognition and action in skilled behaviour*. Amsterdam: Elsevier Science Publishers B.V.

Lesny, I. A. (1980). Developmental dyspraxia-dysgnosia as a cause of congenital children's clumsiness. *Brain and Development, 2,* 69-71.

Lord, R. & Hulme, C. (1988). Visual perception and drawing ability in clumsy and normal children. *British Journal of Developmental Psychology, 6,* 1-9.

Losse, A., Henderson, S. E., Elliman, D., Hall, D., Knight, E., & Jongmans, M. (1991). Clumsiness in children - do they grow out of it? A ten year follow up study. *Developmental Medicine and Child Neurology, 33,* 55-68.

McKinlay, I. (1978). Strategies for clumsy children. *Developmental Medicine and Child Neurology, 20,* 494-501.

Missiuna, C. & Polatajko, H. (1995). Developmental dyspraxia by any other name: Are they all just clumsy children? *American Journal of Occupational Therapy, 9,* 619-627.

Miyahara, M. (1994). Subtypes of students with learning disabilities based upon gross motor functions. *Adapted Physical Activity Quarterly, 11,* 368-382.

Orton, S. T. (1937). *Reading, writing and speech problems in children.* New York: Norton.

Powell, R. P. & Bishop. (1992). Clumsiness and perceptual problems in children with specific language impairment. *Developmental Medicine and Child Neurology, 34,* 755-765.

Schellekens, J. M. H., Scholten, C. A., & Kalverboer, A. F. (1983). Visually guided hand movements in children with minor neurological dysfunction. *Journal of Child Psychology and Psychiatry, 24,* 98-102.

Schmidt R. A. (1988). *Motor control and learning: A behavioural emphasis* (2nd ed.). Champaign, IL: Human Kinetics.

Schoemaker, M. M. & Kalverboer, A. F. (1994). Social and affective problems of children who are clumsy: How early do they begin? *Adapted Physical Activity Quarterly, 11,* 130-140.

Shafer, S. Q., Stokman, C. J., Shaffer, D., Ng, S. K-C., O'Connor, P. A., & Schonfeld, I. S. (1986). Ten-year consistency in neurological test performance of children without focal neurological deficit. *Developmental Medicine and Child Neurology, 28,* 417-427.

Silva, P. A. & Ross, B. (1980). Gross motor development and delays in development in early childhood: Assessment and significance. *Journal of Human Movement Studies, 6,* 211-226.

Stott, D. H., Moyes, F. A., & Henderson, S. E. (1984). *The Henderson Revision of the Test of Motor Impairment.* Guelph, Ontario: Brook Educational Publishing Ltd.

Sugden, D. A. & Keogh, J. F. (1990). *Problems in movement skill development.* Columbia, SC: University of Columbia Press.

Touwen, B. C. L. (1979). *The examination of the child with minor neurological dysfunction.* London: S.I.M.P. with Heinemann Medical.

Touwen, B. C. L. (1993). Longitudinal studies on motor development:

Developmental neurological considerations. In A. F. Kalverboer, B. Hopkins, & R. H. Geuze (Eds.), *Motor development in early and later childhood: Longitudinal approaches*. Cambridge: Cambridge University Press.

Van Dellen, T. & Geuze, R. H. (1988).Motor response processing in clumsy children. *Journal of Child Psychology and Psychiatry, 29*, 489-500.

Wall, A. E. (1982). Physically awkward children: A motor development perspective. In J. P. Das, R. F. Mulcahy & A. E. Wall (Eds.), *Theory and research in learning disabilities*. New York: Plenum Press.

Wall, A. E., Reid, G., & Paton, J. (1990). The syndrome of physical awkwardness. In G. Reid (Ed.), *Problems in movement control*. Amsterdam: Elsevier Science Publishers B.V.

Walton, J. N., Ellis, E., & Court, S. D. M. (1962). Clumsy children: Developmental apraxia and agnosia. *Brain, 85*, 603-612.

World Health Organization. (1989). *The ICD-9 classification of mental and behavioural disorders: Clinical descriptions and diagnostic guidelines*. Geneva: World Health Organization.

World Health Organization. (1992). *The ICD-10 classification of mental and behavioural disorders: Clinical descriptions and diagnostic guidelines*. Geneva: World Health Organization.

World Health Organization. (1994). *The ICD-10 classification of mental and behavioural disorders: Diagnostic criteria for research*. Geneva: World Health Organization.

MARINA M. SCHOEMAKER, BOUWIEN C. M. SMITS-ENGELSMAN AND ALEX F. KALVERBOER

# THE CLASSIFICATION OF SPECIFIC MOTOR DISORDERS: IMPLICATIONS FOR INTERVENTION

## INTRODUCTION

Although problems of motor incoordination have been frequently described in literature, it was not until 1987 that motor disorders of unknown aetiology were included in the Diagnostic and Statistical Manual of Mental Disorders of the American Psychiatric Association (DSM-III-R, American Psychiatric Association [APA], 1987) under the heading Developmental Coordination Disorder (abbreviated DCD). DCD was placed within the subclass of Specific Develop mental Disorders, which included three categories, namely inadequate development of specific academic skills, language and speech skills, and motor skills. In the 1994 version of DSM (APA, 1994), the subclass of Specific Developmental Disorders no longer exists as a separate entity. To date, developmental disorders are part of the section Disorders Usually First Diagnosed in Infancy, Childhood, or Adolescence, and are divided into three new groups: Learning Disorders, Motor Skills Disorder (specified DCD) and Communication Disorders. The essential features of this group of disorders are: an achievement that is substantially below that expected given a person's chronological age, measured intelligence, and age-appropriate education; the disturbance interferes with academic achievement or activities of daily living. Excluded from this group are disorders explicable in terms of neurological or sensory deficits.

A Developmental Coordination Disorder is characterized by a predominance of disturbances in the acquisition of motor skills, resulting in clumsiness, poor performance in sports or poor handwriting. In general, the relevance of a diagnosis in a classification system depends on it's reliability, validity, and clinical utility (Skinner, 1986). Reliability refers to the consistency within and between clinicians to assign individuals to a specific diagnostic category; the validity of a diagnosis is dependent on the reliability and refers to whether specific diagnostic categories can be distinguished from one another. The last feature of a diagnosis is its clinical utility. As previous papers in this volume have addressed



*J. Rispens et al. (eds.),*
*Perspectives on the Classification of Specific Developmental Disorders,* 231–244.

issues concerning the reliability and validity of specific developmental disorders (Rispens & Van Yperen, this volume), and DCD in particular (Henderson & Barnett, this volume), the present chapter attempts to address the utility of the diagnosis of DCD for research and intervention. The advantages and disadvantages of classification will be discussed, as well as the usefulness of the current definition of DCD for clinical practice and research.

## CLASSIFICATION

Classification is the ordering of disorders into mutually exclusive categories based on their intrinsic characteristics. From a clinical point of view, classification has some important benefits (Blashfield, 1984).

First, an adequate classification system can provide the vernacular for professionals in the field to communicate with each other efficiently and effectively. The use of the same term for the same group of children may facilitate communication in both research and clinical practice. This aspect is very relevant to DCD. Before the introduction of a separate category concerning motor disorders in children in DSM, numerous papers appeared on this topic in which many terms were used to describe this kind of children. Henderson and Barnett (this volume) have presented a list of the different terms previously used for children with DCD. The use of different terms hampers the comparison of research findings, as it is unclear whether the same kind of children were involved in different studies. The confusion as to how to label children with motor problems becomes apparent in clinical practice as well. Even now, it is not uncommon that professionals apply different terms for the same group of children depending on their professional schooling preference. For instance, physiotherapists might speak of children with a motor delay, while occupational therapists would label them as children with a sensory integration disorder. Out of dissatisfaction with the confusion about the terms and operational definitions that surrounded children with difficulty coordinating their movements, a consensus meeting was held in London, Ontario in 1994, attended by 43 researchers and professionals in this field from all over the world. One of the aims of this meeting was to reach agreement on the nomenclature for the children under consideration. It was decided that the term Developmental Coordination Disorder be used from now on, as it describes the primary observable feature of the condition ("The London Consensus"; Fox & Polatajko, 1994).

A second benefit of an adequate classification is that it can provide relevant information pertaining to number and kind of symptoms, prognosis, treatment selection, response to treatment, and comorbid conditions. In order to be able to supply this kind of information, the operational definition of DCD has to be reasonably specific. However, the way in which DCD is currently described in DSM is insufficiently specific to make it optimally useful for either diagnosis or prognosis (Deuel, 1992), or intervention purposes. This is partly due to the inclusion of all types of motor performance deficits in one broad category, and partly due to the lack of more specific exclusion criteria.

First, DCD is by no means a homogeneous syndrome as regards the movement difficulties experienced. Large individual differences in both the range, seriousness, and pervasiveness of movement difficulties are common in children with DCD (see also Henderson & Barnett, this volume). The category DCD is a wastebasket of all kinds of motor disorders of unknown aetiology. Secondly, due to the lack of more specific inclusion criteria, comorbidity is a serious problem in this category. The results of an unpublished study by our group illustrate this point. The aim of this study was to make an inventory of the kind of motor and comorbid problems of a group of 24 primary school children (aged 5 to 11) referred for treatment of their motor problems to an arbitrary physiotherapy practice. All the children were classified as having DCD by the physiotherapist, as their problems fell within the boundaries of the operational definition of DCD. Before entering treatment, the motor and other kinds of developmental problems of all the children were diagnosed thoroughly. Table 1 gives a summary of the main problems of these children.

TABLE 1

Summary of percentages of motor and concomitant problems of a group of children (N = 24) diagnosed as having DCD.

| Problem | present | not present |
|---|---|---|
| Movement problems | 100% | - |
| Hyperactivity | 54% | 46% |
| Distractibility | 71% | 29% |
| Problems at school | 67% | 33% |
| Learning difficulties | 67% | 33% |
| Emotional problems | 71% | 29% |
| Family problems | 46% | 54% |

Comorbidity proved to be a common problem in this group of children: all the children in this group experienced motor problems, but a range of concomitant problems was found as well. Some of the children with DCD may be classified in diagnostic categories such as ADHD or Learning Difficulties. A recent study showed that this result is no exception (Smits-Engelsman, 1995). A questionnaire was sent to a large group of physiotherapists to make an inventory of the problems of children referred for DCD in various physiotherapy practices. The same picture emerged as described above: a range of motor and concomitant problems seems to be characteristic of children diagnosed with DCD. These examples illustrate the possible overlap with other diagnostic categories. The various categories of specific developmental disorders are by no means mutually exclusive. It is therefore hardly surprising that the reliability and validity of this diagnosis has been questioned (Rispens & Van Yperen, this volume). However, the lack of reliability and validity has serious consequences for clinical practice, especially if it concerns issues such as treatment selection and response to treatment. In the next paragraphs, we will elaborate on this point.

## TREATMENT SELECTION

With respect to treatment selection, the following remarks can be made. The present description of DCD in DSM-IV does not provide any information about treatment selection. In addition, no research findings allow for the identification of a treatment of choice for children with DCD (Fox & Polatajko, 1994). No explicit standardized treatments are available for children with DCD. Consequently, in clinical practice, treatment selection for children with movement problems is to a large extent dependent upon the nature of the therapist's schooling. Generally, there are no strict boundaries between various treatment programmes in actual practice. Elements from different treatment programmes are often combined into one treatment programme, especially and usually the elements that seem to be most effective are used. Bobath and Bobath (1984) warned against this eclectic approach, because techniques derived from different programmes are based upon different views of the children's problems and might, therefore, not result in a cohesive treatment programme. Results of effect evaluation studies confirm the Bobath's viewpoint. In their meta-analytical study, Kavale and Mattson (1983) found the effects of treatments in which different programmes were combined to be smaller than the effects of treatments based on a single programme. Nevertheless, despite these results, the use of a mixture of techniques is quite widespread. This situation will not change as long as no guidelines have been published about which treatment programme might be most effective with a particular group of children.

## RESPONSE TO TREATMENT

The heterogeneity of children diagnosed with DCD certainly hinders the provision of information about treatment selection. It is not unlikely that certain kinds of motor problems require different kinds of treatment, especially when various of concomitant problems are involved. Treatment of a shy, introvert clumsy child would call for a different approach than the treatment of an aggressive, hyperactive child with movement problems. And what is to be done with an intellectually bright motor delayed child compared with a dull child with movement problems from a deprived background? As studies concerning treatment response in specific groups of children with DCD have only just begun to appear (Schoemaker, Hijlkema, & Kalverboer, 1994; Smits-Engelsman, Schoemaker, Janssen, & Niemeijer, in press), it will take some time before these questions can be answered reliably.

Research findings regarding response to treatment clearly demonstrate the need for carefully selected, homogeneous groups of children. During the past thirty years, several studies have attempted to evaluate the effectiveness of treatment programmes for children with movement difficulties. Reviews of the results conclude that only a small percentage of these studies was reliable due to methodological problems, and most studies reported disappointing results (Densem, Nuthall, Bushnell, & Horn, 1989; Halahan & Cruickshank, 1973; Kavale & Mattson, 1983; Myers & Hammill, 1976; Rispens, 1977). Treatment programmes for children with movement problems have not produced significant changes in motor incoordination. The heterogeneity of the samples included in these studies has frequently been mentioned as one of the problems responsible for this lack of effect. When different types of children are included in one evaluation study, it is not unlikely that some children might benefit more from treatment than others. When group means are used in evaluation studies, the negative and positive results of treatment are summed, and the net effect of intervention will be nil. Thus, studies using heterogeneous groups of children do not detect the significant gains made by some individuals. In order to know which children do benefit from treatment, the use of more homogeneous groups of children is a pre-requisite in evaluation studies. Information about responsiveness to treatment is of increasing importance, at least in the Netherlands, where health care insurance companies supply funding only for treatments that have proven to be effective.

Although review articles about the effectiveness of intervention mainly report disappointing results, professionals in clinical practice, such as physiotherapists and occupational therapists, do claim to achieve positive results in the treatment of at least some children with DCD. To verify this claim, we recently conducted two evaluation studies, in which we tried to avoid the problem of sample heterogeneity (Schoemaker, Hijlkema et al., 1994; Smits-Engelsman et al., in press). In the first study, the effects of physiotherapy were evaluated in a group of children with DCD. Seventeen primary school children were involved in this study: 15 boys and 3 girls aged 6 to 10. The children were selected according to the DCD criteria in DSM-III-R (APA, 1987), but we applied some additional criteria in order to ensure that the group would be as homogeneous as possible. Table 2 presents a list of these exclusion criteria.

In order to evaluate the effectiveness of treatment, a pretest-posttest design was used in this study, but with the added variant that the children with DCD also acted as their own controls. First, two pretest measures were taken at three-month intervals to determine the spontaneous rate of motor development without treatment. After the second pretest, the DCD group received treatment for three months. After these three months, the children were tested again to determine the effectiveness of intervention. A general motor test, the Movement Assessment Battery for Children (Henderson & Sugden, 1992), was used for these purposes. In

TABLE 2

Exclusion criteria for selecting children with DCD for an evaluation study.

exclusion criteria:

* no children from schools for special education
  (thereby excluding children with learning difficulties)
* no children who had been treated previously
* no children with a medical condition (asthma, epilepsy etc.)
* no children with family problems (parental divorce, death of a relative)

contrast to the disappointing results of previous effect evaluation studies, positive effects of treatment were found in this study. Both the gross and the fine motor skills of the children with DCD improved after intervention (for more details about this study see Schoemaker, Hijlkema et al., 1994).

In a second study, we evaluated the effects of physiotherapy in a group of children with DCD, who experienced primarily fine motor problems (i.e. handwriting problems). Two groups of children with DCD were involved in this study: a group of 22 children with DCD who received treatment during three months, and a group of 10 children with DCD who did not receive treatment. The same exclusion criteria as mentioned above were applied. In order to evaluate the effectiveness of treatment, a pretest-posttest design was applied. Again, the Movement Assessment Battery for Children was used for evaluation. In this study too, a positive effect of intervention was found, corroborating the results of our first study. (See Smits-Engelsman et al., in press, for details of this study). Thus, our conclusion is that if more homogeneous groups are used, an adequate therapy may result in demonstrable effects.

However, the exclusion criteria applied in the above mentioned evaluation studies were relatively arbitrary. As long as the operational definition of DCD is not described precisely, each researcher is free to apply his or her own selection criteria. As a consequence, research findings remain difficult to compare, as different groups of children with DCD may be selected in each study. A possible solution to this problem is the subclassification of children with DCD.

## SUBCLASSIFICATION

The fact that the heterogeneity of children with DCD has been disregarded by current classification schemes has been criticized by both Henderson and Barnett (this volume) and Deuel (1992). Consequently, these authors make an appeal for the subclassification of children with movement problems. By subclassification, children with the same intrinsic characteristics are classified in one subgroup. More homogeneous subgroups would facilitate the provision of information about prognosis or intervention alternatives and improve the comparability of research findings. There are two different approaches to subclassification. Deuel proposed a subclassification based upon a clinical inferential approach, whereas Henderson and Barnett opt for empirical classification techniques. Both approaches will be discussed briefly.

In addition, a third approach towards classifying children with movement problems will be introduced.

### *Clinical Inferential Approach*

The clinical inferential approach depends largely on the clinical observations of professionals in the field (Hooper, 1992). The theoretical position, experience, and intuition of the professionals play a major role in this approach (Hoare, 1994). DSM is an example of a classification system based on the clinical inferential approach. This approach was also applied by the Task Force on Nosology of Higher Cerebral Function in Children (David et al., 1981). Because of dissatisfaction with the lack of specificity of the current category DCD in DSM-IV, a general typology of disorders of motor execution was proposed. Motor performance deficits were divided into three categories: clumsiness, adventitious movements, and dyspraxia. Clumsiness is defined as slowness and inefficiency in performing all elemental fine motor movements. Adventitious movements are involuntary movements that occur in combination with any purposeful motor activity. Lastly, dyspraxia is the inability to learn and perform age-appropriate sequences of voluntary movements in the face of preserved coordination, strength and sensation. The categories are divided into subcategories, and a child may display symptoms belonging to more than one general category of deficit and may be classified in more than one subcategory within each category (Deuel, 1992). A comprehensive description of each category is presented together with information about ways to examine the syndromes, differential diagnosis, and the relation with neuropsychiatric disorders.

Another theoretical approach for the differentiation into subtypes of DCD might be sought in the neurological architecture that subserves complex motor behaviour. Problems in execution, coordination, planning, and learning have been shown to relate to divergent neural systems. Lundy-Ekman, Ivry, Keele, and Woollacott (1991) studied clumsy children divided into two groups on the basis of soft signs. The division included a cerebellar and a basal ganglia dysfunction type. The basal ganglia dysfunction group was more variable in force control tasks, while the cerebellar dysfunction group was impaired on timing. However, reciprocal connections between the brain areas involved are complex and preclude simple localisationary explanations. Hence, one might question the validity of the approach of Lundy-Ekman and colleagues (1991) towards classification.

Unfortunately, classification models derived from a clinical inferential approach have some major drawbacks. Although these models might make sense intuitively, the schemes are of questionable validity and limited clinical utility (Hooper, 1992). The information provided in this volume about the reliability, validity and clinical utility of specific developmental disorders in general and DCD in particular underlines this point of criticism. Even though the subclassification proposed by the task force is very comprehensive and conceptually driven, no data on the empirical tests of its reliability or validity have been presented so far.

## *Empirical Classification Techniques*

The development of advanced statistical techniques, such as cluster analysis and factor analysis, has provided possibilities for empirical classification of syndromes. Recently, several studies used this technique in search for subtypes within the group of children with DCD (Hoare, 1994; Lyytinen & Ahonen, 1988; Miyahara, 1993). From a sample of 1138 five-year old children Lyytinen and Ahonen selected 153 children (13.4%) with motor problems. Subsequently, the motor performance of these children was examined on measures of motor control, speed and fluency, temporal-spatial sequencing, motor inhibition, kinaesthesia, and spatiality. The results of a cluster analysis yielded 5 subtypes of motor problems. Hoare, too, identified 5 subtypes within a sample of 6 to 9-year old children with DCD. She selected six variables, partly different from the ones used by Lyytinen and Ahonen, based upon both clinical reports and experimental studies of children with movement difficulties. These variables included measures of visual and kinaesthetic perception, visual-motor integration, manual dexterity and gross motor ability. Miyahara identified four homogeneous subtypes within a group of learning disabled students, based upon gross motor functions as measured by gross motor subtests from the Bruininks-Oseretsky Test of Motor Proficiency, namely running speed and agility, balance, bilateral coordination, strength and upper limb coordination. For more information about the different subtypes found in these studies, the reader is referred to the paper by Henderson and Barnett (this volume). In conclusion, children with DCD represent a heterogeneous group. Cluster analysis results in at least four or five subtypes of children with DCD. However, different subtypes were obtained in each of the studies.

As with the clinical inferential approach, the empirical approach has not been received without criticism. According to Hooper (1992), the adequacy and strength of models derived by empirical classification methods are influenced by many a priori clinical decisions, including those regarding theoretical orientation, sample selection, and variable selection. The results of empirical classification methods are entirely based upon the performances of children on standardized motor tests. Motor tests are generally product oriented, as they only assess the outcome of a movement. However, there are several ways in which a child can achieve a certain outcome. A child can fail to catch a ball for several reasons, such as reacting too late, moving too slowly, or moving in the wrong direction. These aspects of movement performance are completely overlooked by a product oriented approach. Insight into the underlying mechanisms of movement performance requires a more process-oriented approach. This approach would enable us to identify homogeneous subtypes of DCD children with the same underlying motor control problems.

Even then, it is questionable whether standardized tests are sensitive to all aspects of a clinical syndrome (Bishop, this volume). An underlying theory about the motor problems of children with DCD is lacking in the studies previously described. The variables for cluster analysis were chosen relatively arbitrarily. Consequently, different subtypes were obtained in each of the studies, depending on the variables chosen for cluster analysis. Whether the outcome of a cluster analysis has any face validity depends to a large extent on whether the selected variables represent the key characteristics of children with DCD. The clinical inferential approach might be helpful in selecting variables that represent the critical features of a syndrome.

Moreover, categorization does not end with the identification of subtypes. Subsequently, the validity and clinical utility of the identified subtypes must be demonstrated. One approach to validating the subtypes is to investigate the responsiveness to intervention (Hoare, 1994; Henderson & Barnett, this volume). Miyahara (1993) described remediational strategies for each of the four subtypes he identified, but, so far, the effectiveness of these strategies has not been evaluated.

### *The Alternative: A Process-oriented Approach*

A disadvantage of the two classification methods described above is that classification is not based on a sound theoretical model of psychomotor functioning. In our opinion, subclassification should be conceptually driven. A theoretical model based upon scientific knowledge about motor control and mechanisms underlying goal-directed movements is needed to explain the different symptoms of children with DCD. This kind of model was recently developed by Smits-Engelsman (1995). Then, this model should determine the choice of measurement instruments. Writing and drawing tasks are examples of conceptually based instruments. Subsequently, movement performance should be analyzed kinematically by using advanced measuring techniques. These techniques enable us to study the organization of movements by breaking them down into their constituent components, which can be measured separately. The usefulness of a process oriented approach to the classification of motor disorders was demonstrated in two studies (Schoemaker, Schellekens, Kalverboer, & Kooistra, 1994; Smits-Engelsman, Van Galen, & Portier, 1994).

The first study included 18 children who performed poorly on both fine and gross motor tasks (Schoemaker, Schellekens et al., 1994). The second study included only children with primarily fine motor problems (Smits-Engelsman et al., 1994). The children in both studies were selected according to the criteria for DCD in DSM-IV; only mainstream primary school children were involved, aged 6 to 10 years. Both groups of children failed on drawing or writing tasks, because of their inability to draw or write neatly. Thus, the outcome of movement performance was the same in both groups. However, when the process of movement organization during writing or drawing tasks was studied in detail, a different picture of their problems was revealed. Children with DCD who had both gross and fine movement problems wrote more slowly, more dysfluently, and with longer pauses between consecutive strokes than age-matched control children without motor problems. In contrast, children with DCD with fine motor problems wrote with higher velocity and changed direction in the writing trajectory less frequently than age-matched controls without motor problems. Thus, although the outcome was the same in both groups (inaccuracy of drawing or writing), this outcome was reached in a completely different way for each group. This example demonstrates that the essential features of movement organization may remain unrecognized if one relies solely on outcome measures.

Data obtained through more finely tuned, process-oriented measuring instruments need to be included in classification studies in order to obtain subtypes that are both valid and clinically useful. Then, intervention strategies must be developed to treat identified subtypes of movement problems. The validity of these subtypes may be investigated subsequently by the evaluation of the effects of different intervention strategies. In the next chapter, the process oriented classification method will be discussed in more detail (Smits- Engelsman, Van Galen, & Schoemaker, this volume).

## CONCLUDING REMARKS

The formal acknowledgement of children with primarily motor problems as a separate clinical group has been a major breakthrough in caregiving for these children. However, the inclusion of this group of children in formal classification systems, such as DSM, is only the first step. Now, the classification requires intern validation. Including examination of its reliability, homogeneity, and robustness. Both the reliability and the homogeneity of DCD as a diagnostic category have been questioned in the present paper on the basis of current research findings. In order to improve the reliability of the category, the operational definition of DCD has to be described more precisely. The inclusion and exclusion criteria of the category have to be specified in order to prevent overlap with other diagnostic criteria.

In addition, the clinical implications of the co-occurrence of different syndromes within one child has to be outlined. Is DCD in a bright child comparable to symptoms of DCD in intellectually backward children? In order to improve the homogeneity of children with DCD, the search for subtypes using a process-oriented classification approach has been advocated. Subsequently, the reliability and validity of the identified subtypes has to be investigated, for instance by the investigation of the response of homogeneous subtypes to different treatment approaches. In conclusion, classification is an ongoing process of theory formulation and both internal and external validation based upon the results of empirical studies.

## REFERENCES

American Psychiatric Association. (1987). *Diagnostic and statistical manual of mental disorders* (3rd. ed., rev.). Washington, DC: American Psychiatric Association.

American Psychiatric Association. (1994). *Diagnostic and statistical manual of mental disorders* (4th. ed.). Washington, DC: American Psychiatric Association.

Blashfield, R. K. (1984). *Classification of psychopathology*. New York: Plenum.

Bobath, K. & Bobath, B. (1984). The neuro-developmental treatment. In D. Scrutton (Ed.), *Management of motor disorders of children with cerebral palsy*. Oxford: Blackwell Scientific Publications Ltd.

David, R., Deuel, R., Ferry, P., Gascon, G., Golden, G., Rapin, I., Rosenberger, P., & Shaywitz, B. (1981). *Proposed nosology of disorders of higher cerebral function in children* (Task Force on Nosology of Disorders of Higher Cerebral Function in Children). Minneapolis, MN: Child Neurology Society.

Densem, J. F., Nuthall, G. A., Bushnell, J., & Horn, J. (1989). Effectiveness of a sensory integrative therapy program for children with perceptual-motor deficits. *Journal of Learning Disabilities, 22*(4), 221-229.

Deuel, R. K. (1992). Motor skill disorders. In S. R. Hooper, G. W. Hynd, & R. E. Mattison (Eds.), *Developmental disorders: Diagnostic criteria and clinical assessment* (pp. 239-275). Hillsdale, NJ: Lawrence Erlbaum Associates Publishers.

Fox, A. M. & Polatajko, H. J. (1994, October). *"The London Consensus" from Children and Clumsiness*. International consensus meeting, London, Ontario, Canada.

Hallahan, D. P. & Cruickshank, W. M. (1973). *Psycho-educational foundations of learning disabilities*. New Jersey: Prentice Hall.

Henderson, S. E. & Sugden, D. A. (1992). *The Movement Assessment Battery for Children*. San Antonio, TX: The Psychological Corporation.

Hoare, D. (1994). Subtypes of developmental coordination disorder. *Adapted Physical Activity Quarterly, 11*(2), 158-169.

Hooper, S. R. (1992). The classification of developmental disorders: An overview. In S. R. Hooper, G. W. Hynd, & R. E. Mattison (Eds.), *Developmental disorders: Diagnostic criteria and clinical assessment* (pp. 1-21). Hillsdale, NJ: Lawrence Erlbaum Associates Publishers.

Kavale, K. & Mattson, P. D. (1983). "One jumped off the balance beam": Meta-analysis of perceptual-motor training. *Journal of Learning Disabilities, 16*(3), 165-173.

Lundy-Ekman, L., Ivry, R., Keele, S., & Woollacott, M. (1991). Timing and force
control deficits in clumsy children. *Journal of Cognitive Neuroscience, 3*, 367-376.

Lyytinen, H. & Ahonen, T. (1988). Developmental motor problems in children: A 6-year longitudinal study. *Journal of Clinical and Experimental Psychology, 10*, 57 (abstract).

Miyahara, M. (1993). *Subtypes of learning disabled children and youths based upon gross motor functions*. Unpublished PhD thesis, University of California, LA.

Myers, P. I. & Hammill, D. D. (1976). *Methods for learning disorders*. New York: John Wiley & Sons.

Rispens, J. (1977). Funktietrainingsprogramma's: ondanks alles... toch maar doen? *Pedagogische Studien, 54*, 98-109.

Schoemaker, M. M., Hijlkema, M. G. J., & Kalverboer, A. F. (1994). Physiotherapy for clumsy children: An evaluation study. *Developmental Medicine and Child Neurology, 36*, 143-155.

Schoemaker, M. M., Schellekens, J. M. H., Kalverboer, A. F., & Kooistra, L. (1994). Pattern drawing by clumsy children: A problem of movement control? In M. L. Simner, W. Hulstijn, & P. Girouard (Eds.), *Contemporary issues in the forensic, developmental, and neurological aspects of handwriting*. (Monograph of the Association of Forensic Document Examiners, Vol. 1) (pp. 45-64). Toronto, Canada: Association of Forensic Document Examiners.

Skinner, H. A. (1986). Construct validation approach to psychiatric classification. In T. Millon & G. L. Klerman (Eds.), *Contemporary directions in psychopathology* (pp. 307-330). New York: Guilford.

Smits-Engelsman, B. C. M., Van Galen, G. P., & Portier, S. J. (1994). Psychomotor aspects of poor handwriting in children. In M. L. Simner, W. Hulstijn, & P. Girouard (Eds.), *Contemporary issues in the forensic, developmental, and neurological aspects of handwriting*. (Monograph of the Association of Forensic Document Examiners, Vol. 1) (pp. 17-44). Toronto, Canada: Association of Forensic Document Examiners.

Smits-Engelsman, B. C. M. (1995). *Theory-based diagnosis of fine motor coordination development and deficiencies using handwriting tasks*. Unpublished PhD thesis, University of Nijmegen, Nijmegen, the Netherlands.

Smits-Engelsman, B. C. M., Schoemaker, M. M., Jansen, M. P. H. T., & Niemeijer, A. S. (in press). Fysiotherapie bij schrijfproblemen: een effect evaluatie. *Nederlands Tijdschrift voor Fysiotherapie*.

BOUWIEN C. M. SMITS-ENGELSMAN, GERARD P. VAN GALEN, AND MARINA M. SCHOEMAKER

# THEORY-BASED DIAGNOSIS AND SUBCLASSIFICATION IN THE DEVELOPMENTAL COORDINATION DISORDER

## INTRODUCTION

The American Psychiatric Association's Diagnostic and Statistical Manual of Mental Disorders (DSM-IV, American Psychiatric Association [APA], 1994) provides a variety of classifications of disorders arising in childhood. One of these is the Developmental Coordination Disorder (DCD). Developmental Coordination Disorder appears in infancy, childhood or adolescence and is characterized by a predominance of disturbances in the acquisition of motor skills. Such disturbances may be part of a more general delay in development or a failure in skill acquisition. A further restriction is that these deficiencies are not due to demonstrable physical or neurological disorders, a Pervasive Developmental Disorder, Mental Retardation, or deficient educational opportunities.

In this chapter a process-oriented account of the motor problems in DCD is proposed. The purpose is to relate the motor deficiencies to a recently developed psychological model of psychomotor functioning (Van Galen, 1991). This model is used as a basis for conceptually based measuring instruments for the assessment of DCD and for a process-oriented subclassification of DCD. The purpose of the present chapter is to give an overview of our research on DCD using the conceptually founded measuring instruments and to relate categories of motor deficiencies to the psychological model that underlies the protocol.

## HETEROGENEITY IN THE CHARACTERISTICS OF DEVELOPMENTAL COORDINATION DISORDER

This section examines the heterogeneity in age-related symptoms, aetiology and research designs pertaining to DCD. Confusion in operationalizing the definition of DCD forms a major reason for dissatisfaction with the current classification. DCD lacks specificity, which is caused by the inclusion of various types of motor deficits



*J. Rispens et al. (eds.),*
*Perspectives on the Classification of Specific Developmental Disorders*, 245–264.

into one broad category. While clinical features seen the in Developmental Coordination Disorder may represent functional levels which are normal for younger children, there is no implication that children with these disorders will catch up in development. The word delay in the definition of DCD may suggest that in time full development (recovery) may occur, but, most cases tend to become chronic (Geuze & Boerger, 1993; Gillberg, Gillberg, & Groth, 1989; Gillberg & Gillberg, 1989; Hadders-Algra, Huisjes, & Touwen, 1988; Losse et al., 1991). Moreover, the fact that the condition persists does not imply that age-specific symptoms remain unchanged over time, or that the kind of problems experienced by the children in activities of daily life remain the same. Diagnoses from the group of developmental disorders often predict both behavioural and school achievement problems years later.

As to aetiology, the motor problems in DCD probably do not have a common and singular basis. It is important to realize that equality of the outcome does not implicate the singularity of the underlying psychomotor processes. The same levels of (poor) motor performance may have different aetiologies and different loci of deficit and may not be based on a homogenous uni-dimensional problem. As a consequence of the well proved flexibility of the Central Nervous System different combinations of factors may result in the same functional outcome (e.g. poor handwriting) because there are different routes by which the psychomotor system can arrive at the same end result or functional state. The reciprocal connections between involved brain areas are complex and preclude simple localisations. Furthermore, in the case of deficiencies, various adaptive processes may accompany individual motor development. The situation becomes even more complicated when it is recognized that for the same tasks different brain areas are actively involved depending on whether tasks are novel or overlearned. Therefore any causal linkage between overt motor deficiencies and underlying neurological architecture is ambiguous.

Understanding the motor coordination process is vital for the evaluation of the development and treatment of DCD children. Motor development and developmental motor disorders have been research topics for many years. However, it is not easy to compare results of studies on DCD and DCD related syndromes (MND, MBD, ADHD, Clumsy children), because of the variety of subjects and designs. Comparison of research findings is hampered by the lack of agreement in the definition of this disability (Fox & Polatajko, 1994). Consequently, it is unclear whether the same kind of children are involved in different studies (Schoemaker, Smits-Engelsman, & Kalverboer, this volume). Although DCD related problems are studied quite frequently, research is sometimes characterized by a lack of theoretical framework to guide the designs. In this chapter a theory-based assessment protocol for DCD will be described.

## PROBLEMS IN THE CLINICAL UTILITY OF THE DIAGNOSIS DCD

An adequate differential diagnosis should contribute to relevant information about prognosis, intervention planning and comorbidity. However, the diagnosis DCD as described in DSM-IV is insufficiently specific to make it optimally useful for these purposes (Deuel, 1992). A complication of the diagnosis DCD is that the group of children that meet the criteria of DCD often manifest a variety of motor problems, i.e. problems in general motor proficiency or problems in specific academic motor skills such as writing and drawing. A further complication is that DCD symptoms may appear singly or in combination, or may overlap other disorders.

Nevertheless, the broad range of clinical presentations of DCD challenges the clinician to find ways for differentiating DCD from normal age-related variations and from disturbances due to a general medical or psychiatric condition. Because many symptoms of DCD are relatively non-specific, it is essential for differential diagnoses to pinpoint significant features that characterize the disorder in more specific terms. It is the primary aim of the present article to provide a more adequate terminology, supported with our recent empirical data, in an effort to differentiate between a dystactical and a dyspractical variant in DCD. In methodological terms, our approach is a theory-based framework for assessment (Smits-Engelsman, 1995) that is based on a process-oriented account of the motor behaviour problems. The basic assumption to this approach is that motor behaviour is the concerted outcome of qualitatively different underlying processes (or processing modules) such as motor programming, size control, and muscle initiation. Clinical conditions may affect any or a combination of these subprocesses. For diagnostic purposes it is essential to know which subprocesses are involved. Details of the theory will be discussed in the following paragraph. The theoretical framework has become the basis for conceptually based measuring instruments used in the proposed protocol for psychomotor assessment. This protocol not only helps to determine the overall level of motor development, but also links the motor problems to underlying psychomotor processes. For intervention purposes the approach implies that process tailored treatment and learning strategies can be selected. The applicability - in clinical practice has been tested for the last five years by the pediatric physical therapists educated at our school (Smits-Engelsman et al., 1994). Validity aspects of the protocol have been examined in experimental studies that will be summarized further on in the chapter (Smits-Engelsman & Schoemaker, 1994, 1995; Smits-Engelsman, Van Galen, & Schoemaker, 1995).

## A THEORETICAL MODEL OF MOTOR BEHAVIOUR

The theoretical model of motor behaviour is based on scientific knowledge about motor control processes underlying goal-directed movements or skills. The model is especially useful to study skills that are acquired through practice. The process-oriented model of motor behaviour starts from the principle that skilled actions are based on intentions and cognitive representations of the action goals. The process of movement production is divided into a number of subprocesses, which are supposed to take place in separated functional modules. According to the modular nature of the model the demonstrated movement responses are the concerted result of the processing of movement representations through distinct motor modules. At higher levels of the hierarchy the stored representations are fairly abstract, whereas the representations at lower levels are assumed to be more concrete in order to be able to finally evoke the necessary muscle twitches for the required response. The model is hierarchical in the sense that more abstract, central operations precede the more peripheral, biomechanical operations. Nevertheless, all modules can be engaged simultaneously. The higher modules are merely thought to be further ahead of the current part of the movement processing than the lower modules.

The highest levels of the model are directly related to cognitive aspects of the action planning and refer to intentions, cognitive structures (i.e. linguistic structures) and attentional processes needed to monitor voluntary actions. The processing modules which are typically thought to be responsible for the processing of motor aspects of the task are:

(1) - motor programming, i.e. the retrieval of an action pattern from a long-term motor memory. For example, when asked to

write a capital letter E, subjects activate a general sequence of drawing strokes, irrespective of their size and irrespective of the musculature which will be used in their realization.
(2) - parameterization, a processing step by which the overall force level and tempo of the task performance is regulated.
(3) - muscular initiation, the process of motor unit recruitment resulting in a tension, developed by the muscle fibers, appropriate for a task in a given biomechanical context. The gradation of the tension depends on the variation in the number and types of motor units activated and on the frequency of stimulation. Thus the initiation process causes the motor units to contract and relax at different rates which results in a certain level of smoothness of the muscle pull.

### *Learning and Skill Acquisition*

When considering problems in learning and skill achievement, another important feature in DCD-children, some aspects in the model must be further clarified. The first important feature is modularity. Different processing modules are involved in different aspects of the movement production. Thus, dissimilar dysfunctions will show qualitatively different motoscopic patterns. Dysfunction of the more central programming levels of control will be characterized by poor performance in terms of coordination failures, breaking up of the movement patterns and general slowness. A dysfunction of the more peripheral muscular initiation processes will be evidenced by tuning problems and movement patterns that are structurally correct, but spatially variant.

Although the architecture of the modules is serial in the sense that the output of each stage forms the input for the next lower stage, it is not necessarily 'hard-wired'. During the execution of an overlearned movement the modules may be engaged in a different connectivity in other tasks (Van Galen, 1991). In the case of learning a movement more modules will become engaged in processing activities simultaneously. Because the processing units at the higher levels are larger than the units at the lower levels, buffering the information is necessary during a particular processing stage. If a skill becomes mastered, more parallel or concurrent processing goes on in all modules concerned, as far as the memory characteristics of individual modules permit (Schomaker & Van Galen, in press). Another feature that has been experimentally proven is that through practice the size of processing units can increase. This phenomenon is called chunking (Hulstijn & Van Galen, 1988; Portier, Van Galen, & Meulenbroek, 1990).

The model as described so far can explain characteristics of motor learning. Early in learning the learner must attend to outside cues (instructions, examples) to understand the nature of the task and how it should be performed. There is heavy involvement of conscious cognitive processing. Once a stable motor program has been established and internalized, a decrease of visual dependency occurs and proprioceptive monitoring takes over the guiding process. Subsequently, after the instructions have been learned and the task is understood well, inputs are more directly linked to the appropriate action. As a result, processing resources become available for other forms of information processing. Error rates decrease as does performance time. In this phase, the skill becomes more automatized and most of the regulation is done through feedforward. Interference from outside demands is reduced and attentional requirements are decreased. This will allow the subject to perform a skilled task concurrently with other activities. There is a broadening of the range of applicability of the task. Gradual improvements and refinements will be made by the expert performer. By this time, most steps of the motor process are integrated, enabling the system to use its resources to monitor and adapt to internal and external changes quickly and with high flexibility. This adaptability and flexibility is a suitable measure for the degree of skilfullness. Consequently, the examination protocol for children with DCD symptoms must include tasks in which the number of processes to be integrated is varied, the availability of input changes, and the (un)predictability of the environment varies.

## A PROPOSED PROTOCOL FOR DIAGNOSIS IN CHILDREN WITH DCD SYMPTOMS

In order to grasp of the full range of diagnostic problems a broad examination protocol for children with DCD symptoms is proposed, consisting of quantitative, qualitative and process-oriented measures (Table 1). In the following paragraphs, the minimal requirements of a protocol are discussed. Subsequently, an account will be given of five related studies in which these methods were applied.

The psychomotor assessment protocol must differentiate DCD from normal age related variations. Hence, in every investigation of the DCD syndrome a motometric analysis of gross and fine motor proficiency, using norm-referenced tests, must be accomplished in order to identify what the child can do compared to the norm groups of his or her age and cultural background. By using norm-referenced tests the normal developmental changes in the motor performance that occur throughout childhood are taken into account.

Further examination of individual test items may contribute to a motor (dys)function profile by which the examiner can decide which of the possible varieties of motor problems in particular is manifest in a child. Children with the same motometric scores can be characterized by very different profiles (general low levels of performance on all items versus a more specific motor disorder as manifested by very low levels of performance on one or two items e.g. for balance items only).

TABLE 1

General Psychomotor Assessment Protocol for DCD

| | |
|---|---|
| **1** | **Psychomotor assessment** |
| 1.1 | Quantitative or motometric examination |
| 1.1.1 | General motor proficiency tests |
| 1.1.2 | Fine motor proficiency tests |
| 1.2 | Qualitative or motoscopic examination |
| 1.2.1 | Fundamental motor patterns |
| 1.2.2 | Manipulative movement patterns |
| **2** | **Questionnaires and reports on associated problems** |
| 2.1 | Motor behaviour |
| 2.2 | Classroom behaviour |
| 2.3 | School achievement, learning problems |
| 2.4 | Behaviour at home |
| **3** | **Self reports on personality traits** |
| 3.1 | Fear of failure, depression |
| 3.2 | Attributions |
| **4** | **Experimental extension with process-oriented tasks** |
| 4.1 | Attention/Cognition |
| 4.2 | Planning/Strategies |
| 4.3 | Programming |
| 4.4 | Force control |
| 4.5 | Distal tuning |
| 4.6 | Dependency on feedback |

General skills, as measured by psychomotor tests, mostly have fixed standards that are considered typical for the skills. For instance, the minimal standard for running requires only that the feet move forward alternately and that a push-off from the support foot be followed by a brief period of nonsupport. This standard is fulfilled both by the first successful running attempt of a two-year-old as well as by the world champion 100 meter sprint, even though the kinesiological stage of the motor patterns is qualitatively different (initial versus mature pattern). Evaluation of the quality of movements, however, is age-dependent. Movements that are considered qualitatively normal at younger ages become retardation signs when they are still apparent at older ages. Therefore, knowledge of the prototypical development of motor patterns is a pre-requisite to differentiate between a suspected motor delay (retardation signs) and a possible neurological dysfunction (qualitative abnormal signs). Evaluating retardation signs is more difficult than abnormal signs for the clinician, because proper age-norms are still lacking for many of the motor patterns seen in locomotor and manipulative functions.

To examine motor proficiency in a more qualitative way, the examiner should report *how* the child moves. For this endeavour, kinematic features of movements can be recorded in a research setting. However, in clinical practice qualitative data can also be obtained through a structured observation and ordinal rating of fundamental and manipulative movement patterns. Studies by Wickstrom (1983) and Gallahue (1993) on e.g. running, jumping, kicking, ball catching and throwing can form a basis for these structured qualitative evaluations. Also, the impact of input availability and aspects of motor learning on the movements should be described.

In addition, neurodevelopmental items (e.g. walking on heels and tiptoe, standing on one foot, diadochokinesis) should be reported in a more qualitative way. The degree of dyskinesia, discreetness of movements in proximo-distal direction can be observed and rated. For instance, during a diadochokinesis test, which consists of quickly pronating and supinating the hand and forearm, not only the number of rotations is counted but, also the extent the elbow moves is observed, because it reflects the degree of differentiation or discreetness of hand and arm movements. The accompanying movements (mainly mirror movements) in the opposite arm are also recorded and compared to age norms if available. For instance, at the age of eight pronation and supination of the forearm is generally smooth and the amount of associated movements has decreased. The combined motometric and motoscopic examination supplies the examiner with more details about movement strategies, maturation, and noisiness of the motor system (overflow, dyskinesia, and associative movements) (Lazarus & Todor, 1987; van der Knaap et al., 1991).

Another complication for the consistent use of the DCD diagnosis is that DCD symptoms may appear *singly or in combination* and they may show overlap with other disorders. Van Leeuwen and Slot (1991) reported that 30% of the children who were referred for pediatric psychiatric assessment were found to be clumsy, i.e. these children had performance levels on a test of motor proficiency that were more than two standard deviations below the average. Because DCD symptoms might be assumed to have a multiple aetiology it is useful to relate research outcomes to data from broad inventories of school, social and family problems. To this end validated questionnaires for teachers and/or parents on motor performance, classroom behaviour, school achievement, learning difficulties, and behaviour at home can be utilized. In this same perspective, attention should be paid to data from self reports or interviews of the child to assess personality traits, such as selfesteem, fear of failure, coping strategies, depression and personal attributions.

### *Applications of the Assessment Protocol*

Generally speaking, there are three main groups of children with DCD symptoms for which this protocol can be implemented. First, there is a group under suspicion of a developmental delay without an obvious neurological disorder. The main issue in this group is differentiation between normal age-related variations (non-DCD), a neurological dysfunction (non-DCD) or a general motor delay (probably DCD). Secondly, the group of children referred because of complaints by parents and teachers about learning and behavioural difficulties. In this group, the likelihood is explored whether a motor control dysfunction might restrict the child's options to interact and adapt to his or her environment. The third group with which this assessment protocol may be used, consist of children whose ability to perform skilled movement is impaired and who have disturbances in the acquisition of motor skills (DCD). For differential diagnosis and subsequent intervention planning, it is necessary to gain insight into the movement related information processing underlying the poor motor performance, the amount of effort it takes the child to learn a motor task and the reasons why the child experiences difficulties in learning motor tasks.

## SUBCLASSIFICATION OF DCD

A growing body of evidence testifies to the heterogeneity of the DCD population or subtypes of the disorder (Ahonen, 1990; Hoare, 1994; Hoare & Larkin, 1989). Different approaches for subclassification, namely the clinical inferential and the empirical (statistical) approach, have been discussed by Schoemaker et al. in this volume. An alternative approach, which is pursued in the present article, is to relate categories of motor deficiencies to a model of psychomotor functioning using our theory-based assessment protocol. The advantage of this process-oriented account is that explanations for the diversity of behavioural and other problems related to DCD directly relate to dimensions of motor behaviour. In order to define significant features that characterize a DCD subtype, the approach is to find out which of the basic psychomotor processes underlies the disturbed (motor) behaviour. In our experimental research, an extension of the protocol with process-oriented tasks (Table 1) was used to find out which of the basic psychomotor processes are deficient in a group of DCD children. The method, called 'process loading task method', is characterized by the application of handwriting and drawing tasks that represent different components of the general psychomotor model. An advantage of using writing or drawing tasks for this purpose is that modern equipment such as computer monitored XY-tablets have opened up possibilities to investigate, in a very precise manner, the psychomotor processes which form the basis of these skills. The goal of the method is to find out which of the basic psychomotor processes are deficient in DCD children. Essential to our method is that tasks have been designed to affect one of the processing modules of the theoretical model selectively and that process-specific dysfunctions can be made detectable. Evidence may be gathered that within the DCD population subtypes exist which may be characterized by deficiencies in different psychomotor processes.

### *Towards a Process-Oriented Subclassification of DCD*

Although existing research reports point to the heterogeneity of the DCD population (see Schoemaker et al., this volume), few studies have pursued a systematic differentiation from a consistent psychomotor viewpoint. In the present article we attempt to bridge this gap by using a theory-based framework for a diagnosis in terms of the process(es) of the deficit in DCD. Writing and drawing tasks are among the most sensitive tests to reveal psychomotor disturbances. It is the complexity of the processes involved as well as the delicacy of the motor control that they require which make these kinds of tasks sensitive indicators of psychomotor deficiencies. The assumption in this research account is that kinematic features measured during handwriting can reflect psychomotor demands of the tasks. There is in fact a considerable body of knowledge, that provides evidence that the kinematics of handwriting movements reflect the underlying psychomotor processes (e.g. Van Galen, 1991; Van Galen, Smyth, Meulenbroek, & Hylkema, 1989; Van Mier, Hulstijn, & Petersen, 1991).

The information presented in the subsequent section is a summary of five studies that report on our own research on DCD and poor handwriting (Schoemaker, Schellekens, Kalverboer & Kooistra 1994; Smits-Engelsman, 1995; Smits-Engelsman, Van Galen, & Portier, 1994a, 1994b; Van Galen, Portier, Smits-Engelsman, & Schomaker, 1993). In these studies computer-assisted recording of children's performance in experimental writing tasks was used to validate the results of the general psychomotor assessment protocol. The task demands in the experimental writing tasks were chosen in such a way that they independently loaded upon the alleged components of the motor system. The results of these studies will be briefly reviewed in order to substantiate a particular hypothesis on subtypes of DCD.

### *Study 1. Poor Handwriting and DCD: Evidence for a Dystactical Variant*

In a nationwide investigation, psychomotor and other psychological characteristics were collected of a representative sample (N=746) of Dutch children between the ages of 7 and 10. At the behavioural level, the common feature of the group of children under study was that they failed to make sufficient progress in fine motor tasks at school, in particular in handwriting. These handwriting problems were typically of a motor nature and were not caused by insufficient spelling or other psycholinguistic skills. Smits-Engelsman et al. (1994a) selected from this sample (N=746) two matched groups of poor (N=24) and proficient writers (N=24), who participated in a handwriting experiment in which spatial and kinematic features of handwriting performance were measured. The group of poor writers in this study met the diagnostic criteria described in DSM-IV (APA, 1994). The group is characterized by significantly lower performance in fine motor coordination test items, given the chronological age (milestones are achieved too late) and intellectual capacity, as well as by inadequate development of specific academic motor skills like writing and drawing which interferes with activities of daily living. These symptoms are not due to a known physical disorder such as neurological or sensory deficits.

The experimental paradigm was designed to test whether the poor writers had special difficulty with any of the process-related task variables. The specific task demands were letter repetition versus alternation (variable 1: loads upon motor programming), small versus large letter size (variable 2: loads upon parameterization), required spatial accuracy (variable 3: loads upon muscular initiation) and an attentional task variable which asked the subjects to translate a number code into the letters forming a non-word which was then written (variable 4: loads upon cognitive processing). The aim of the study was to relate writing problems to one of these psychomotor processing stages. The results indicated that poor writers contrasted most clearly and selectively with the better performers in that they failed to accommodate for the spatial accuracy constraints of experimental tasks (variable 3). The poor writers evidenced no specific problems, neither in letter form retrieval (variable 1) nor in size control (variable 2). Also, there were no signs that they had more cognitive problems with the performance of the task (variable 4). The group of subjects under study was characterized by poor writing performance without overall gross motor disorder, and had problems that are localized in muscular initiation processes. Movements of the less proficient children were cruder (more spatial errors), were produced with higher movement velocities and were particularly sensitive to increased spatial accuracy demands (variable 3).

These findings suggest that the group under investigation is characterized by a predominance of problems in muscular initiation displayed by various irregularities in movement control. Therefore, the term proposed for the condition of this group is 'dystactical DCD'.

### *Study 2. Poor Handwriting and Neuromotor Noise: Further Evidence*

In a parallel study, Van Galen et al. (1993) applied a new measure to estimate the noisiness of a child's movements. This new method was developed to gain insight into the process of controlling the accuracy of movements (Van Galen & Schomaker, 1992). A basic assumption of the method is that one of the causes of spatial inaccuracy lies in the inherent variability of the motor output system. This so-called neuromotor noise is considered to be a dynamic influence on the spatial variability of movement. The method is based on the application of Power Spectral Density Analysis (PSDA) to estimate the relative contribution of noise to the total energy which is present in a recorded movement signal. PSDA of the velocity profile of comparable handwriting tasks was used to estimate the degree of neuromotor noise in movement profiles of poor and proficient writers. The technique revealed that handwriting movements of poor writers were substantially more *noisy* than those of proficient writers, with a consistent peaking of the noise energy in that region of the spectrum which is representative for neuromotor tremor. Also, poorly writing subjects were less successful in adapting the level of noise to the variable accuracy demands of the tasks. In line with the outcome of study 1 it may be concluded that in this group of children, the muscular initiation system can be characterized as being noisy and failing to make fine adaptations to the spatial demands in motor tasks.

### *Study 3. Dystactical Handwriting Problems: Longitudinal Aspects*

In a longitudinal study on the persistence of deficiencies of fine motor skills, Smits-Engelsman et al. (1994b) analyzed task proficiency in eight poor and eight proficient writers (matched for age and grade) from the group in the previous study, after an interval of one year. Significant interactions between proficiency level (poor versus good writers) and development were found for spatial features only (overshoots and undershoots). The results showed differences between the poor and the good writers in developmental pace for the effects of size variation. One year later, poor writers made relatively more overshoots in the larger letter condition and more undershoots in the small letter condition. In contrast, good writers showed a fairly consistent improvement of writing performance. The poor writers did not catch up, nor did their performance improve much in the one year period. Therefore, the alternative hypothesis that poor handwriting is caused by a maturational lag was rejected.

On the basis of these results, it is concluded that poor handwriting in this group of subjects is not caused by a developmental delay, but that the condition implies a particular, specific combination of symptoms. In performance terms, the most typical feature of poor handwriting is the failure to control spatial accuracy demands. As to the underlying theoretical explanation, two related aspects seem to be relevant. One is that poor writers are characterized by a deficient muscular initiation process. The other aspect implies that these subjects, probably because of their failing muscular initiation, are less effective in the management of the natural neuromotor noise in their movement systems. At the behavioural level, this deficit might explain the inconsistent and dystactical appearance of their writing and drawing performance.

### *Study 4. Support from the General Psychomotor Assessment Procedures*

The following study reports on the results of our general assessment protocol for assessing the motor capabilities of the children of study 1 (Smits-Engelsman, 1995). One of the questions to be answered in the study was whether a specific dysfunctioning of one or more of the component psychomotor processes, as observed in the computer-recorded handwriting movements, could be validated by the results of the general psychomotor assessment protocol. The results of the assessment protocol showed that the group of DCD children under investigation was most typically characterized by a high degree of involuntary associated movements (dyskinesia), a lower level of discreetness of movements, spatial inconsistencies, and fine motor deficits. Their movements seemed to be less articulated or less inhibited, or both. Indeed, these clinical observations seem to corroborate the hypothesis that, in terms of the psychomotor model, the deficit in the group of children with fine motor problems and poor handwriting is most probably caused by an ill-functioning muscular initiation stage. It was concluded that both the experimental task-loading method as well as the assessment protocol evoke the picture of poor spatial control of fine motor tasks. As a possible sequel, an underachievement of muscular initiation processes is the most likely explanation for the poor motor functioning in this particular group. It was proposed, therefore, that these children be classified as dystactical DCD.

### *Study 5. Graphic Performance of a Different Group of DCD Children: Evidence for a Dyspractical Variant*

In the last study to be discussed here, Schoemaker et al. (1994) used a comparable theoretical and methodological approach in an effect evaluation of physical therapy in DCD children. The children participating in the study were assigned to the experimental group on the basis of their poor *general motor proficiency*. Subjects were selected if they performed below the 5th percentile on a Psychomotor Assessment protocol (Test of Motor Impairment, Stott, Moyes, & Henderson, 1984). This score indicates a serious impairment of motor functioning. Experimental subjects were matched to controls for age and gender. The scores of DCD children were significantly poorer than their controls in visuomotor tasks, in ball catching and throwing, as well as in static and dynamic balancing tasks (hopping and jumping). The authors varied the complexity in drawing tasks and measured spatial accuracy. Whereas in the above mentioned studies (study 1-4) DCD children did not differ in RT compared to controls, the DCD children in study 5 drew more slowly and this effect became greater as figure complexity increased. In the more complex tasks, the children under study showed less fluent graphomotor trajectories with more velocity peaks per segment. Although DCD children showed a higher incidence of spatial undershoots and overshoots (twice as many), no differential speed-accuracy trade-off was found. Both DCD and control groups showed approximately the same increase in errors under accuracy and time-pressure conditions. In addition to the greater number of dysfluencies, the movement patterns of the DCD children in this study were characterized by longer pause durations. This led to movement trajectories with a large number of small intra-movement steps. Schoemaker et al. assumed that during these pauses, additional programming took place and concluded that DCD children in this study use a different movement strategy than other children. They seem to have fewer possibilities to prepare for an oncoming drawing task to the full extent and in enough detail to carry out a fluent execution. As a result, they prepare the tasks only globally during the reaction time interval and postpone further programming until the execution phase proper. It is this serial processing strategy which disrupts fluent movement execution. Results showed that figure complexity was the load which contributed most distinctly to the observed group differences. A preliminary conclusion might be that the group of DCD children in the latter study suffer from motor programming problems. Problems in programming purposeful movements, in the absence of peripheral causes, are called dyspraxia. Therefore, the term dyspractical is proposed for this variant of DCD.

## CONCLUSIONS ON SUBCLASSIFICATION

The results of our studies strongly suggest that at least two subgroups may be discriminated within the general population of children who satisfy the criteria for DCD (DSM-IV, APA, 1994). The first group, which practically coincides with the experimental groups in the first four studies, suffers from muscle initiation and distal tuning problems, and is exemplified by a higher than normal movement speed and, furthermore, by structurally correct but spatially and dynamically noisy movement patterns. These findings imply that the group under investigation is characterized by a predominance of *dystactical* problems: too rapid movements, too many errors, too little adaptation to increased accuracy demands, and too much neuromotor noise. At the same time, we concluded that a second group exists (Schoemaker et al., 1994) which is characterized by poor performance in terms of motor programming problems, coordination failures and general slowness. On empirical grounds, we therefore proposed the conceptualization of at least two subtypes of DCD. Firstly, a *dystactical* variant, which involves impairment of the metrization of movement, motor impersistence, and motor restlessness. It is hypothesized that the noisiness of movement is larger in this subtype, but the source of this noisiness is as yet unknown. Secondly, a *dyspractical* variant is proposed, which in particular involves information processing and planning problems, and which is associated with slowness and dysfluency. Although little is known about the underlying causes of the motor deficiencies in DCD children there is some evidence to suggest that construction and/or activation of the central motor program may be problematic in the dyspractic DCD subtype. On the other hand, implementation of the motor program to the environmental constraints may be most problematic in the dystactical DCD subtype.

## GENERAL CONCLUSIONS

The purpose of the present chapter was to give an overview of our research on DCD and to relate motor development and categories of motor deficiencies to a psychological model of psychomotor functioning. This framework has become the basis for conceptually founded measuring instruments used in the proposed psychomotor assessment protocol. The design of the experimental handwriting tasks was guided by basic scientific knowledge of motor control and the mechanisms which underlie goal directed behaviour. Our studies suggest that the process-oriented approach can account for some of the diversity of motor behaviour problems shown in DCD. The framework has proven its clinical utility as a basis for the choice of measurement instruments for diagnosing children with DCD symptoms. As to intervention planning, it can provide relevant information on the different kinds of performance problems and assists in the choice of intervention programs for the different types of motor performance deficits. By applying the framework we arrived at a process-oriented subclassification of DCD, which is potentially useful for purposes of research and clinical practice. From the combined results of the five studies it is concluded that theory-based diagnosis is a useful strategy to classify the underlying dysfunctions in the Developmental Coordination Disorder. Important, too, is that the findings are supported by clinical observations. A further practical implication is that if the same protocol for classification would be used by different researchers, the results of DCD studies will become more comparable and terminological ambiguities may be resolved. Furthermore, validity aspects of the proposed subclassification should be empirically tested in future intervention studies. Finally, it is our sincere hope that theory-driven diagnostic procedures will lead to the selection and successfull application of more effective intervention programms.

## REFERENCES

Ahonen, T. (1990). *Developmental coordination disorders in children: A developmental neuropsychological follow-up study*. Jyvaskyla: PhD Thesis, University of Jyvaskyla.

American Psychiatric Association. (1994). *Diagnostic and statistical manual of mental disorders* (4th ed.). Washington, DC: American Psychiatric Association.

Deuel, R. K. (1992). Motor skill disorders. In S. R. Hooper, G. W. Hynd, & R. E. Mattison (Eds.), *Developmental disorders: Diagnostic criteria and clinical assessment* (pp. 239-275). Hillsdale, NJ: Lawrence Erlbaum Associates, Publishers.

Fox, A. M. & Polatajko, H. J. (1994, October). *"The London Consensus" from Children and Clumsiness*. International consensus meeting, London, Ontario, Canada.

Gallahue, D. L. (1993). *Developmental physical education for today's children*. Dubuque, IA: Brown & Benchmark.

Geuze, R. H. & Boerger, H. (1993). Children who are clumsy: Five years later. *Adapted Physical Activity Quarterly, 10*(1), 10-21.

Gillberg, I. C. & Gillberg, C. (1989). Children with preschool minor neurodevelopmental disorders, IV: Behaviour and school achievement at age 13. *Developmental Medicine and Child Neurology, 31*, 3-13.

Gillberg, I. C., Gillberg, C., & Groth, J. (1989). Children with pre-school minor neurodevelopmental disorders, V: Neurodevelopmental profiles at age 13. *Developmental Medicine and Child Neurology, 31*, 14-25.

Hadders-Algra, M., Huisjes, H. J., & Touwen, B. C. L. (1988). Perinatal risk factors and minor neurological dysfunction: Significance for behaviour and school achievement at nine years. *Developmental Medicine and Child Neurology, 30*, 482-491.

Hoare, D. & Larkin, D. (1989). Subtypes of dyspraxia in children. [Abstract]. In S. A. Dunlop & M. D. Grounds (Eds.), *Transactions of the tenth annual neuroscience colloquium of Western Australia*. Fremantle, W.A.

Hoare, D. (1994). Subtypes of Developmental Coordination Disorder. *Adapted Physical Activity Quarterly, 11*, 158-169.

Hulstijn, W. & Van Galen, G. P. (1988). Levels of motor programming in writing familiar and unfamiliar symbols. In A. M. Colley & J. R. Beech (Eds.), *Cognition and action in skilled behaviour* (pp. 65-85). Amsterdam: North Holland.

Knaap, M. S. van der, Valk, J., Bakker, C. J., Schooneveld, M., Faber, J. A. J., Willemse, J., & Gooskens, R. H. J. M. (1991). Myelination as an expression of the functional maturity of the brain. *Developmental Medicine and Child Neurology, 33*, 849-857.

Lazarus, J. A. C. & Todor, J. I. (1987). Age differences in the magnitude of associated movement. *Developmental Medicine and Child Neurology, 29*, 726-733.

Losse, A., Henderson, S. E., Ellisman, D., Hall, D., Knight, E., & Jongemans, M. (1991). Clumsiness in children. Do they grow out of it: A ten year follow-up study. *Developmental Medicine and Child Neurology, 33*, 55-68.

Portier, S. J., Van Galen, G. P., & Meulenbroek, R. G. J. (1990). Practice and the dynamics of handwriting performance: Evidence for a shift of motor programming load. *Journal of Motor Behaviour, 22*, 474-492.

Schoemaker, M. M., Schellekens, J. M. H., Kalverboer, A. F., & Kooistra, L. (1994). Pattern drawing by clumsy children: A problem of movement control. In M. L. Simner, W. Hulstijn, & P. L. Girouard (Eds.), *Contemporary issues in forensic, developmental and neurological aspects of handwriting* (Monograph of the Association of Forensic Document Examiners, Vol. 1) (pp. 43-64). Toronto: Association of Forensic Document Examiners.

Schomaker, L. R. B. & Van Galen, G. P. (in press). Computer modeling of handwriting. In T. Dijkstra & K. Desmedt (Eds.), *Computational linguistics*. Hamel Hampstead: Harvester Wheatsheaf.

Smits-Engelsman, B. C. M. (1995). *Theory-based diagnosis of motor development and deficiencies using handwriting tasks*. Thesis, University of Nijmegen, Nijmegen, the Netherlands.

Smits-Engelsman, B. C. M. & Schoemaker, M. M. (1994, June). *Effects of physical therapy on psychomotor aspects of poor handwriting*. Proceedings of The International Conference Improving The Quality Of Physical Therapy, Den Bosch, The Netherlands.

Smits-Engelsman, B. C. M. & Schoemaker, M. M. (1995). *Theory-based evaluation of the effects of physical therapy on the underlying psychomotor processing*. Proceedings of World Confederation for Physical Therapy Congres 1995, Washington, DC.

Smits-Engelsman, B. C. M., Van Galen, G. P., & Schoemaker, M. M. (1995). *Effects of physical therapy on psychomotor features of poor handwriting*. Proceedings of the Seventh Handwriting Conference of the International Graphonomics Society, London, Ontario, Canada.

Smits-Engelsman, B. C. M., Van Galen, G. P., & Portier, S. J. (1994a). Psychomotor aspects of poor handwriting in children. In M. L. Simner, W. Hulstijn & P. L. Girouard (Eds.), *Contemporary issues in forensic, developmental and neurological aspects of handwriting* (Monograph of the Association of Forensic Document Examiners, Vol. 1) (pp. 17-44). Toronto: Association of Forensic Document Examiners.

Smits-Engelsman, B. C. M., Van Galen, G. P., & Portier, S. J. (1994b). Psychomotor development of handwriting proficiency: A cross-sectional and longitudinal study on developmental features of handwriting. In C. Faure, P. Keuss, G. Lorette, & A. Vinter (Eds.), *Advances in handwriting and drawing. A multidisciplinary approach* (pp. 187-205). Paris: Europia Press.

Smits-Engelsman, B. C. M., Van de Lint-van de Poel, A., Van der Net, J. J., Van der Grient, M., Twigt, J., & Van Groeningen, A. P. M. (1994) Onderwijsleerplan kinderfysiotherapie. *Tijdschrift Nederlandse Vereniging voor Fysiotherapie in de Kinder- en Jeugdgezondheidszorg, 10*, 4-18.

Stott, D. H., Moyes, F. A., & Henderson, S.E . (1984). *The Henderson Revision of the Test of Motor Impairment*. San Antonio, TX: Psychological Corporation.

Van Galen, G. P. (1991). Handwriting: Issues for a psychomotor theory. *Human Movement Science, 10*, 165-191.

Van Galen, G. P. & Schomaker, L. R. B. (1992). Fitts' law as a low-pass filter effect of muscle stiffness. *Human Movement Science, 11*, 11-22.

Van Galen, G. P., Portier, S. J., Smits- Engelsman, B. C. M., & Schomaker, L. R. B. (1993). Neuromotor noise and deviant movement strategies as an explanatory ground for poor handwriting in children. *Acta Psychologica, 82*, 161-178.

Van Galen, G. P., Smyth, M. M., Meulenbroek, R. G. J., & Hylkema, H. (1989). The role of short-term memory and the motor buffer in handwriting under visual and non-visual guidance. In R. Plamondon, C. Y. Suen, & M. L. Simner (Eds.), *Computer recognition and human production of handwriting* (pp. 253-272). Singapore: World Scientific.

Van Leeuwen, H. M. P. & Slot, H. M. (1991). De coordinatie-ontwikkelings-stoornis: Een nieuwe diagnostische categorie in de DSM-III-R. *Tijdschrift voor Psychiatrie, 33*, 592-606.

Van Mier, H., Hulstijn, W., & Petersen, S. E. (1991). Changes in motor planning during the acquisition of movement patterns in a continuous task. *Acta Psychologica, 82*, 291-312.

Wickstrom, R. L. (1983). *Fundamental motor patterns*. Philadelphia, PA: Lea and Febiger.

ALEX F. KALVERBOER

# ON THE RELEVANCE OF SPECIFIC CLASSIFICATIONS OF DISORDERS WITH PARTICULAR FOCUS ON DCD, DEVELOPMENTAL COORDINATION DISORDER

## INTRODUCTION

In DSM-IV (APA, 1994) factors such as growing insight in clinical conditions based on scientific studies, and the need to adapt the system to a large variety of cultures are mentioned as reasons for the ongoing process of adapting classification systems. Not explicitly mentioned but maybe also a possible motivation for change is the continuously growing need for 'specificity' of categories. There has to be a proper balance between the two requirements: generality or globality on the one hand, and specificity on the other. The optimal level of generality depends of the function(s) that category has to serve. Broadly speaking, there are two important 'functional domains', namely:

- the clinical domain: here the category serves to identify children, characterized by a particular set of 'clinical' phenomena, which may be the basis for 'clinical' decisions with respect to the individual child. Categories become either too specific or too global if they do not sufficiently match the sorts of decisions clinicians have to take with respect to guidance, treatment, measurements with respect to remedial teaching, special school placement or institutionalisation, etc.;
- the scientific domain: here the category serves as a basis for the understanding of 'the underlying nature' of that particular condition. It should allow for a scientific (= empirical) approach to possible mechanisms at various 'levels of explanation': e.g. at the level of the organism/the nervous system: its anatomy, biochemistry, neurotransmission, neurophysiology or neurological functions or at the level of psychological functions: its way of processing information and the planning and execution of its behaviour or at the level of its social relationships and structures. Ideally in this connotation, a category is a source and stimulus



*J. Rispens et al. (eds.),*
*Perspectives on the Classification of Specific Developmental Disorders*, 265–278.

for theory-building. There is a mismatch with the scientific study of diseases if the circumscription is so vague or ambiguous that it is meaningless to postulate particular mechanisms which can be empirically studied and which can be hypothesized to be core mechanisms in that particular condition.

Both functions, the clinical and the scientific, can 'fertilize' each other: improved precision in clinical descriptions and an increase in knowledge with respect to aetiology and prognosis is crucial for progress in the study of mechanisms, whereas an increase in scientifically-based knowledge on core mechanisms may be a help and even essential for the development of more adequate procedures for diagnosis and treatment.

The aim of this chapter is to discuss the category of DCD from the perspective of that tension in the classifications of clinical entities between 'specificity' on the one hand and 'globality' on the other. I propose that there is not one general solution for this classification dilemma. Instead, I suggest that categories may have different functions, each of which requires a different level of preciseness.

## MECHANISMS OF CLUMSINESS

### *Various Levels of Explanation*

Studies on DCD can focus on mechanisms at various 'levels of explanation' (Kalverboer, 1989; Rose, 1976), as there are:

a. the level of endocrinology (e.g. how do hormone deficits affect motor functioning, e.g. in congenital hypothyroidism);
b. the level of neuroanatomy/neurophysiology (e.g. which role do cerebellar or basal ganglia processes play in movement control and timing);
c. the level of sensory and motor systems in direct relation to C.N.S. development;
d. the level of psychological functions, such as:
    - sensory-motor/perceptuomotor functions (e.g. which is the role of kinaesthesis, proprioception (see Laszlo & Bairstow, 1983) or vision in movement control and timing?) and
    - visual memory and rehearsal strategies;
e. the level of adaptive behavioral patterns, like complex motor skills, play or exploratory activity;
f. the level of interactional processes (e.g. how does clumsiness affect interaction/communication in school/family conditions);
g. the level of relational systems (e.g. how are relationships with

peers affected by children's motor problems);

h. the level of social institutions, e.g. in how far should schools consider these problems?

This discussion mainly focuses on levels c. to f., with some excursions to other levels of explanation. Important questions at levels c. and d. concern whether clumsy children suffer from a central or a peripheral deficit, in other words: whether problems mainly concern the preparation or the execution of movements. Empirical studies show few differences between clumsy children and controls in the execution of simple goal-directed movements (Van Dellen & Geuze, 1990). Problems arise in more complex motor tasks (such as drawing or writing tasks). The more complex

TABLE 1

'Levels' of analysis (adapted from Rose, 1976).

| | 'Levels' | Specification |
|---|---|---|
| In context (holistic) | 1) Sociological | *social institutions:* like family, neighbourhood, school, health services, etc. |
| | 2) Psychological | a) *relational systems:* like parent-child, child-group, etc.<br>b) *interactional processes:* in family, school, etc.<br>c) *behavioral systems:* adaptive behavioral patterns, like (complex) skills, play, behaviour, exploratory activities, contact behaviour, etc.<br>d) *psychological basic functions:* like attention, long and short memory, perceptuo-motor and cognitive functions, in general: structural and energetic aspects of information processing, incl. psycho-physiology. |
| | 3) Neurological/ neurophysiological | *sensory and motor systems:* optimality of the central nervous system EEG, EMG, etc. |
| Out of context (reductionistic) | 4) Biochemical | neurotransmission |
| | 5) Anatomical | functionally organized systems in the CNS/ mechanical characteristics of the organism |

the task, the better it discriminates between clumsy children and controls. Thus, if a sequence of movements is required, the durations of pauses are longer and more variable in clumsy children than in controls (Schoemaker, 1992). Van Dellen and Geuze (1988) and Schoemaker both found a response selection deficit in clumsy children, whereas Geuze and Van Dellen (1990) also report response preparation problems in an anticipation task. Generally no specific movement **execution** problems related to task demands are reported in clumsy children, although movement execution is generally slower (possible due to a lower quality of the preparation process?). Also the organization of eye-hand coordination (e.g in perceptuo-motor tasks, such as putting blocks in holes) may be less optimal in clumsy children as compared to controls (Kalverboer & Brouwer, 1983, von Hofsten & Rösblad, 1988). Rösblad and von Hofsten (1994) studied the role of visual information in repetitive goal-directed arm movements in DCD children (task: picking up beads, one at the time, from one cup and carrying them to another). Children with motor impairments, as a group, seemed to be more dependent on visual information about the target for end-point accuracy than children without motor impairment. For the transportation phase of the movement, visual feedback of the hand was not important for either group of children. They found that DCD children move more slowly from cup to cup than controls; this confirms findings in earlier studies of an impaired capacity for anticipatory control. Until now there is only one study on the role of ophthalmic factors in DCD: Mon-Williams, Pascal, and Wann (1994) do not find any significant difference in visual status between (N=29) DCD-children and a random (N=29) control group. The authors conclude that no simple ophthalmic difficulty can explain such children's movement control problems. Finally, Dwyer and McKenzie (1994) report an impairment of visual memory in clumsy children in a task in which children had to reproduce geometric patterns. No difference in accuracy of reproductions was found on immediate recall. After a 15 day delay however, clumsy children's reproductions were markedly less accurate, whereas those of the control children were unchanged. Reason for the authors to suggest a visual rehearsal strategy deficit.

## *Timing, Variability and Inconsistency*

During the last decade there is a growing interest in the timing and variability of movements in various conditions. Problems of timing may impair the adaptive quality of movements and have adverse effects on automatization processes. Inconsistency or lack of persistence of movements has been frequently reported in children with mild neurological impairment (Birch, 1964; Touwen, 1979). It may directly interfere with the smooth execution of movements, as is required in e.g. handwriting or fine motor skills. A distinction should be made between unadaptive and adaptive variability. The ability to flexibly adapt movements to changing environmental demands is characteristic for an optimally functioning nervous system. E.g. the inability to smoothly go from one rhythm to another may indicate mild neurological impairment. In timing experiments (tapping tasks) Geuze and Kalverboer (1987) found more 'unadaptive' variability in clumsy children than in controls (clumsy children not being able to consistently maintain equal time intervals between taps and showing more problems in changing from one rhythm to another). Geuze and Kalverboer (1994) compared clumsy and dyslectic children and a control group (age range 7-12 years) in a tapping task in which children had to maintain an imposed rhythm in three conditions:

- A unimanual condition, in which only one hand was involved, with one tap to every beep;
- An alternating bimanual condition, in which one finger responded to the first beep, the other finger to the next beep, and so on;
- A 2:1 or 1:2 asymmetrical condition, in which one finger, the left or the right, responded to every beep while the other finger responded to every second beep.

Subjects performed the unimanual tasks with the left and the right hand at two speed levels: a fast condition with a 560-ms interval length and a slow condition with a 1,120-ms interval length. This set up enabled direct comparison with the bimanual coordination conditions in which the fingers also produced intervals of 560 ms or 1,120 ms. The performance measure taken was the variability of tapping after the pacing signal had ceased. Comparing the three groups, the clumsy children showed a slightly increased variability across all tasks but no sign of lateralized performance differences. In contrast, dyslexics showed increased variability only in one task, involving the right hand. Timing variability in dyslexia did not seem to be simply a problem of hemispheric laterality (only in one task a right hand superiority was found) or interhemisphere communication (the latter explanation was suggested in Wolff, Michel, Ovrut, & Drake study, 1990). Ivry and Keele (1989) used a model proposed by Wing and Kristofferson (1973) to separate the total variability into a central component (thought to be of cerebellar origin) and a motor delay component. Pursuing this idea Lundy-Ekman, Ivry, Keele, and Woollacott (1991) and Williams, Woollacott, and Ivry (1992) found in a cerebellar-clumsy group and not in a basal ganglia-clumsy group a central timing deficit (inconsistency in timing) whereas the latter group was more variable in controlling the amplitude of isometric force pulses, thought to be indicative for motor delay variability. However, application of the Wing and Kristofferson's model presented these researchers and also researchers in our laboratory with the problem that many of the analyzed interval sequences (ca. 30%) yielded negative variances. This weakens the strong relation between cerebellar function and timing suggested in the above studies.

In the meantime we have applied another way of analyzing data in relation to central versus peripheral deficits in children, treated early for Congenital Hypothyroidism (Kooistra, Snijders, Schellekens, Kalverboer, & Geuze, in press), which avoids this problem of negative variance. In this study of children treated early for CH, the estimate of the motor delay variance was six times higher than in controls (suggesting basal ganglia involvement), whereas the estimate of the clock variance did not significantly differ between CH and controls (not supporting a cerebellar timing deficit hypo-thesis). Peripheral mechanisms seem to play a major role in CH motor problems, although cerebellar mechanisms may also contribute to these children's problems. It should be noted that in all experimental studies on timing and variability a large part of the clumsy group does **not** differ at all from controls on the dependent variables (Geuze & Kalverboer, 1994). This is true for most comparisons between clinical groups, such as ADHD and clumsiness, and controls on a variety of variables at different 'levels of explanation'. It indicates how careful one has to be with predictions about individual children on the basis of comparisons of groups.

In an ongoing longitudinal study in our laboratories by Visser, Geuze, and Kalverboer (submitted), the focus is on the complicating effects of physical growth on motor development in clumsy children and controls. Such effects may depend of the quality of the 'propriocepsis', which must provide the organism with the information necessary to modify the internal representation of body characteristics. First results will be reported in due course. Dependent variables will concern the spatial and temporal accuracy of movements in various conditions, in which possibilities for proprioceptive and visual control are manipulated. In the context of this growth effect study a first comparison was made between clumsy and control children (N=25 and 23, 11-14 years old) (Visser et al., submitted). DCD children in our sample seemed to have extreme problems in the consistent application of force, especially when high rates of force were required (possibly due to 'slow recruitment of muscle fibres'), but not with timing per sé, as was indicated by the duration of muscle contractions. This finding suggests primarily basal ganglia involvement.

In summary, experimental studies on movement control mechanisms may enhance our insight in clumsy children's problems. They can improve our possibilities for therapy evaluation.

## *Some Remarks on Therapy and Therapy Evaluation*

As clumsiness may negatively affect the child's intellectual and socio-emotional development and is evidently more than a temporary problem (Losse et al., 1991, Geuze & Börger, 1993), in many instances treatment is indicated. There is a wealth of procedures for guidance and treatment of children with developmental problems, including DCD, but a scarcity of systematic studies for the effect- evaluation of such programs (see for a critical review Schoemaker, 1992). Consequently, it is still largely unclear how far treatment is effective and what the most important determinants of effectiveness are. Evaluative studies are methodologically complicated, and they may present us with many practical and ethical problems (Schoemaker & Kalverboer, 1990). However, they are badly needed in order for us to know how waste of energy and money can be avoided and optimal profit can be obtained.

Some basic requirements for such studies can be formulated:

a) There should be some insight, explicitly formulated, in the relationship between:
   - the characteristics of the group (= the profile of problems in motor development and their concomittants);
   - characteristics of the process of treatment/guidance and;
   - aspects to be measured in the effect-evaluation.

   Ideally, such studies are designed on the basis of some theory or a body of well established (clinical) knowledge.

b) The effects on the concomittants (e.g. socio-emotional problems) of clumsiness should be considered.

Two therapy evaluating studies, which were executed in our laboratory, are relevant here:

- a study by Kooistra et al. (1994) on the effects of early hormone substitution therapy on motor and cognitive development in children with CH (Congenital Hypothyroidism) and
- a study by Schoemaker, Schellekens & Kalverboer (1994) on the effect of physiotherapy on handwriting in clumsy children.

Our follow up study of early treated CH aimed at the effect evaluation of early hormone substitution treatment in Congenital Hypothyroidism. Untreated, such children may, besides mental retardation, also develop severe motor impairment with phenomena such as hypotonia, disorders in the lateralisation of functions and motor coordination problems, frequently with signs of clumsiness. Early treatment prevents such severe abnormalities. However, a substantial number of early treated CH-patients still have problems in motor development.

Our study, using instruments such as the TOMI and the Beery test, showed that children with low neonatal thyroxine concentrations (< 50 nmol/L), particularly those with thyroid agenesis, had substantial motor problems and borderline intelligence scores as late as 9½ years of age. Specific aspects of their motor functioning, especially balance, seemed to deteriorate, notwithstanding continuation of (well-controlled) treatment. A further refined analysis of possible deficits in timing experiments suggested that peripheral mechanisms play a major role in CH motor problems (see later). The combination of standardized and well-validated tests for motor development/impairment with experimental procedures, aimed at underlying 'mechanisms' (like disorders in planning or execution of movements or problems in force control or duration of muscle contractions) is a most valuable approach to the evaluation of treatment effects. It provides us with a differentiated clinical profile of motor dysfunctions and gives insight into underlying mechanisms. Results can be fed back to the paediatricians and endocrinologists responsible for early treatment, who can modify treatment procedures on the basis of such results (this is what happened in the Netherlands).

A study by Schoemaker et al. (1994) on the effects of short-term physiotherapy on the handwriting proficiency of clumsy children demonstrated that kinematic analysis of the organisation of strokes in drawings, made by children on a XY digitizer, was more sensitive to treatment effects than outcome-oriented measures of motor functioning alone. It gives fine-grained information on the components of movement organisation in which deficits may occur. Didactical procedures can focus on such deficiencies. Therefore, I strongly agree with the statement in Schoemaker et al. (1994, p. 147) 'theory driven evaluations are now called for to investigate the mediating factors underlying treatment effectiveness'. Such an approach requires not only sets of well validated instruments for clinical assessment and experimental analyses, but also a clear description of the treatment process. Aspects that may mediate particular effects should be systematically related to outcome measures. Only in this way can a rationale for therapeutic interventions be obtained.

### *Concomittants of Clumsiness in the Social/Emotional Domain*

Studies on clumsy children's social/communicative behaviour in school and family situations (based on teachers' and parents' descriptions) have shown that clumsy children tend to have marginal positions in their peer groups, often being described by their teachers as 'isolated' and 'submissive' (Kalverboer, de Vries, & Van Dellen, 1990). Some of these children lack self-confidence, possibly as a reaction to difficulties they have with the execution of socially important skills. They are also described as often teased. However, 'likes to tease' was also more frequently applied to the clumsy children. Mechanisms behind these problems may be varied and frequently coincide. Candidates are:
- insecurity as a direct effect of lack of movement control and failure to learn important skills (Cermak, 1985);
- a poor body scheme, resulting in a poorly defined concept of self (Ayres, 1980). A similar explanation postulates an excessive fear reaction on the basis of vestibular processing deficits;
- avoidance reactions, or ostracizing reactions from peers/ classmates;
- as a reaction the clumsy child may further isolate him/herself or show overt or hidden aggressive reactions (Keogh, Sugden, Reynard, & Calkins, 1979);

Evidently, the interplay of underlying factors may be different in each child. Still our 1990-statement holds (Kalverboer et al., 1990, p. 267): 'As long as longitudinal studies by researchers who take a transactional position is lacking, the formulation of general rules is mere speculation. It is largely unknown whether and how social concomitants of clumsiness may change in the course of development and what the underlying mechanisms are. Such longitudinal research is needed to provide us with a better body of knowledge for optimizing psycho-social guidance in these children. In any case, insecurity and lack of self-confidence may affect children's task performance in real life situations as well as in experimental conditions. Consequently, in clinical research, the selection of experimental and control groups only on the basis of specific target phenomena may lead to misinterpretations of results. Social concomitants should be part of the research diagnostic criteria, applied in the selection and description of groups to study'. At present we are involved in studies on bullying and being bullied in clumsy and hyperactive children. First results indicate that clumsiness substantially contributes to the risk of being the victim of bullying by peers/classmates. Hyperactives are frequently victims as well as bullyers.

Intriguing are 'language problems', frequently reported in clumsy children by parents as well as teachers (see also reports on articulary apraxia as a feature of clumsiness, Walton, Ellis and Court, 1962). Direct observations of such children's communicative behaviour may help to further clarify these relationships.

## CONCLUDING REMARKS AND FUTURE LINES OF RESEARCH

Clumsiness or Developmental Coordination Disorder is a serious clinical condition which requires the attention of (neuro-) paediatricians, child-psychiatrists and -psychologists, neurologists, but not the least of family doctors, parents and teachers. In the last two decades, scientific knowledge has greatly increased. This is true with respect to basic-fundamental processes in movement development as well as with respect to the clinical features of clumsiness, its concomittants, the child's future perspectives and the procedures for diagnosis, guidance and treatment. Important further requirements are:

- research focused on the links between the clinical, behavioral and functional phenomena of DCD and the underlying neurology;
- the application in clinical practice of the scientific knowledge about underlying mechanisms which is available to obtain a better rationale for diagnostics and treatment;
- improvement of our instruments for diagnosis and therapy-evaluation.

Longitudinal, individual-oriented experimental and clinical studies will be particularly important in increasing our insight in DCD.

Evidently, it is a great advantage that DCD is now recognized as a clinical entity in the DSM-system (how internally inconsistent this system still may be). However, this is no more than a start. First it should be stated that the DSM-system is largely a-theorctical and does not give any guideline for future programs for research and practice. Such guidelines have to be formulated by the people in the field and the laboratories and supported by the politicians. However, the question has to be posed whether the category DCD meets minimal requirements of an adequate balance between specificity and globality? It may be questioned whether requirements with respect to 'homogeneousness' on the one hand and to an adequate description of a clinical condition on the other, are intrinsically compatible. In fact, clinical conditions concern individuals, characterised by a set of complex characteristics, none of which can be described in terms of just one dimension. Adopting a 'categorization-approach' instead of a dimensional approach, which DSM does, implies that primarily the 'central tendency' not the 'individual variability' is covered. Therefore, it is unavoidable that different individuals, covered by the same term, may widely differ which respect to phenomenology, aetiology and pathogenesis. Maybe, it is preferable to reformulate the specificity/globality question as follows: are the 'central tendencies' as subordinated under the umbrella term DCD, sufficiently valid, in view of their clinical and scientific applicability? Our conclusion is that, for both functions, the DCD category has serious flows.

Although DSM has explicitly chosen a **categorical** system (which type of classification inevitably suffers from 'internal inconsistencies within categories') instead of a more precise, dimensional system, there is, clinically and scientifically, an increasing tendency to 'purify' clinical entities, such as Clumsiness, now DCD. For good reasons: we will never make much progress in our understanding of the mechanisms, playing a role at various levels of explanation in a particular clinical condition, if that condition itself is too broadly and vaguely described. To give an example, it makes little sense to detect that a wastebasket of the most diverse children, all labelled MBD, or ADHD or Clumsy, is characterised by say: problems in a particular stage of information processing or in the regulation of the behavioral state or in a particular neurotransmission system if one cannot answer the question: which particular children in this wastebasket manifest these problems and to which aspect(s) of these complex clinical entities, MBD, ADHD, Clumsiness, do these findings relate? The more concise the clinical circumscription of phenomena, the more empirical research can be clinically relevant (see Kalverboer, 1978). Another point in case is the study of early risk factors, playing a role in the aetiology of particular clinical problems, such as dyslexia or ADHD. Here again, it is almost meaningless to search for such risk factors if the clinical entities, thought to be related to those factors are too 'internally inconsistent', which is the case for dyslexia, ADHD and a large variety of other clinical disorders (Kalverboer, 1988).

Finally, procedures for guidance and treatment can only be developed and properly evaluated, if meaningful relationships can be postulated between facets of such procedures on the one hand and well described core phenomena in the children which are guided or treated on the other. Effects of therapy can only be adequately evaluated if the clinical condition at the start of this 'manipulation' has been clearly described in operational terms, so that changes in dependent measures can be specifically related to particular facets of the clinical condition and the therapeutic procedure.

In conclusion: one category, like DCD, can not meet all the requirements, clinical and scientific, which are worthwhile to be formulated. Specific refinements or specifications have to be defined in view of the particular aim of the user. E.g. to study therapy effects relatively broad categories may suffice, given that specific aspects of the behavioral patterns (target behaviours) can be related to particular aspects of the therapy: a profile approach, as applied by Hoare (1994), may be the most proper way to proceed. However, to study basic mechanisms, e.g. with respect to information processing deficits or involvement of particular neurotransmissions systems, such broad clinical categories do not suffice. Then specific subgroups have to be identified based on available theory which allow for specifying hypotheses concerning mechanisms. How, after all, such mechanisms may contribute to the broadly defined clinical condition, has to be carefully assessed in relation to the individual profile of deficits.

## REFERENCES

American Psychiatric Association. (1994). *Diagnostic and statistical manual of mental disorders* (4th ed.). Washington, DC: American Psychiatric Association.

Ayres, A. J. (1980). *Sensory integration and the child*. Los Angeles: Western Psychological Services.

Birch, H. G. (1964). *Brain damage in children*. Baltimore: Williams & Wilkins.

Cermak, S. (1985). Developmental dyspraxia. In E. A. Roy (Ed.), *Neuropsychological studies of apraxia and related disorders*. Amsterdam: Elsevier, North-Holland.

Dwyer, C. & McKenzie, B. E. (1994). Impairment of visual memory in children who are clumsy. *Adapted Physical Activity Quarterly, 11*(2), 179-189.

Geuze, R. H. & Börger, H. (1993). Children who are clumsy: Five years later. *Adapted Physical Activity Quarterly, 10*, 10-21.

Geuze, R. H. & Dellen, T. Van (1990). Auditory precue processing during a movement sequence in clumsy children. *Journal of Human Movement Studies, 19*, 11-24.

Geuze, R. H. & Kalverboer, A. F. (1987). Inconsistency and adaptation in timing of clumsy children. *Journal of Human Movement Studies, 13*(8), 421-432.

Geuze, R. H. & Kalverboer, A. F. (1994). Tapping a rhythm: A problem of timing for children who are clumsy and dyslexic? *Adapted Physical Activity Quarterly, 11*, 203-213.

Hoare, D. (1994). Subtypes of Developmental Coordination Disorder. *Adapted Physical Activity Quarterly, 11*(2), 158-169.

Hofsten, C. von & Rösblad, B. (1988). The integration of sensory information in the development of precise manual pointing. *Neuropsychologia, 26*, 805-821.

Ivry, R. B. & Keele, S. W. (1989). Timing functions of the cerebellum. *Journal of Cognitive Neuroscience, 1*, 136-152.

Kalverboer, A. F. (1978). M.B.D.: Discussion of the concept. In A. F. Kalverboer, J. Mendlewicz, & H. M. van Praag (Eds), *Advances in Biological Psychiatry, Vol. 01 : M.B.D.: Facts and fiction*. Basel: Karger.

Kalverboer, A. F. (1988). Follow-up of biological high-risk groups. In M. Rutter (Ed.), *Studies of psychosocial risk: The power of longitudinal data* (pp. 114-137). Cambridge: Cambridge University Press.

Kalverboer, A. F. (1989). Merits and limitations of the information processing approach for the study of attentional deficit disorder. In L. M. Bloomingdale & J. M. Swanson (Eds.), *Attention deficit disorder, Vol. 4: Current concepts and emerging trends in attentional and behavioral disorders of childhood* (pp. 273-282). Oxford: Pergamon Press.

Kalverboer, A. F. & Brouwer, W. H. (1983). Visuo-motor behaviour in preschool children in relation to sex and neurological status: An experimental study on the effect of 'time-pressure'. *Journal of Child Psychology and Psychiatry, 24*(1), 65-88.

Kalverboer, A. F., Vries, H. de & Dellen, T. Van (1990). Social behaviour in clumsy children as rated by parents and teachers. In A. F. Kalverboer (Ed.), *Developmental biopsychology: Experimental and observational studies in children at risk* (pp. 257-269). Ann Arbor: University of Michigan Press.

Keogh, J. F., Sugden, D. A., Reynard, C. L., & Calkins, J. A. (1979). Identification of clumsy children: Comparisons and comments. *Journal of Human Movement Studies, 5*, 32-41.

Kooistra, L., Snijders, T. A. B., Schellekens, J. M. H., Kalverboer, A. F., & Geuze, R. H. (in press). Timing variability in children with early treated Congenital Hypothyroidism. *Acta Psychologica*.

Kooistra, L., Laane, C., Vulsma, T., Schellekens, J. M. H., Meere, J. J. van der, & Kalverboer, A. F. (1994). Motor and cognitive development in children with congenital hypothyroidism: A long-term evaluation of the effects of neonatal treatment. *The Journal of Paediatrics*, June 94, 903-909.

Laszlo, J. I. & Bairstow, P. J. (1983). Kinaesthesis: Its measurement, training and relationship to motor control. *Quarterly Journal of Experimental Psychology, 35*a, 411-421.

Losse, A., Henderson, S. E., Elliman, D., Hall, D., Knight, E., & Jongmans, M. (1991). Clumsiness in children - Do they grow out of it? A 10-year follow-up study. *Developmental Medicine and Child Neurology, 33*, 55-68.

Lundy-Ekman, L., Ivry, R., Keele, S., & Woollacott, M. (1991). Timing and force control deficits in clumsy children. *Journal of Cognitive Neuroscience, 3*, 367-376.

Mon-Williams, M. A., Pascal, E., & Wann, J. P. (1994). Ophthalmic factors in Developmental Coordination Disorder. *Adapted Physical Activity Quarterly, 11*(2), 170-178. (Special Issue: Developmental Coordination Disorder).

Rösblad, B. & Hofsten, C. von (1994). Repetitive goal-directed arm movements in children with Developmental Coordination Disorders: Role of visual information. *Adapted Physical Activity Quarterly, 11*(2), 190-202 (Special Issue: Developmental Coordination Disorder).

Rose, S. (1976). *The conscious brain*. London: Penguin.

Schoemaker, M. M. (1992). *Physiotherapy for clumsy children: An effect evaluation study*. Thesis, State University of Groningen, Groningen, the Netherlands: Stichting Kinderstudies.

Schoemaker, M. M. & Kalverboer, A. F. (1990). Treatment of clumsy children. In A. F. Kalverboer (Ed.), *Developmental biopsychology: Experimental and observational studies in children at risk* (pp. 241-255). Ann Arbor: University of Michigan Press.

Schoemaker, M. M., Schellekens, J. M. H., & Kalverboer, A. F. (1994). Effects of short-term physiotherapy on the handwriting proficiency of clumsy children. In C. Faurzé, P. Keuss, G. Lorette, & A. Vinter (Eds), *Advances in handwriting and drawing: A multidisciplinary approach* (pp. 463-476). Paris: Europia Press.

Touwen, B. C. L. (1979). *Examination of the child with minor neurological dysfunction*. London: Spastics International Medical Publications.

Van Dellen, T. & Geuze, R. H. (1988). Motor response processing in clumsy children. *Journal of Child Psychology and Psychiatry, 29*, 489-500.

Van Dellen, T. & Geuze, R. H. (1990). Experimental studies on motor control in clumsy children. In A. F. Kalverboer (Ed.), *Developmental biopsychology: Experimental and observational studies in children at risk* (pp. 187-206). Ann Arbor: University of Michigan Press.

Visser, J., Geuze, R. H., & Kalverboer, A. F. (submitted). Variability in force, timing and impulse in isometric responses: Effects of age and motor competence.

Walton, J. N., Ellis, E., Court, S. D. M. (1962). Clumsy children: Developmental apraxia and agnosia. *Brain, 85*, 603-612.

Williams, H. G., Woollacott, M. H., & Ivry, R. (1992). Timing and motor control in clumsy children. *Journal of Motor Behaviour, 24*(2), 165-172.

Wing, A. M. & Kristofferson, A. B. (1973). The timing of interresponse intervals. *Perception & Psychophysics, 13*, 455-460.

Wolff, P. H., Michel, G. F., Ovrut, M., & Drake, C. (1990). Rate and timing precision of motor coordination in developmental dyslexia. *Developmental Psychology, 26*, 349-359.

TOM A. VAN YPEREN, WILLIAM YULE AND JAN RISPENS

# THE FUTURE OF THE CONCEPT OF SPECIFIC DEVELOPMENTAL DISORDERS:

# SUMMARY AND CONCLUSIONS

## INTRODUCTION

The purpose of this book was to critically review the concept of specific developmental disorders (SDD). Although disorders such as dyslexia, dysphasia and clumsiness are wellknown in clinical practice, the corresponding categories in classification systems such as ICD and DSM are far from unproblematic. The chapters in this book provide ample evidence of the shortcomings, that may be characterized as the result of a struggle between theory, empirical data, clinical evidence, and taxonomical considerations.

One of the questions we tried to answer in this volume is whether progress has been made during the last decades. Has research and clinical experience led to a better understanding of the nature of these disorders, and are we moving toward improved descriptions and diagnostic criteria? In this final chapter we briefly summarize the contributions of the various authors of this volume to this discussion. In a concluding section, we offer suggestions for future research and for the further development of the classification schemes.

## A SUMMARY OF FINDINGS

### *The ICD and DSM Categories of SDD Do Not Reflect Consensus*

In their review of the development of DSM and ICD, Rispens and Van Yperen concluded that the categories of SDD in recent versions of ICD and DSM are still controversial. Most of the other chapters in this book support this conclusion. It is evident that there are serious problems regarding the operationalization and the validity of the concept of SDD. Data on the reliability of the categories are scarce and incomplete. Hardly any of the validity studies have been conducted in the context of the official schemes, and most studies used concepts and definitions that differ from t hose in the official



*J. Rispens et al. (eds.),*
*Perspectives on the Classification of Specific Developmental Disorders*, 279–286.

classifications schemes. Hence, our insight in the psychometric qualities of the categories is limited.

These problems have been described in the literature many times, mostly with regard to the category of reading disorders. As a consequence, the concept of dyslexia is subject to much debate and does not reflect a broad consensus between researchers and practicioners. In the various versions of DSM and ICD these critical remarks have been neglected. On the contrary, in these schemes the original concept of SDD was elaborated and refined. Although the most recent version of DSM seems to have abandoned the concept of SDD, the description of the categories still has a clear resemblance with the earlier versions.

However, there is consensus about the heterogeneity of developmental delays in scholastic skills, language, speech, and motor coordination. Hence, it is clear that a distinction between different types of disorders is needed. Yule and Maugham note that there is agreement about the relevance of distinctions that take into account the type of skill involved, and about the distinction between difficulties in acquiring a skill and the loss of the skill. Much less consensus exists with respect to the relevance of the distinction between delays in the domain of particular skills versus a general retardation. Therefore, it makes sense that different types of impairments in scholastic skills, language, speech, and motor coordination are distinguished in DSM and ICD. However, in classification schemes some of these categories should be presented as controversial and subject to further evaluation.

### *The Concept of SDD Cannot Serve as an Umbrella*

The concept of SDD originated from clinical practice and the research on reading disorders. In the successive revisions of ICD and DSM, this concept was extended from specific reading disorders to disorders in writing, math, language, speech and motor coordination. This suggests the existence of a higher order concept of specific developmental disorders. In DSM-III(-R) the developmental disorder is used as a valid description for a number of disorders in different developmental domains. However, empirical evidence for this extension is lacking. Yule and Maugham point to the fact that little is known of the prevalence, antecedents, course, correlates or outcome of specific spelling disorders and disorders in the field of arithmetic. Bishop and Amorosa demonstrate in their chapters that there are no qualitative differences between children with the dianosis specific developmental language disorder and children that have different diagnoses. Henderson and Barnett argue that the notion of a discrepancy has received little attention in the domain of movement disorders. In their view, there is not enough empirical evidence supporting the idea that the specific developmental disorder in motor functioning is a single disorder.

In view of these findings, there is no reason to consider the overall concept of SDD as a valid higher order category. Therefore, we suggest that the approach in DSM-IV, of abandoning the overall concept of SDD should be adopted by ICD. Moreover, both DSM and ICD should critically consider the diagnostic criteria for the specific disorders in mathematics, writing, language, speech, and motor functioning. The substantial similarity of these criteria, and especially the systematic use of the concept of a discrepancy suggests a conceptual unity that cannot be justified. Instead, the diagnostic criteria for the categories of disorders in mathematics, writing, language, speech, and motor functioning should be based on concepts and definitions that are currently used in both research and clinical practice with regard to each of these developmental domains.

It is important to note that abandoning the overall concept of SDD does not mean that the different disorders are not linked. Stanovich and Siegel suggested that reading disorder is to be considered as a specific type of language disorder. Such suggestions of possible theoretical links may help to unravel the underlying causes of different disorders. However, as long as these links are not supported empirically, or do not reflect a broad consensus, no one would suggest that in the next version of a classification system the category of reading impairment should be part of the main category of language disorders. The same holds true for the idea of placing a language disorder under the SDD-umbrella. As long as the notion of the existence of this umbrella lacks general support, there are no reasons to use the concept of SDD as a main category.

### *The Distracting Focus on the Discrepancy Model*

Many discussions were devoted to the question whether the discrepancy model offers an adequate criterion for diagnosing SDD. Stanovich and Siegel noted that the discrepancy debate is, in fact, a distracting issue. They found that IQ discrepancy does not correlate strongly with the primary phenotypic indicators of reading disability. Their conclusion was that research should go beyond the discrepancy model. They argue research on neurological and genetic correlates of reading disability should not be limited to the reading-IQ discrepancy. This idea is supported indirectly by the findings of Remschmidt, Schulte-Körne and Hennighausen. In their chapter they showed that genetic studies also support the assumption of heterogeneity within the group of dyslexics. Underachievers constitute a very heterogeneous group, varying from very bright underachieving children with limited progress in reading, to dull children who have additional profound handicaps in particular developmental areas. It is highly important that in the discussion about the relevance of the concept of discrepancy a distinction is made between subgroups. Rather than focusing on the pros and cons of the idea of a discrepancy, it would be more fruitful to explore the relevance of various alternative distinctions.

This does not mean that a distinction between groups of children with developmental delays based on IQ is irrelevant. Subgroups based on differences in IQ reflect genuine differences in capacities. In studying particular skills and cognitive processes, there are good reasons for separating children with mental retardation (Wechsler IQ $< 70$), from average children ($70 \leq$ IQ 130) and gifted children (IQ $\geq 130$). Within the group of average IQ, we may continue to experiment with different criteria for defining the reading disorder, including the discrepancy model. The discrepancy model should be used as only one of the ways to explore the characteristics of backward readers with normal IQ. Applying different types of criteria may ultimately shed light on the relevance of the notion of a discrepancy.

### *Confusion about the Purposes of Classification Categories*

The various chapters of our book allow at least one solid conclusion, namely that, given the current state of knowledge, the categories of SDD do not suffice for treatment selection. The categories may offer concepts that fit the clinical idea that specific developmental disorders is actually a class of disorders.The categories may also serve research purposes. However, these categories are not sufficiently adequate to determine which children require special services.

This is an important point that needs to be stressed over and over again. Most categories in the ICD and DSM sections for mental disorders are meant to describe problems, not treatments. In some cases, the type of treatment that is appropriate follows from the type of problem. But in most cases this relation is less clear. In the case of SDD, this relation is problematic, due to the heterogeneity of the disorders in the category and the lack of qualitative differences between children with SDD and children with disorders that are classified in other categories.

Also, as Yule and Maugham state, even though ICD and DSM have adopted the discrepancy model as a legitimate model for the purpose of research, this does not mean that the categories are a legitimate basis for admitting or denying specific services to certain children. In their opinion it would be scandalous if authorities use the ICD and DSM classifications to regulate access to additional resources for children. Yule and Maugham's comment shows that it is of vital importance to be aware of the proper purposes of the categories in ICD and DSM, before using them in practice.

### *The Need for Unity in Definitions*

Several chapters stressed the need for more unity in the concepts, definitions, and operationalizations used in classification research and practice. The reader will have noticed as a striking example that various authors in this book used different terms and abbreviations for the same topics. At the same time they agreed that there is a chaos in the terminology and that contradictory research outcomes may stem from this confusion. This situation illustrates that the study of the categories of SDD in ICD and DSM has been caught in a paradox. In order to investigate the validity of particular concepts on a broad scale, standard definitions as in international systems like ICD and DSM are needed. Only with the use of standard definitions systematic accumulation of comparable data is to be expected. This does not mean that these definitions should not be studied critically. Van Yperen noted that, since we have no standard for testing the accuracy of classification criteria, the quest for the core characteristics of SDD requires experimentation with formulae, tests, and cut-offs. Alternative definitions may lead to valuable results, but only if researchers are explicit about how these definitions deviate from international standards. The current chaotic situation in research on scholastic skills, language, speech, and motor coordination, does not lead to an effective accumulation of data for two reasons. First, the alternative definitions vary too much. A second reason may be that ICD and DSM do not provide international standards to define SDD in scholastic skills, *and* language, *and* speech, *and* motor functioning that are acceptable to most researchers in these areas. Therefore, we conclude that it is essential that ICD and DSM reflect the state of the art in each of these areas more accurately.

### *The Need for Theory*

Several authors have called for theory driven research on SDD that tests different hypotheses about the essential characteristics of the disorder. This call can only be answered if it is clear whether ICD and DSM offer categories based on aetiological or on phenomenological distinctions. This important point should receive attention in the further development of ICD and DSM. Yule and Maugham note that an aetiologically based system will be the eventual aim, but that until processes are better understood, we have to make do with a system based on phenomenological distinctions. Most authors argue that we need to go beyond this type of defining developmental disorders. Stanovich and Siegel demonstrated that the concept of dyslexia is based on the idea of an aetiologically distinct type of reading disability associated with moderate to high IQ. Smits-Engelsman, Van Galen and Schoemaker make a point for a theoretical model that accounts for some of the motor behaviour problems shown in DCD. Kalverboer states that the identification of specific subgroups must be based on current theory.

It is clear that the definition of the categories of specific developmental disorders includes both phenomenological and aetiological distinctions. In the classification of disorders in the development of skills this seems unavoidable, particularly when factors such as severe neurological trauma, obvious physical defects or severe abuse or neglect are known to cause abnormalities in the developmental areas of motor skills, language, speech, or scholastic skills. With this knowledge, it would be absurd to consider all impairments in scholastic skills, language, speech or motor skills as belonging to the same type merely because they have parallel phenomenological characteristics. This is not to say that definitions of categories or subcategories should rely exclusively on aetiological considerations. The relevance of the categories can be increased by including considerations with regard to treatment selection as well. Categories that refer to disorders that are aetiologically distinct, but bear no relevance for treatment selection may be interesting for research, but not for clinical practice.

It is time that we agree on the fact that ICD and DSM are not schemes solely based on the phenomenology of disorders, but that aetiological considerations and hypotheses about underlying cognitive processes also play a part. Although agreement on this issue may lead to disagreement as to how to define and describe SDD in ICD and DSM, it would be stimulating to search for consensus about the hypotheses that are relevant for further research. Moreover, it would acknowledge the fact that current classification schemes cannot be built on signs and symptoms alone. They are also built on concepts, like SDD, that may give raise to many questions, but are at the same time generally considered as valuable.

## THE FUTURE

### *A Research Agenda*

There is clearly a great need for further research on several issues, such as the best way to subdivide the heterogeneous pool of impairments in scholastic skills, language, speech, and motor disorders, as well as the course, cause, prevalence and relevance for differential treatment of each type of disorder. At the same time, it is necessary to develop reliable and valid instruments to assess the various aspects of the skills involved, especially with regard to the developmental domains of language, speech and motor functioning.

In view of our findings, it would be less urgent to investigate the relevance of the higher order concept of SDD. The research should focus on the best way to define and subdivide disorders within each of the developmental domains, and not be distracted by ideas and discussions that may be relevant for one disorder, but not for the other. This pertains in particular to the discrepancy concept. It may be useful to continue experiments with this concept with regard to the disorders in scholastic skills and the language disorders, but it may not be relevant for the disorders in motor coordination.

What we also need is more insight in the treatments that are offered, and the factors that influence the efficacy of these treatments. The tradition has been to identify subgroups that are phenomenologically distinct, and that may have a different aetiology. Research in the coming years should be dedicated to identifying subgroups that are related to differences in treatment. In this way, the relevance of classification research for clinical practice may be enhanced.

## *On the Next Revision of ICD and DSM*

Should the categories for SDD be removed from DSM and ICD? We already concluded that ICD should follow the same course as DSM and abandon the higher order concept of SDD. Furthermore we suggest to use the concept in different ways, depending on the domain of developmental disorders to which it is applied (i.e. to use it as a lower order concept of SDD of scholastic skills, language, speech, or motor functioning). Amorosa even proposed to discard the lower order concept in the domain of language disorders. She suggests six categories for the classification of language and speech: [0] No speech or language; [1] Disorders of speech production; [2] Fluency disorder (stuttering, cluttering); [3] Expressive language disorder; [4] Receptive language disorder; [5] Use of speech and language in communication. These language disorders are classified independently from other conditions that are diagnosed on other axes. This proposal implies that the categories for SDD would be abandoned entirely. The focus is on categories that are phenomenologically distinct and are relevant for treatment selection. The current SDD diagnoses can only be reconstructed by combining information that has been classified on different axes. The discrepancy model does not play a role in her proposed classification.

Van Yperen suggests not to abandon the lower order SDD concept, but to place the SDD category in an ordering of categories that is roughly similar to that of Amorosa. The only difference is that each of the linguistically defined main categories contains subcategories for disorders with distinct aetiologies or specific natures. These subcategories correspond with the constructs of the specific developmental disorder, the environmentally determined disorder, and the disorder due to mental retardation, neurological trauma, or other physical abnormalities. For research purposes, the SDD category can be operationalized in terms of a discrepancy, but also models are possible as well.

The proposals by Amorosa and Van Yperen can be extended to the other developmental domains as well. The key issue, however, is to what degree adaptions of ICD and DSM can be founded on consensus and empirical research. In this respect, the next revision of ICD and DSM should be more open to alternative definitions and models. In some developmental domains this may lead to abandoning the SDD category. If this is the result of research and debate, so be it.